Foundations of Physical Education, Exercise, and Sport Sciences

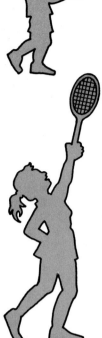

Foundations of Physical Education, Exercise, and Sport Sciences

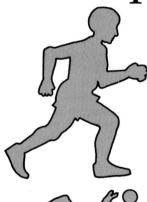

WILLIAM C. ADAMS, Ph.D.

Professor, Department of Physical Education
University of California
Davis, California

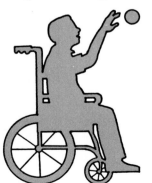

LEA & FEBIGER

1991

Philadelphia • London

Lea & Febiger
200 Chester Field Parkway
Malvern, Pennsylvania   19355-9725
U.S.A.
(215) 251-2230
1-800-444-1785

Lea & Febiger (UK) Ltd.
145a Croydon Road
Beckenham, Kent BR3 3RB
U.K.

Reprints of chapters may be purchased from Lea & Febiger in quantities of 100 or more.

Library of Congress Cataloging-in-Publication Data

Adams, William C. (William Carter), 1933–
    Foundations of physical education, exercise, and sport sciences /
William C. Adams.
        p.   cm.
    Includes bibliographical references and index.
    ISBN 0-8121-1359-4
    1. Physical education and training.   2. Exercise—Physiological
aspects.   3. Sports sciences.
GV341.A324   1990
613.7′1—dc20   90-37084
                                                                      CIP

PRINTED IN THE UNITED STATES OF AMERICA

Print number: 5   4   3   2   1

DEDICATION

TO

Charlotte, without whose original suggestion
and continued encouragement this book
would not have been written

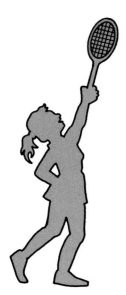

PREFACE

During the past quarter century, physical education has increasingly become an academic discipline, though it retains a strong professional context. Further, a dramatically enhanced societal awareness of the role of structured physical activity programs now extends well beyond the traditional educational institutional setting. The development as an academic discipline has resulted in an increasing tendency for scholars to specialize in one of the subdisciplines basic to the study of human movement, such as biomechanics, exercise physiology, motor learning, or sport psychology. Concurrently, the application of structured physical activity programs has become more pluralistic and diverse. This is particularly evidenced by the increasing attention to the role of physical activity and fitness in the achievement of health and well-being, which has now become more firmly established in schools, colleges, and universities, as well as in community organizational settings, health clubs, the corporate sector, and in clinical settings. Indeed, the title of the text, "Foundations of Physical Education, Exercise, and Sport Sciences," implies that the term physical education is now recognizably inadequate to describe the expanded role of human movement studies and its societal application in the late 20th century.

There are numerous introductory textbooks in physical education, many of which have treated the academic body of knowledge somewhat superficially, focusing instead primarily on pedagogical and professional aspects, including the identification and description of attendant career opportunities. In this text, the latter are treated in brief, with the primary thrust entailing a thorough examination of the basic knowledge of the field. Accordingly, material from the basic subdisciplines has been selected and organized to whet the appetite of students interested in the broad field of physical education, exercise and sport science at an early stage in their college matriculation, as well as to establish an integrating element that provides an awareness of the many linkages that exist between these specialized areas of study. In this manner, growth in one's broad perspective of the field can be more effectively enhanced with completion of advanced coursework in one or more of the specialized areas covered in each chapter.

In essence, the text represents a holistic approach to the multidimensional study of human movement, in that it also examines the principal applications of this fundamental knowledge base to particular subpopulations, especially in terms of developmental and health maintenance and enhancement aspects. This intent stems from the accumulating impressive evidence that physical activity and physical fitness contribute to good health. It includes documented evidence about human physical activity and health related behavior, as well as application of this information to one's own life and to those of others that one influences in family, or in other social or professional life settings. Thus, while subdisciplines such as biomechanics, exercise physiology, and sport psychology can be studied for inherent basic knowledge, they provide a more important societal impact via their effective application.

While the most important basic concepts in physical education, exercise and sport science are identified in the text, they are not examined in detail appropriate to a challenging upper division course. Indeed, in many institutions, physical education majors take an entire course in each of the subject areas covered in the nine chapters herein. This, then, is an introductory text that gives the college student interested in the study of human movement and its place in modern society, a broad perspective of the field. As such, it is not intended solely as the introductory theory course for the physical education major, but also for students enrolled in a general education course in a liberal arts and sciences curriculum which permits an elective in this field of increasing societal importance.

The order of material presented has been arranged to achieve the objectives identified above. The first chapter is prefatory, but broad and integrative, in that it deals with the history of human organized physical activity programs and modern man's continued need for vigorous physical activity. The integrative concept basic to this presentation is anthropologic, including both physical and cultural dimensions. Distinction between the roles of science in the continued growth of the knowledge base in human movement, and of the philosophic process in ferreting out elements of its comprehensive meaning in terms of benefit to modern man, is also made. In the next four chapters basic concepts, supported by data from the scientific literature, are presented in the primary subdisciplines of the field: (1) biomechanics, (2) exercise physiology, (3) motor learning, and exercise and sport psychology, and (4) the sociology of sport and physical education. In addition to a theoretical overview, numerous examples of various aspects of physical education, exercise and sport applications are given. In the next two chapters, the relationship between physical activity and (1) growth and development to adulthood, and (2) the aging process, are examined. Next, the concepts of health, well-being and fitness are surveyed, with emphasis on the development of chronic "life-style" disease. In the final chapter, the role of enhanced physical activity in alleviating the effect of several important chronic diseases is examined.

There are several features of this text which should be useful to one teaching an introductory course in physical education. Each chapter begins with an introduction that provides a summary statement of the scope of material to be covered. Further, each chapter ends with an enumerated summary emphasizing major points. Throughout the text, basic concepts are identified and developed via citation of original research or carefully chosen substantiation advanced in specialized textbooks of the field. The latter, especially those listed in the bibliography of each chapter, afford a ready source for the student interested in a more detailed treatment.

A basic premise employed in this text is that even beginning students in the field should be presented with data in some detail that substantiate fundamental assertions. Accordingly, tables and graphs have been plentifully employed to aid in presenting salient data substantiating major concepts. Selected photographs have also been incorporated to improve presentation of material and emphasize key points. While the number of basic concepts and the magnitude of data presented may seem initially formidable, this text can prove particularly useful to the instructor who wishes to present an introductory course utilizing a text similar in approach to those readily available for introductory courses in traditional academic disciplines, such as anthropology, physics, physiology, psychology, and sociology. An accompanying caveat is that some departments might find it better to use this text in a team-taught course employing a specialist in one or more of the major areas covered, though one person must clearly assume primary responsibility for assuring effective integration.

I acknowledge the valued input of numerous undergraduate students, whose relatively uninhibited questions and viewpoints provided additional insight over the past 25 years in the development of the prototype course for which this text has been written. Thanks is extended to numerous colleagues—at the University of California, Davis, and elsewhere—who intentionally, and sometimes unwittingly, provided feedback over the years relative to the purpose, scope, and usefulness of an introductory foundations course primarily focused on the academic knowledge base of the field. The selection and organization of the material in the text represents my original work, but it is with pleasure that I acknowledge the contribution of others' ideas, as well as much of the data presented in the text, which represents an impressive collection of scholarly productivity by many colleagues in physical education, exercise and sport science. Errors and omissions, however, are my sole responsibility.

I am grateful for the original illustrations prepared by Geoffrey Adams, Candace Ireton, and William J. Penny, Ph.D. Appreciation is gratefully extended to organizations and publications which made illustrations, photographs, tables, and other material available. Finally, I am deeply indebted for the wide ranging contributions of Candace Ireton, which included all administrative aspects of preparing the manuscript for forwarding to the publisher, editing of the original manuscript, word processing, preparing outlines following review of original source material, as well as preparing original drafts of several pages of text. It is hard to visualize how this project could have reached fruition without her manifold contribution.

Davis, California   William C. Adams

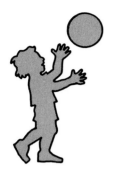

CONTENTS

1

Anthropologic, Historic and Philosophic Foundations of Physical Education

2

Biomechanics of Human Movement

3

Exercise Physiology

4

Psychologic Foundations: Motor Learning, Exercise, and Sport Psychology

5

Sociology of Sport and Physical Education

6

Physical Activity, Growth, and Development

7
Exercise and Aging

8
The Modern Concept of Health

9

Exercise and Chronic Disease

1 ANTHROPOLOGIC, HISTORIC, AND PHILOSOPHIC FOUNDATIONS OF PHYSICAL EDUCATION

INTRODUCTION

Until the late 1960s, physical education in the United States was almost exclusively considered a profession. That is, the field possessed a scientific and philosophic basis, employed specialized skills, and performed a service to society. It offered physical activity instructional programs in educational institutions which were designed to make contributions to the mental, social, emotional, and physical development of students (i.e., education through the physical[83]). Further, it developed and administered programs of professional training for teachers and coaches to conduct these physical activity instructional programs in sport, dance, and exercise.

Physical education in the United States has developed and expanded during the past quarter century in two principal ways: (1) it is increasingly an academic discipline (though it retains a strong professional context) with a growing body of knowledge whose central focus is human movement (i.e., man engaged in physical activity); and (2) via the dramatically enhanced societal awareness of the optimal health/fitness role of structured physical activity programs that now extend well beyond the traditional educational setting. The latter has been spurred primarily by societal forces outside of the profession, including increased leisure time, enhanced discretionary income, federal public health sup-

port,[76,77] and expanded media exposure.[66,68] The application of structured physical activity programs has become more pluralistic and diverse, including those for preschool children, middle-age adults, and senior citizens, in addition to the traditional programs in educational institutions. This is particularly evidenced by the increased role of fitness based programs in the achievement of health and well-being, now widely available in community organizational settings, health clubs, the corporate sector, and clinical settings.[35] This growth outside of the educational setting has provided an expanded array of career options for physical education majors beyond traditional teaching and coaching careers, including health/fitness instruction, physical therapy, athletic training, sports administration, sports communication, and sports marketing.[39]

Physical education's growth as an academic discipline has been a resultant of the enhanced role of science and research in higher education, and the need of the profession for more sound information and theories upon which to develop and administer its programmatic offerings.[61] A number of specialty areas of knowledge have developed, but there is disagreement among physical educators as to which are properly regarded as subdisciplines. Biomechanics, exercise physiology, motor learning and sport psychology, and sport sociology are generally accepted subdisciplines. Other specialty areas with less well-developed knowledge bases include: (1) history and philosophy of physical education and sport; and (2) physical education and sport pedagogy. The latter is concerned with the systematic study and development of facts and theories relevant to physical education and sport program curriculum content, teaching methods, organization and administration, and teacher preparation.[65]

The continuously increasing knowledge base in each of the academic subdisciplines within college physical education departments has resulted in an increased tendency for specialization. Less concern has been evidenced for the profession's continuing need for educating professionals who can provide effective integration of this information, together with well-organized delivery (teaching) of structured physical activity programs to an increasingly varied clientele.[25] Hence, there is a pressing need for effective interaction and communication between these seemingly diverse but effectively interdependent elements. That is, the academic subdisciplines in physical education have a binding commitment to devote some of their effort to providing information that can be utilized to develop structured physical activity programs of higher quality. Concurrently, those who develop the pedagogical skills of professional physical educators must be aware of the latest information from the various academic subdisciplines which can be implemented most effectively.

Recent expansion of structured physical activity instructional programs beyond the traditional educational institution setting has resulted in a change of emphasis in the way physical education is defined in terms of its objectives for individual participants. There is now more emphasis on physical education as a life-long process involving education both *of* and *through* the physical, or as Metheny states, "learning to move and moving to learn."[44] In addition to the previously identified holistic developmental objectives for educational institution participants, modern programs seek to enhance the opportunity for one to achieve optimal development of motor skills and physical fitness commensurate with health

and well-being, together with knowledge and attitudes likely to enhance one's electing a physically active lifestyle.

The broadened societal setting for structured physical activity programs, and the decreased emphasis on professional preparation of teachers and coaches, together with the increased emphasis on the study of human movement as an academic discipline, has led to an identity crisis for physical education departments.[61] As Cheffers and Evaul state: "If human movement is the discipline that incorporates a body of knowledge about human beings in motion, then physical education is a profession that applies that knowledge."[13:xii] This observation suggests that physical education may not be the best descriptor, at least alone, for a university department increasingly dedicated to the scientific study of human movement. Janz et al.[36] surveyed all 680 4-year institutions offering degree programs in physical education to determine (1) if they had changed their name, and (2) if so, whether a new common name for the profession was evident. They found that 33% of the institutions responding had changed their name during the period from 1976 to 1988, with one-half of them having done so in the last 3 years. Sixty-five percent included physical education in their new title, linking it most frequently with the terms health, leisure studies, or sport studies. The primary reasons given for retaining physical education in the new name chosen were that the latter more accurately described areas of specialization, while maintaining an overall title that was easily recognized. Of those departments electing to change their names without retaining physical education in the title, most were large institutions granting master's and/or doctoral degrees. Primary reasons cited for electing this option included: (1) more accurately describes areas of specialization; (2) reflects curricular priorities; (3) enhances image in academia; and (4) enhances grant funding opportunities. The authors concluded that the trend toward name change has not resulted in a commonly accepted departmental name, although kinesiology, human performance, human movement, kinetics, sport science, and exercise science were names cited most often.

The choice of title for this text reflects my contention that physical education is no longer an adequate term to describe this modern, highly diverse field. However, it has over a century of tradition in professional and public acceptance and understanding, and appears to remain an appropriate descriptor for physical activity instructional and professional training programs.[27,61] Thus, it is retained, while exercise and sport sciences are added to encompass an overarching focus of the primary academic subdisciplines of the field.

While history and philosophy of physical education and sport are important extensions of their traditional humanities disciplines, they are accounted for in the text title only by inference in the term physical education. Fundamental information and concepts from these knowledge bases, together with examination of the anthropologic perspective of human movement (both cultural and physical) constitute the remainder of this chapter.

ANTHROPOLOGIC PERSPECTIVE

Anthropology, literally is the study of man. It is the science dealing with the interaction of man's culture, biology, and environment. Anthropologists are concerned with study of the individual human, but also with the comparison of societies of people both contemporary and historic. Of particular importance is how groups adjust biologically and culturally to their environments. Accordingly, the two major subareas of study are physical and cultural anthropology. While early cultural anthropologists observed and recorded the ways of life of "primitive peoples," many now study the impact of modern technologic societies on cultural changes necessitated by this complex environmental change in man's life. Biologic demands of the environment are a primary concern of the physical anthropologist, particularly with respect to the long history of human evolution. Since man adapts biologically via the relatively slow process of evolution,

the highly technologic, urban environment we now live in may well place demands on us that we are biologically ill-prepared to handle.[80] Biologic evolution has facilitated man's capacity for assimilating a complex culture, and the two are interrelated in man's ability to cope successfully with the environment.

Culture is sometimes defined in a narrow sense to indicate a society's level of accomplishment in literature, music, and art. Anthropologists consider it in a much broader context to include "the complex whole of knowledge, beliefs, morals, law, custom, art and any other capabilities and habits acquired by man as a member of society."[23:7] As such, it is not inherited biologically as is so much of the body structure, function and personality predisposition. Instead, culture is learned from other humans, and not only by children from their parents, as in biologic heredity. Indeed, man is born very much an animal, in that his behavior is characterized by involuntary reflex actions, such as crying, blinking, and sucking. However, man is also born with unique potentialities, including the capability of analyzing and describing, of thinking, and of recording and communicating thoughts. He is the most plastic and adaptable creature on Earth, and hence is able to survive and flourish in widely varied environments. Because he is the most educable creature, his cultural heritage has become vastly more complex than even the highest forms of sub-human animals. At birth, however, the infant is not yet a personality, i.e., ideas, interests, fears, and desires are not yet formed; one's occupation, economic and social status are still to be shaped by experience. Sorokin compared the infant's development to a phonograph, when he asserted:

He is like a phonograph, capable of playing any record. A well-constructed phonograph, to be sure, plays any record better than a poorly constructed phonograph. But what records it will play—whether a Beethoven symphony or jazz—does not depend upon the phonograph. Similarly a person born with a superior constitution may develop a better mind and play his "sociocultural records" better than one born with inferior hereditary endowments; but what "sociocultural records" he will play usually depends rather little upon the organic or biological factors.[71:5]

The interrelations between the biologic and cultural components of human evolution are best understood in terms of how they serve the same basic function—adaptation to man's environments, though in a subtly distinct way. Dobzhansky[23] contends that most contemporary evolutionists are of the opinion that adaptation of a living species to its environment is the chief agency impelling and directing biologic evolution. Further, this process takes place through natural selection, which promotes the survival and reproduction of the carriers of some genetic components and inhibits others. Dobzhansky further states:

The construction of man's body and the conformation of his intellect developed as they did because they made our species biologically highly successful. The genetic basis of man's capacity to acquire, develop or modify, and transmit culture emerged because of the adaptive advantages which this capacity conferred on its possessors. Culture is, however, an instrument of adaptation which is vastly more efficient than the biological processes which led to its inception and advancement. It is more efficient among other things because it is more rapid—changed genes are transmitted only to the direct descendants of the individuals in whom they first appear; to replace the old genes, the carriers of the new ones must gradually outbreed and supplant the former. Changed culture may be transmitted to anybody regardless of biological parentage, or borrowed ready-made from other peoples.[23:20]

It is a mistake then to consider culture as an independent variable subject to genetic transmission, which then would exhibit natural selection akin to a social Darwinism effect.[23]

MAN'S EVOLUTION AND
PHYSICAL ACTIVITY

Man's biologic evolution extends over millions of years, with the first true man, *Homo erectus*, living as a hunter and food gatherer over a substantial geographic area at least 1½ million years ago.[80] *Homo sapiens* existed 35,000 to 50,000 years ago in much the same environmental demand relative to physical activity necessary for provision of an adequate food supply. Astrand[1] contends that early man's successful evolution necessitated hours of walking each day in order to get enough food. The motivation for this habitual activity was not love for exercise but plain hunger. More recently, perhaps 10,000 years ago, plants were domesticated and man became more an agrarian, stationary farmer.[80] However, this also required hours each day of vigorous physical activity, which has only recently (within the last 100 years in the United States) been replaced as the predominant lifestyle characteristic of our increasingly industrialized and high-technological society. Astrand[1] has contrasted this century as representing only 1 centimeter in a 460 kilometer journey of the evolution of life on earth. Another important aspect of this recent change is that man previously lived in small groups, with a less complex culture to assimilate and probably with less emotional stress.[80] Kraus and Raab summarize the significance of this basic change in human lifestyle:

A tremendous transition has taken place in the biologically short period of time that has transpired from primitive man to the present highly civilized and domesticated citizen: a transition from an active and physically strenuous life, subject to privations and hardships of climate, to an extremely well protected but caged existence. It seems unlikely that such a change of environment and mode of living can take place without major reactions of the organism. While adaptability to new circumstances is one of the outstanding qualities of the human body, as well as the human mind, it can function only within certain limits. It is likely that overly dramatic changes of living habits may throw the organism off balance.[38:4]

One should appreciate that from the standpoint of biologic evolution, man has been propelled ahead thousands of years. His nervous system, emotions, vital organs, and muscular system appear far behind in their power of adaptation when compared to recent advances in science and technology.[41]

BRIEF OVERVIEW OF TECHNOLOGIC DEVEL-
OPMENT IMPACT ON MAN'S PHYSICAL AC-
TIVITY LEVEL. Contemporary American society is in a state of rapid change brought
about primarily by the impact of science
and technologic development, and its wide
diffusion in our culture. Their effects on
our work and leisure patterns have been
manifold, and there is also evidence of enhanced difficulty in behavioral adjustment
to an increasingly complex societal input.
In addition, economic innovation, particularly the impact of Keynesian economics,
has produced a credit system that has resulted in a greatly expanded demand for
goods and services. These significant
changes in our way of life have hardly produced the utopia some had imagined when
20th century man became increasingly re-
lieved of hard physical labor. Bates has
aptly summarized the apparent dilemma
arising from these changes:

We now have . . . an abundance of goods and
services for nearly everyone which even the
privileged few could not command a century
ago. We have a wide variety of machines to
replace physical labor, giving leisure time to all
ranks of society . . . We are well into the "space
age," and the fantasies of yesterday's science
fiction become the realities of tomorrow. Yet our
time has also been called the "age of anxiety."
We have goods and services, but we don't quite
know what to do with them. We have leisure,
but we are not sure how to use it for the greatest
satisfactions . . . we calm our nerves with great
quantities of tranquilizers and alcohol; we can
scarely provide room enough in our hospitals
for the mentally ill. Utopia is here—and we are
afraid . . . The problem of our age, then, is to
gain the wisdom we need to use our growing
power intelligently.[3:107]

Automation. Automation is a technologic
advance that has produced at least four significant changes with which modern-day
America must contend: (1) Less physical
effort is required for workers to complete
their occupational tasks; (2) many are
obliged to perform monotonous assembly
line work; (3) more jobs in the service category, involving hours of sitting at a desk
or behind a counter, have been created;
and (4) a vast majority of our populace has
increasingly larger amounts of leisure time
available, though there is conflicting information as to whether this trend is plateauing.[18,58]

Industrialization and Urbanization. Industrialization, urbanization, and prosperity
are other resultants of this country's scientific and technologic advance. They have
made man's life less physically rigorous in
working and securing goods and services,
yet at the same time, apparently have occurred so rapidly that he has been unable
to make a satisfactory adjustment. Industrial progress means more production
which, in turn, usually results in a higher
standard of living. Thus, people have not
only more leisure, but more money to
spend on leisure. As more jobs have arisen
in our urban industrial centers, much of
our rural population has migrated there.
This urban "population explosion" with
the accompanying space demands for
housing, parking lots, and industrial enterprises seriously jeopardizes open play
space for all age groups at an increasing
rate. In addition, our living tempo has
greatly increased and we hurry from place
to place meeting one deadline after another.[58]

Today, most Americans ride wherever
they go, and use an endless variety of machines to accomplish chores in and around
the home. We employ power-driven tools
for housework, leisure time handiwork,
and even for exercising! Certainly, it is well
to stop and ask the question: Is there really
drudgery inherent in our play and leisure
activities? Another important related concern regarding leisure is its worthy use.
This concept has been studied in some detail by Nash,[47] and is presented in graphic
summary form in Figure 1–1. There are
four levels above a zero category. Nash
rates the field of entertainment and amuse-
ment, such as television, radio and popular
movies, all as an antidote to boredom,
nearest zero. Next on the scale is the level
of emotional participation, followed by active participation and creative participation. Nash feels that it is desirable and necessary to participate in leisure experience
at all of these levels. However, he cautions
that too many activities low on the scale
are dulling. Below zero on the scale is depicted as a level of anti-social behavior as
reflected in delinquency and crime.

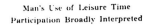

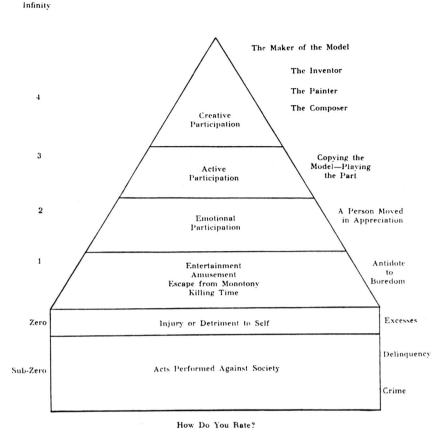

FIG. 1–1. Scale for rating man's use of leisure time-participation broadly interpreted. (From Nash, J.B.: Philosophy of Recreation and Leisure. St. Louis: Mosby, 1953, p. 89.)

It should be noted that physical activity can make a contribution at three levels: (1) as an antidote to boredom through observation of sport (level 1); (2) as an emotional experience gained through the support of a team or sports group (level 2); and (3) as a provision for active participation in a variety of activities (level 3). Physical activity also has the potential to contribute at the creative level for a few individuals. However, this potential is not unique to physical activity participation, as it applies to many other life activities.

There is ready evidence in our society of many individuals who spend the vast majority of their leisure time in non-creative, sedentary activities that are often merely an antidote to boredom (level 1). However,

there is increasing evidence of a growing number of people who are becoming more actively involved in leisure time pursuits, including fitness activities and sports participation.[74] While the latter represent only two kinds of many worthwhile leisure time pursuits, their value is further enhanced because of our largely activity-void jobs.

HEALTH EFFECTS OF INSUFFICIENT PHYSICAL ACTIVITY—HYPOKINETIC DISEASE. The first American public health revolution—bringing infectious disease under control—has been largely successful, in that today they account for only 1% of total deaths. However, efforts to deal with the vast increase in chronic disease and mortality have only recently showed notable progress, primarily as a result of a 36% decrease in heart disease deaths in 1983 compared to 1968.[55] There is increasing evidence that a lack of sufficient physical activity in our sedentary population plays a major role in the development of many chronic disease states.[46] Kraus and Raab contend that this effect appears directly mediated through underuse of the skeletal musculature, stating:

The system that has been put all but out of commission, the striated musculature, constitutes a major part of our body weight and has an important role which exceeds the mere function of locomotion. Action of the striated muscle influences directly and indirectly circulation, metabolism, and endocrine balance. It directly affects the structure of our bones, our posture, and the positions of our bodies. Last but not least, the striated muscles serve as an outlet for our emotions and nervous responses, the means by which we react and respond to stimuli and emotional stresses. Obliteration of an important safety valve and constant suppression of natural responses forced on us without the opening of vicarious outlets, might well upset the original balance to which the body of primitive man has been adapted.[38:4]

Chronic diseases, including heart disease, cancer, and stroke, now account for more than 70% of deaths in the United States each year.[76] Causes of heart disease, stroke, diabetes, hypertension, obesity, osteoporosis, low back pain, and psychosomatic disorders are multiple, but insufficient activity is involved, either directly or indirectly, in each.[7,67] Kraus and Raab's conceptualization of how hypokinetic disease mediates internal diseases, musculoskeletal and psychiatric problems, is illustrated in Figure 1–2.

In addition to increasing incidence of chronic disease, the middle-aged and elderly individuals experience a progressive loss in physiologic function and physical performance capacity. As shown in Figure 1–3, the average rate of loss differs for various parameters. Bortz[9] has observed qualitative similarities in many body structure and physiologic function changes that are common to aging and inactivity (disuse). It is estimated that 50% of reduced maximum aerobic capacity in the elderly is due to chronologic aging and the other 50% to substantially reduced activity.[33,50,69] The elderly also become less mobile, more infirm, and less confident and autonomous due, in part, to substantially reduced activity levels characteristic of advancing age.[46]

PHYSICAL ACTIVITY LEVELS IN AMERICAN CHILDREN AND ADULTS. The U.S. Public Health Office of Disease Prevention and Health Promotion included a school physical education and leisure time physical activity survey in the National Children and Youth Fitness Study of 1982 to 1984.[60] Though 80% of students, grades 5 through 12, were enrolled in physical education, there was a drop off from 95% in grades 5 and 6 to about 50% in grades 11 and 12. Among students enrolled, only 36% participated in physical education on a daily basis, although the average of 3.6 periods per week, encompassing 141 minutes, is reasonable for achieving well conceptualized educational and fitness objectives. The typical student was found to spend about 80% of his physical activity time (approximately 10 hours per week) outside physical education class. However, only about 50% participated in large muscle dynamic movement at an intensity of 60% of maximal aerobic capacity, 3 or more times weekly, for at least 20 minutes per session—considered to be an appropriate physical activity level essential for an effectively functioning cardiorespiratory system.[60] In 1985, the President's Council on Physical Fitness and Sports completed a 10-year follow-up study of the National School Population Fitness Survey.[54] Mean scores on physical performance tests for children, ages 6 to 17 years, were not significantly different from those observed in 1965 and 1975. However, there was also a low level of performance by large numbers of boys and girls on cardiorespiratory endurance tests. It was concluded that increased emphasis on regular fitness related activities is required to improve youth fitness levels.[54]

Stephens[74] has analyzed U.S. adult physical activity patterns reported in several national surveys using similar techniques completed between 1971 and 1985. It was found that 27% of adults, ages 18 to 75

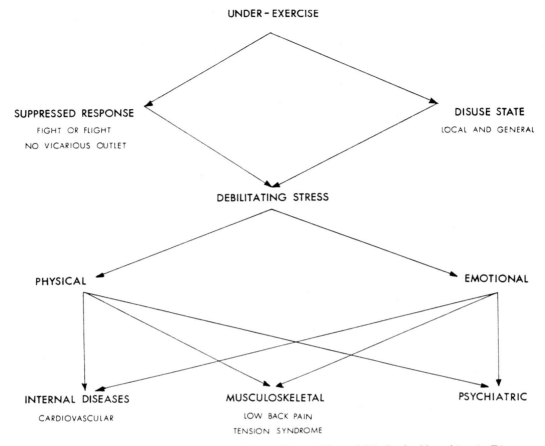

FIG. 1–2. Effects of hypokinetic disease. (From Kraus, H. and W. Raab: Hypokinetic Disease. Springfield: Charles C Thomas, 1960, p. 7.)

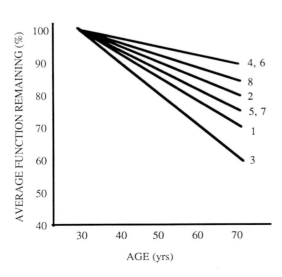

FIG. 1–3. Loss of physiological function and performance capacity from age 30 to 70 years. 1) Cardiac output; 2) Maximum heart rate; 3) Maximal oxygen uptake; 4) Basal metabolic rate; 5) Hand grip strength; 6) Nerve conduction velocity; 7) Bone—females; 8) Bone—males. Data from Astrand, P.-O., and K. Rodahl: Textbook of Work Physiology: Physiological Bases of Exercise (3rd ed.). New York: McGraw-Hill, 1986, p. 409; Garn, S.M.: Bone loss in aging. In The Physiology and Pathology of Aging. Edited by R. Goldman and M. Rockstein. New York: Academic Press, 1975, p. 43; and Shock, N.: The physiology of aging. Sci. Amer. *206*(1):110–112, 1962.

years, were sedentary in 1985, down from 41% in 1971. Women, especially those in the age range, 35 to 49 years, showed the greatest reduction in sedentary lifestyle, from 52 to 29%. Older adults, 65 to 75 years (men and women combined) showed a decrease from 50 to 39%. On the other hand, these surveys indicated that the upper socioeconomic class was notably more active, with managers and professionals highest, white-collar workers intermediate, and blue collar workers least active during leisure time. There was no significant difference between Caucasians and blacks in leisure time physical activity when age and socioeconomic status were accounted for. However, suburban residents engaged more in leisure time physical activity than did those living in rural areas or large cities. Of particular importance was the consistent increase since 1978 in the percent of adults who are vigorously active according to a daily dose considered sufficient to provide cardiovascular benefit.[32] This is roughly equivalent to 2½ miles of jogging or fast walking, and as shown in Figure 1–4, reveals a steady increase at all ages for both sexes (lines) and for both sexes (bars) from 1978 to 1985. Increased adult leisure time physical activity levels have been paralleled by a substantial drop in heart disease deaths—36% from 1968 to 1983. Goldman and Cook[29] have estimated that over 60% of this decrease can be attributed to reduction in cigarette smoking, less animal fats in the diet, and more exercise.

There appears to be conflicting evidence as to whether the public interest and participation in fitness activities are steadily increasing or beginning to level off. Figure 1–5 indicates a near consistent projected increase through 1990, following the last

actual amount of consumer sales of fitness equipment (1983). Further, at a time when personal expenditure for paid admissions to spectator sports rose from $3.5 billion to $4.5 billion (1972 to 1984), annual sales of sports and fitness magazines rose from 12½ to 22 million copies.[74] However, the number of participants in certified competitive distance running events plateaued between 1983 and 1985, after a more than 10-fold increase during the previous decade.[74] Shephard[63] has reported a clear tendency for the steady increase in Canadian adult physical activity levels in the 1970s to plateau between 1981 to 1985.

HISTORIC FOUNDATIONS

Anthropologists have discovered some cultural universals in otherwise widely diverse phenomena. These include dance, games, education, and other activities fundamentally associated with physical education and recreation.[48] Cassidy[12] has astutely observed that the place of physical activity in any culture is determined by what the predominant philosophy is relative to the way one's body should be treated—whether trained, denied, disciplined, developed, or educated. Historic examination of the role of organized physical activity programs reveals that various cultures have placed widely disparate value on the physical being and the corresponding resultant emphasis on physical education. In the following historic review, it will be evident that a wide variety of organized physical activity programs have been developed to meet prevalent cultural aims emanating from the existent educational, political, religious, and economic

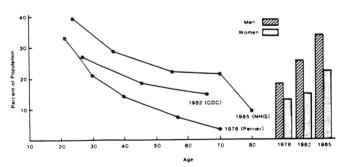

FIG. 1–4. Percent of U.S. adult population who are vigorously active, 1978–1985 (3+ kcal/kg/day of leisure time activity). (From Stephens, T.: Secular trends in adult physical activity: exercise boom or bust. Res. Quart. Exer. Sport. 58:94–105, 1987.)

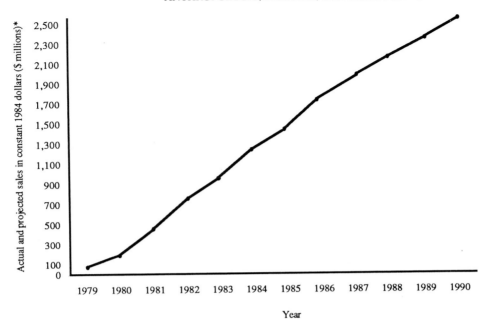

FIG. 1–5. Consumer sales of fitness equipment 1979 to 1990. *Base figure for 1983 is from National Sporting Goods Association and is in 1983 dollars. (From Physician and Sportsmed. *13*(5):140–141, 1985.)

conditions. However, there is also collective evidence of similarities observed from time to time throughout history, as well as in recent U.S. programs.

EARLY ORIGINS OF PHYSICAL EDUCATION

It should not be surprising that prior to recorded history, there is archeologic evidence of man using stones, spears, bow and arrows, and other hunting implements. The physical skills required for obtaining food and shelter, as well as running, jumping, and climbing to survive in a hostile environment, were clearly of sufficient importance to necessitate early development of an informal educational process. This probably took the form of children being taught physical survival skills, primarily by their parents. It also seems likely that younger children mimicked basic physical survival skills performed by older children and adults in their physical play activities. Siedentop[66] contends that studies by Margaret Mead of the Manus, a primitive people of New Guinea illustrate the relatively informal but nonetheless systematic nature of the Manu child's acquisition of aquatic skills. Mead states:

As soon as the baby can toddle uncertainly, he is put down into the water at low tide when parts of the lagoon are high and others only a few inches under water. Here the baby sits and plays in the water or takes a few hesitating steps in the yielding spongy mud . . . As he grows older, he is allowed to wade about at low tide. His elders keep a sharp lookout that he does not stray into deep water until he is old enough to swim. But the supervision is unobtrusive . . . His whole play world is so arranged that he is permitted to make small mistakes from which he may learn better judgment and greater circumspection, but he is never allowed to make mistakes which are serious enough to permanently frighten him, or inhibit his activity.[43:25]

Siedentop reports that "the Manu child was swimming on his own by the age of three. This educational climate also allowed him to learn how to dive, to handle a small canoe, and finally to control the large canoes that he would use as an adult member of the tribe. The entire process appeared to be very informal and unplanned."[66:11] Nonetheless, the results emanating from the educational methodology utilized in this learning environment clearly constitute an interesting form of very effective physical education.

PHYSICAL EDUCATION IN ANCIENT CIVILIZATIONS

Beginning about 10,000 years ago, man became progressively less dependent on hunting and foraging for food in an often nomadic existence, as the result of initiating growing crops and domesticating animals.[80] This change eventually produced a small economically privileged class in Egypt and China before 1,000 B.C. However, for the masses, up to the Industrial Age in Western Europe beginning in the 19th century, basic life demands necessitated the acquisition and utilization of heavy muscular activity skills. In Egypt, there is evidence of upper classes participating in wrestling, tumbling, basic jumping, swimming and kicking games, as well as in ball games. There was more universal participation in hunting and fishing.

During the early years of the Chou dynasty (1100 to 250 B.C.), physical education in China experienced an early enlightened awareness for the potential of contributing not only to enhancement of physical prowess, but also to the learning of accepted moral beliefs and rituals of tradition. These school programs for children of the privileged class continued until about 500 B.C., when the teachings of Confucius and Buddhism resulted in a decline in the role of physical education. Because of its topographic isolation which deterred aggression from outside forces, China had little motivation to employ organized physical training programs to maintain a strong armed force. In ancient India the dominant religion—Hinduism—taught that one must subjugate the body and ignore worldly concerns in order to achieve elevation of the soul. While there was heavy exercise entailed in maintaining an arduous agrarian existence, there was little impetus for vigorous physical activity amongst the privileged class.

In ancient Greece, beginning about 900 B.C., several city-states arose, Sparta and Athens being the principal ones. Sparta was ruled by a select group approximating 5% of the population who developed a highly specialized military training and educational program organized to create citizens who would devote their lives to the service of the city-state. At age 7 years, boys left their parents to initiate training for active military service which ended at age 30. Training of the Spartan youth consisted of a military conditioning program of wrestling, boxing, gymnastics, swimming, running, and the throwing of the discus and javelin. Dancing was used as a means of welding the young soldiers into military units through rhythmic patterns of attack movements.[82] Though Spartan girls did not attend specialized training schools, they were provided regular state supervised physical training, which included dancing, running, jumping, mountain climbing, and ball games. Enhanced physical fitness for motherhood was stressed in the belief that strong women would bear healthier progeny who could perpetuate the powerful armed forces desired by the rulers of the state.

In Athens, the initial focus on enhancing the young adult males' physical prowess was similar to that in Sparta. However, between 700 and 600 B.C., the Athenians initiated a cultural change which permitted the 18-year-old male, following 2 years of intensive military training, an opportunity to become an artist, philosopher, or otherwise privileged citizen. While the Athenian culture recognized several levels of social status, only about 10% of the citizens were provided extensive education that consisted of instruction in gymnastics (physical education), literature, mathematics, and music. If the young man wished to continue physical education at the palaestra (gymnasium), he was encouraged to perfect skills in a wide range of activities, including jumping, running, wrestling, and throwing the discus and javelin. Athenians viewed the human body as an object of great beauty to be perfected by exercise in symmetry and harmony. Further, Plato and Aristotle contended that physical education was important to provide the foundation for mental development and elevation of the human spirit.[82]

The ancient Greeks held festivals that included art, music, and a wide range of athletic contests. They were held to honor the gods, with the Olympic Games honoring Zeus, initiated in 776 B.C., being the most important. The Olympics were held every 4 years and citizens of all social strata were eligible to compete. Great honor was accorded winners of the numerous athletic contests at this event, which was of such importance to the several city-states that wars were allegedly interrupted while the Olympics were in progress.[56] By the 4th century B.C., Plato and Aristotle wrote that the Athenian ideal was changing, as education became more intellectualized in the direction of literature, philosophy, and art. Physical education became of lesser importance, though the most highly skilled athletes were encouraged to become professionals. The Olympic Games remained popular, but active participation by large numbers was increasingly replaced by growing numbers of spectators and fewer, more highly specialized professional athletes. The Games did continue on a regular basis until 394 A.D. when they were abolished by a Roman emperor.[82]

Like Sparta, the Roman government utilized physical activity regimens to facilitate military training of the male citizens. The Roman youth developed strength through physical conditioning and also the marching stamina, courage and fighting ability by which they became the pride of the Republic.[82] By the time the Romans conquered the Greek states, their physical education programs were in decline and the palaestra was not assimilated by the Romans as were other aspects of Greek culture. The only exercise program which the mass of Roman citizenry participated in was at the elaborate public baths, where large open-air swimming pools were available. A rather wide array of sports were popular, including ball games, running, jumping, throwing the discus and javelin, wrestling, acrobatics, and swimming. However, few citizens actively participated, preferring instead to watch professional athletes.[56] By far the favorite spectator events were chariot races, gladiatorial combat, and the fighting of animals by professional athletes and slaves. These festival events were held in the Circus Maximus (capacity of 250,000) and the Colosseum (capacity of 90,000). Given the obsession of Romans with military might, brutality in sport might have been an expected resultant. By 350 A.D., the Roman army consisted largely of mercenaries and half the days of the year were devoted to holiday festivals.[79]

PHYSICAL EDUCATION IN
THE MIDDLE AGES

During this period of approximately 1,000 years, there was relatively little attention given to physical education. This occurred primarily because of two philosophical beliefs: (1) asceticism, and (2) scholasticism. Asceticism arose early as a consequence of the evolving Christian society which rejected the moral decadence of Rome. Religious leaders and converts lived a life of extreme self-denial and self-discipline in the monasteries, where they sought to concern themselves with spiritual development to the exclusion of concern for the physical—even in terms of factors related to personal health. Formal education was not of importance through much of the medieval period, though the knowledge of previous civilizations was preserved in the monasteries. Scholasticism developed later from an increase in importance attached to the writings of early Christian scholars and the rediscovery of Aristotle's writings. However, emphasis was placed on the importance of developing the mind through disciplined study to the neglect of the body.

The feudal society that developed did epitomize the use of physical education in the elaborate training program for knighthood. This opportunity was available to only a select few young males of the feudal aristocracy. Thus, for much of the middle ages, the masses called serfs, who tilled the soil for the noblemen, found their opportunity for physical activity limited almost exclusively to manual labor. Gradually, though, with increased trade, growth in cities' population, and development of a more numerous middle class, sports and games became more widely accepted.[79]

PHYSICAL EDUCATION DURING THE RENAISSANCE AND REFORMATION

In this period extending from about 1350 to 1650, many changes occurred in Western Europe which resulted in an enhanced role for physical education. Renaissance, a French word meaning "rebirth," connoted reawakening of scholars to the classical learning of ancient Greece, and important advancements in literature and fine arts, to be followed by invention of the printing press and initiation of modern science. Principal among the effects of the Renaissance on physical education was humanism, a philosophy that emanated from the writings of Athenian Greeks and ascribed importance to the meaning and value of human life. This represented a distinct departure from the previously prevalent impact of asceticism. Renaissance art reflected a renewed awareness of the individualism of man as the artist focused attention on details of the human form being depicted. Michelangelo is reported to have dissected cadavers to discover the mechanics of movement before painting his great athletic figures.[82]

Renaissance educators no longer felt bound to the restrictive elements cast by scholasticism during the Middle Ages. They built upon a rekindled awareness of the Athenian Greek ideal of an education, concerned both with the mind and body, to develop a program that cultivated a broad-minded intellect, appreciation of the arts, and concern for one's fellow man and civic responsibility. Substantially greater attention was given to the importance of physical exercise and its potential for providing more for man than the physical skills and training required for military objectives.[79] While archery, fencing, riding, and other military-like activities were utilized, other activities including bowling, dancing, swimming, and tennis, reflected the heightened interest in developing the human potential. One of the early exponents of this profound change was the Italian educator, da Feltre, in the early 15th century, who established a school that provided the epitome of physical education exemplified in the training of the medieval knight in combination with study of the classic Greek and Latin scholars. This rejuvenation of the Athenian Greek ideal was later accepted with important contributions to modern Western European and United States physical education by eminent philosophers of the time—Milton and Locke in England, and Rousseau in France.[79]

In addition to important changes in the dominant philosophy of life from asceticism and scholasticism to humanism, the reduced effect of asceticism on physical education was furthered during the Reformation by Martin Luther, who advocated physical activity during leisure as opposed to gambling, drinking, and other sedentary pursuits.[79]

PHYSICAL EDUCATION IN EARLY MODERN WESTERN EUROPE

Important contributions to the further advancement of physical education were made in the late 18th and the 19th century in Western Europe, many of which were to exert a profound effect on early American physical education programs during the late 19th century. Accordingly, this review will be limited to significant developments in Germany, Sweden, and Great Britain from 1760 to 1860.

Johann Basedow was a German schoolteacher, who after reading Rousseau's educational naturalism philosophy in *Emile*, developed the first modern physical education program in 1774. His school admitted children from all classes of society and made physical education an integral part of the overall curriculum. Activities taught included climbing various objects, dancing, jumping, fencing, running, skating, and wrestling. This effort aroused considerable interest and resulted in the establishment of a number of similar schools in Germany, including one in which Johann Guts-Muth taught physical education for 50 years. His program, conducted on a daily basis, initially utilized similar activities as those employed by Basedow, but was expanded to include new games, new exercise apparatus, and a more structured program. He wrote numerous papers and books on physical education, including two classics, *Gymnastics for the Young* (1793) and *Games* (1796).[82]

Friedrich Jahn initiated the Turnverein movement in Germany during the early 19th century. His principal motivation in developing this program was the belief that it would provide the means by which the many loosely bound independent German states could become a strong national force to resist the advances by the French armies of Napoleon. His program was designed to enhance the physical and moral vigor of the young German male adult participants. Most activities were done outdoors, and first consisted primarily of hiking, climbing, running, jumping, vaulting, wrestling, and group calisthenics. Later, basic gymnastics events, similar to those used today, were added.[82] Jahn's Turnverein movement eventually expanded in the mid-19th century to include programs adapted to the needs of older adults, as well as for women and children. In 1870, there were 1,500 Turner societies, which grew to 4,000 in 1890, and 10,000 in 1920.[11]

Nationalism was also the principal motive of Per Henrik Ling in developing a physical education program that would aid in recapturing Swedish dignity and physical vigor of its youth following disastrous loss of territory in wars with Russia during the late 1700s and early 1800s. He developed a system primarily designed to ensure strong, courageous soldiers for the military. However, he also felt that his system of gymnastics, which was devised after extensive study of anatomy and physiology, had aesthetic, educational, and health enhancement value. It was based on apparatus work, including swinging ladders and rings, rope climbing, vaulting bars, and stall bars, while performing complex exercise patterns. Careful attention was given to progression, and exercise routines were generally done in unison in large groups.[82]

The development of physical education in England was quite different through the mid-19th century than in Germany, Sweden, and other western European countries. First, there was a measure of isolation afforded by the English Channel and a strong navy, which enabled England to follow a more independent course. Also, since England had a long history of political unity, it did not have a similar need for programs of physical education that encouraged nationalism.[82] Finally, England had a long history of participation in sports and games, dating from early medieval times, and little interest developed in the highly structured and formalized German and Swedish gymnastics programs until the early 20th century.

While the humanist movement during the Renaissance stirred interest in the potential for physical education of English youth, there was a strong scholasticism influence existent which held that the playing of games and sports had little educational merit in schools and universities.[79] This is an interesting contrast to the early popularity of sports at the prestigious private preparatory schools and their espoused value in Wellington's English army's prolonged but eventually successful confrontation with Napoleon's forces in 1808 to 1814.[16] The strong English public's interest in sports and games also drew notable deterrent efforts from government and the church as to which sports and games could be participated in by the common man.[82] This concern seems, in part, well advised, when one considers the following account of English football (now rugby), the forerunner of American football.

Football, apparently introduced by Roman legions, was played by villagers in England during the Middle Ages, and sometimes a whole village was pitted en masse against another. The game during the Renaissance was viewed as bloody and brutal, and both Henry VIII and Queen Elizabeth I legislated against it. Nonetheless, the game persisted and, in a less brutal form, was introduced into the sports programs of the prestigious private schools during the 18th century.[82:20]

HISTORIC DEVELOPMENT OF PHYSICAL EDUCATION IN THE UNITED STATES

The primary objectives of this section of historic review are: (1) to trace the evolve-ment of physical education in the United States, identifying major events in its development; and (2) to identify the principal political, economic, and sociocultural conditions that have influenced this development. Little is known of physical education programs employed by early native Americans, though it would appear that they reflected objectives of physical survival, as well as dance during festival occasions, and the encouragement of play amongst children in activities simulating future utilitarian activities.[56]

COLONIAL PERIOD (1600 TO 1780). Conditions in early colonial America were not conducive to the development of physical recreation or education. Early Pilgrim colonists, largely of British heritage, experienced great hardship in coping with a hostile environment that necessitated substantial effort in the heavy physical labor of a primitive agrarian life. This precluded any perceived need for recreational physical activity during the minimal amount of leisure time that existed. Further, the dominant Puritan religious belief held that one should be disciplined and austere, thus avoiding pleasurable recreation, as play was seen to be the "work of the devil."[82] Some schools were developed in the 1630s, but they enrolled only children from the few emerging privileged and wealthy families. Further, the curriculum consisted of the three Rs in elementary school, which was supplemented with classics in the secondary school, thus evidencing a strong scholasticism emphasis. It was thought that any serious scholar should be above interest in rowdy, boisterous games.[79]

By the early 18th century, participation in physical recreation involving sports and games occurred widely amongst two groups of people. The Dutch, who settled in New York, brought with them a rich heritage of recreational participation in dances, games, and sports. In addition, many were members of the Dutch Reform Church, which did not adhere to the strict Protestant beliefs opposed to play and recreation. Thus, as economic conditions improved during the late 17th century, more leisure time became available and physical recreation became more prevalent.[82] In Vir-

ginia, settled primarily by Anglicans, there was less religious restraint than with the Puritans. Further, climatic conditions were not so harsh and the richer soil made the agrarian existence less demanding. Employment of slave labor permitted the increasingly numerous aristocracy with greater leisure, and participation in riding, hunting, fishing, swimming, and dancing, as well as early forms of golf and tennis, was prevalent on country estates by the late 18th century.[79]

THE NATIONAL PERIOD (1780 TO 1860). During this 80-year period, several important, but gradual changes in economic conditions and cultural attitudes occurred that strengthened the role of sports, recreation, and physical education. The popularity of sports and games as physical recreation increased steadily due to reduced Puritanical doctrine constraint and the increased leisure time available from the adoption of more efficient agricultural methods, technologic advancements, and the beginnings of urbanization.[79] With the growing middle class, a new public secondary school (called an academy) movement occurred along the Eastern seaboard. The influence of scholasticism was much less evident in this curriculum which sought to provide terminal education for a more effective adult life. In addition to some instruction in hygiene, this more progressive educational view encouraged participation in sports and games after regular school hours for physical health enhancement.[79]

In the mid-1820s, the German gymnastics system developed by Jahn was introduced first by Charles Beck in a small private secondary school in Massachusetts and then 2 years later at Harvard University by Charles Follen. The impact of their efforts was not immediately influential, as few other physical education programs developed in schools and colleges until the late 1850s.[82] An interesting byproduct of this initial effort to incorporate Jahn's German gymnastic system in American school and college curricula was its adaptation for young women to a system of more simple and lighter calisthenic exercise done to music. This new American gymnastics system was developed by Catherine Beecher in 1829, and was designed to produce grace of motion, good carriage, and sound health. Beecher's efforts were premature in America, for her program conflicted with prevalent feminine ideals of the period and failed to win wide acceptance.[82]

There were no organized physical education programs in colleges before 1860, and public schools showed little interest in physical education until the mid-1850s, when some cities allowed a few minutes of calisthenics in the daily curriculum.[79] However, two other important developments occurred during the 15 years preceding the Civil War that set the stage for important advances in school and college physical education. The most important was the initiation of the Turner gymnastics movement in Cincinnati in 1848, and its rapid spread consequent to the substantial German emigration during this period. By 1861, there were 150 Turner societies and 10,000 participants in the United States.[56] Another factor, whose impact did not become substantial in schools and colleges until the turn of the century was the increased popularity, organization of, and participation in sports. This included numerous community baseball teams by 1860, bowling clubs, lacrosse, and swimming.[56] In addition, participation in sports increased steadily on college campuses following daily class sessions, in a manner similar to current intramural and club sports. This early era of sports participation and competition developed amongst students to satisfy their perceived need for physical recreation and competition in their leisure hours. College administrators and faculty paid little attention to this student activity, but by 1860 initial intercollegiate competition had occurred—primarily among Ivy League institutions—in rowing, baseball, and football.[79]

CIVIL WAR UNTIL WORLD WAR I. Following the obvious influence of military training on the physical preparedness of young adult males during the Civil War, much of the previously developed cultural impact on physical education continued to evolve in a reasonably predictable, though somewhat more rapidly expanding pattern during the next 50 years. The major political,

economic, and sociocultural influences on physical education included: (1) increased federal authority, (2) increased technologic and industrial advances which further increased leisure time, (3) over 13 million emigrants between 1865 and 1900, (4) further expansion of concern for a more effective education of a vastly increased middle class, and (5) medical concern for hygiene and the need for exercise in an increasingly urban society.

The latter stemmed from a resurgence of concern for preventive medicine, which originated with Hippocrates (460 to 370 B.C.), was formalized by Galen (129 to 210 A.D.), and has undergone varying degrees of influence since.[6] Hygiene was the term used to describe the preventive medicine concept in the 19th century, and was considered a significant aspect of the science and art of medicine until the advent of antibiotics and the shift in focus to curative medicine. Some medical writers even referred to hygiene as physical education, which included concern not only for appropriate amounts of exercise, but also other "knowledge about one's body," such as breathing fresh air, eating proper foods, and getting adequate sleep. Advice was given concerning one's "responsibility for personal health," "self-management," and "self-improvement," all of which are aspects of the current resurgence of public concern for preventive medicine.[6]

Several medical doctors, who believed that physical education was vital to reaching one's health potential, made important contributions during the 25 years following the Civil War. In 1861, Dr. Dio Lewis, a well-known temperance and health lecturer, developed a new gymnastics system which utilized lighter implements than the Jahn system, and was designed to develop agility, carriage, flexibility, and grace, rather than virtually sole emphasis on strength. Dr. Lewis wrote books, lectured widely, and in 1868 established the first 2 year training program for gymnastics teachers. This development facilitated the spread of his system into secondary schools.[56] Dr. Edward Hitchcock became the first director of a college physical education department, established in 1861 at Amherst College. Hitchcock's method of physical education employed a gymnastics system similar to Lewis's, but he was the first to make systematic body measurements on his students at the beginning and end of each school year. These data were used to identify particular areas of weakness and to assess the effect of individualized exercise programs.[56]

Dudley Sargent received his M.D. degree from Yale University following a 3-year program. He was one of 12 in his medical school class who had a college degree. Some had not even finished high school—such was the state of medical education at the time.[5] Dr. Sargent became director of physical training at the Hemenway Gymnasium at Harvard University (the interior and exterior of which are depicted in Figure 1–6). His program included taking body measurements on all students and giving them basic heart and lung function tests, as well as strength tests that he had devised. Then he prescribed exercises for each student, using many different pieces of apparatus which he invented to meet special physical development needs.[56] He established a summer workshop training program to prepare teachers to use his system for physical education programs in the schools and at colleges that began to initiate programs.[5] Both Hitchcock and Sargent were instrumental in the formation in 1885 of the American Association for the Advancement of Physical Education, a forerunner of the current American Alliance for Health, Physical Education, Recreation and Dance, which remains the primary professional organization for physical education and related professions.

By 1889, there was substantial disagreement as to whether Hitchcock's or Sargent's gymnastic system, the German system which enjoyed strong support from the Turnvereins in most large cities, or the more recently introduced Swedish system, was the best for the emerging American physical education profession to adopt. This debate peaked at the Boston Conference, at which each system was thoroughly described and discussed. At the conclusion of the meeting, it was the predominant feeling of those not personally involved in any one of the systems that no one program fully met the needs of the American nation. It is important also to realize that there was no prominent spokesman at the conference for "sports and games, which had existed since the days of colonial America and were then participated in at the schools and colleges as student-sponsored programs."[82:39]

Sports and games were enjoying increasing popularity, particularly in the increasing number of large urban areas, where the development of numerous neighborhood playgrounds had occurred. The college student-sponsored athletic programs, however, had developed in opposition from administrators and faculty. Part of this opposition in the years just following the Civil War was due to the prevalent academic opinion that community sports participation was associated with a class of person who was otherwise not highly motivated and with low morals. However, by the 1890s various national organizations had been established and rules were set to govern competition. In 1893, the University of Chicago became the first to form a faculty committee to administer intercollegiate sports. At the same time, Amos Alonzo Stagg became director of its Department of Physical Culture, which entailed supervision of physical education for men and physical education for women (both of which consisted of gymnastics instruction), as well as athletics.[56] However, few other institutions combined athletics with physical education until well after the turn of the century.

College and university physical education departments and gymnasiums for activity instruction spread from the Eastern seaboard to Oberlin College (Ohio) in 1885 and to a dozen Mid-western state universities before 1900. The Universities of California, Texas, Utah, and Washington followed Oberlin within a decade.[56] By 1905, 114 institutions of higher education had gymnasiums, with approximately the same number having a physical education department. Nearly 80% required physical education (usually for 2 years), consisting of a gymnastics program, required of all students.[79]

Organized physical education as part of the curriculum first appeared in the ele-

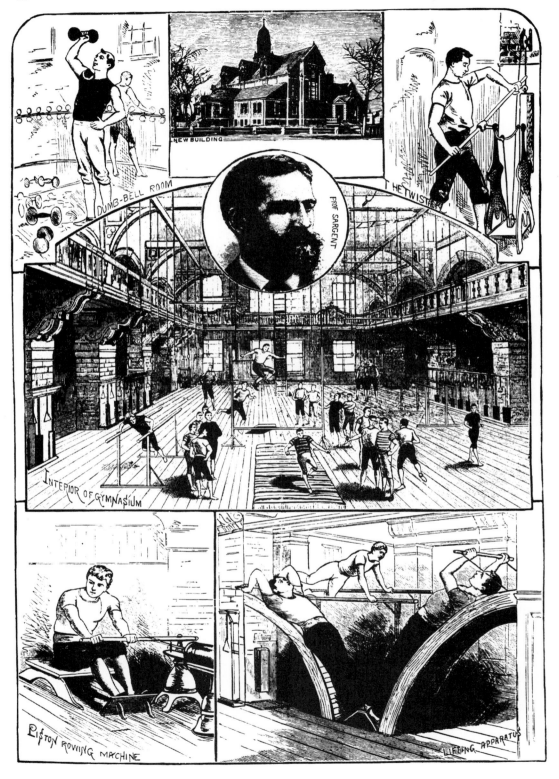

FIG. 1–6. The Hemenway Gymnasium at Harvard University, 1885, programs under the direction of Dr. Dudley Sargent. Note the outside view (top, center) and the expansive depiction of the interior (center). (From Schrader, C.L.: The old Hemenway Gymnasium. JOHPE. *19*(7):476, 1948.) (Reprinted by permission of Harvard University Archives.)

mentary and secondary schools of Boston, St. Louis, and Cincinnati in the mid-1850s. However, this amounted to little more than a few minutes of calisthenics led by the classroom teacher. By the late 1870s and through the 1880s, many large cities hired physical education specialists to conduct programs, most of which consisted primarily of the German system of gymnastics.[56] A survey in 1905 of school physical education programs in 52 cities indicated that gymnastics instruction averaged 15 minutes per day in elementary schools and for two periods weekly in secondary schools. The need for physical education for city school children's physical development and health was widely accepted by 1900, but virtually none of the schools in small towns and rural areas had physical education programs until after World War I. Sports activities in schools before World War I were limited to some intramural and field day competitions starting shortly after 1900, and isolated student initiated and organized interscholastic athletics in several of the largest cities. Students often solicited help from interested adult community members, as there were no teachers or coaches trained in sports.[82]

Indeed, many of the first teachers of gymnastics in schools and colleges often had little more than their own gymnastics participatory experience, together with a summer workshop or a one year college program. Except for Dr. Sargent's summer teacher training program, there was little creditable physical education teacher preparation until the development of a 2-year program at the Young Men's Christian Association (YMCA) International Training School in Springfield, Massachusetts (later Springfield College) in 1887. By 1910, there were over 50 colleges and universities with a 2-year program in physical education. The curriculum included anatomy and physiology, developmental psychology, development of skills in various complex gymnastics and calisthenics routines, and courses on how to organize the teaching of gymnastic skills and routines effectively. By the end of World War I there were approximately 10,000 men and women in the United States professionally trained in physical education.[56] Perhaps, as sug-

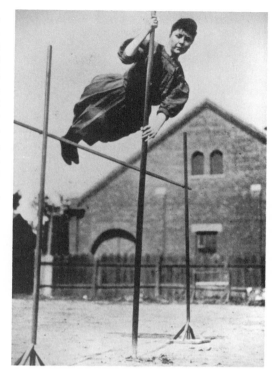

FIG. 1–7. A University of Nebraska woman successfully completes a pole vault in 1905 without benefit of modern athletic attire, training methods, or a cushioned landing surface. (Photograph reprinted by permission of the University of Nebraska Archives.)

gested in Figure 1–7, this impetus inspired an unusually visionary female to attempt a clearly successful pole vault in 1905, while attired in rather restrictive clothing for the achievement of optimal athletic performance.

WORLD WAR I THROUGH WORLD WAR II. This period of physical education history was shaped primarily by the following: (1) the need for increased emphasis on physical fitness in school and college physical education programs during the war years; (2) an economic roller coaster in between, ranging from unprecedented economic prosperity to the Great Depression years, with even greater amounts of leisure time; (3) cultural changes, including increased societal complexity and a substantial liberalization of the dominant educational philosophy. These and other less important factors led to a basic reshaping and increased scope of programmatic offerings. During this period, physical education became a legitimate profession with concomitant improvement in the quality of its programmatic offerings.[56,79]

The occurrence of WW I revealed that approximately 30% of American young adult males called to military duty by the Selective Service Act of 1917, were rejected for physical reasons (including chronic disease, various physical handicaps, and deficiencies in the eyes and teeth). This led to an immediate concerted effort to increase the emphasis on physical training in schools and colleges. This concern for improved fitness of American youth helped provide a dramatic increase in the number of states which passed legislation requiring physical education in public schools in the years during and immediately following the war. Ohio was the first to initiate an effective state requirement in 1892, but by 1913, only 6 others had followed. Twenty-five more passed such legislation between 1915 and 1921, and by 1930, the total was 39.[82]

In the years just prior to WW I, there was evidence of a new physical education evolving that was attuned to important changes in psychology leading to a powerful movement in education progressivism.[56] The leading exponent of this new approach to education was John Dewey, who asserted that one learns best from an interest in doing, and that traditional education should be revised to give the child opportunity to learn material in situations attuned to real-life, thus enabling one to cope better with their application. Though some physical educators, notably Dr. Thomas Wood at Stanford University and later at Columbia University, had developed a concept of the "new" physical education that would theoretically achieve expanded educational objectives beyond that envisioned in prevalent gymnastics programs, this effort had little impact until the mid-1920s.

Prior to 1920, the principal values seen in the gymnastics oriented physical education programs were enhancement of physical capacity and health, and as a release from demanding mental concentration on the study of traditional subject matter. The "new" physical education was envisioned to develop the whole individual—socially, emotionally, and mentally, as well as physically. Dr. Jesse F. Williams was particularly influential in communicating this significant expansion of the purpose of physical education, as evidenced by 8 editions of his classic text, *The Principles of Physical Education*, published over a 37-year period.[83] Physical activities were to remain the medium by which the expanded values of physical education would be communicated. They would continue to include selected gymnastic progressions based upon educational objectives, but also be composed of sports and games, rhythmic, and self-testing activities. Weston astutely summarizes this major change:

Thus, after a century of experimentation with essentially foreign programs of physical education and with programs incorporating foreign elements, a program indigenous to the American people became a reality. It was based upon the social, economic, and political conditions of the United States. The philosophy, principles, objectives, and activities of the new program differed greatly from those of earlier programs and were firmly based upon the latest advances in biology and medicine, sociology and psychology, and education.[82:73]

The technological advance attendant to the Industrial Revolution continued through the first three decades of the 20th century, resulting in a vastly increased urban society with a higher standard of living, and substantially greater leisure time. The Playground and Recreation Association of America was founded in 1906 under the guidance and direction of several prominent physical educators. It facilitated an effective response to the rapidly expanded need for the development of individual and group leisure time activities. The impact of the Great Depression led first to the slashing of recreation budgets, but by 1933, the federal government was working with recreation leaders to finance a vast expansion in public recreation facilities and equipment. This program was extremely successful in providing expanded meaningful recreational opportunities for the large number of unemployed, and was thought beneficial in keeping their morale up.[82] School and college physical education programs, however, experienced significant cutbacks, with about 40% of school programs being cut between 1932 and 1934. Increased interest in recreation had indirect influences on physical education in the schools, including: (1) further popularization of games and sports, (2) further emphasis on social and moral objectives, in addition to physical health, (3) increased awareness of the importance of play as a natural part of growth and as an integral part of the child's education, and (4) increased emphasis on leisure time education in schools.

The nation's interest in sports and games increased substantially in the post WW I years, resulting in not only increased use in community recreation, interscholastic and intercollegiate athletic competition, but also in their becoming an essential part of intramural and physical education instructional programs.[82] The latter contributed to the merger of physical education and athletic programs in schools and colleges, beginning in the 1920s. Also, there was a transition from student organized and administered athletics to a more highly competitive interscholastic and intercollegiate program gradually brought under faculty control, beginning just prior to WW I. The school and college athletic program became a division of the physical education department, though the merger was often an uneasy one as social and economic pressures on athletics occurred increasingly. This was especially true at the college level where programs were frequently developed to satisfy a sports-conscious community and organized more as a business enterprise than primarily attendant to educational objectives of the participants.[82] The National Collegiate Athletic Association (NCAA) was organized in 1905 to provide consistent rules of governance for intercollegiate athletics, but has experienced less than auspicious success in controlling educationally undesirable "big-time" athletic practices. Interscholastic athletic competition has not been immune to similar problems but, in general, has better provided the opportunity for wholesome competition amongst the most physically gifted

students with less distraction from societal influences.[82]

Professional leadership in physical education changed dramatically during the 1920s, as most directors of college physical education programs were no longer medical doctors. By 1927, 87% of department heads held either the Ph.D. or Ed.D. degree. Teacher training programs were expanded from 2 to 4 years during the two decades following WW I, and by 1950, there were nearly 400 institutions of higher education with a 4-year major in physical education. Graduate instruction leading to a doctoral degree was initiated in 1924 at Columbia University and New York University. By 1930, there were 28 colleges and universities offering at least master's degree programs in physical education.[82]

With this development, a substantial increase in research occurred. Initial research was quite varied in a rapidly expanding profession seeking to provide the highest quality instructional programs possible. Early areas of concern included: (1) the development of numerous tests and measurements to assess physical fitness and athletic potential, as well as the effects of various exercise training and sports participation programs; (2) investigations of how sports skills were best taught and learned; and (3) investigation of sports participation effects, via rating scales, on sportsmanship, social, and moral values.[82] In 1930, the profession's expanded need for a means of communicating its growing research knowledge was recognized with publication of the *Research Quarterly*.

Growth in allied professions, first in health and later in recreation, resulted in renaming the American Physical Education Association. In 1937, the organization was renamed the American Association for Health and Physical Education, with "Recreation" added to the title the following year. In 1979, "Dance" was added to the title to form the American Alliance for Health, Physical Education, Recreation, and Dance (AAHPERD), which remains the principal umbrella organization for these allied educational professions.

The primary effect of WW II on school and college physical education programs was a temporary reversal from a primarily sports and games centered program to one with a heavy emphasis on physical fitness. This occurred as a result of initial Selective Service medical examination and armed service fitness tests, which showed many young adult males to be in relatively poor physical condition. Also, girls and women were called upon to assume manual occupational roles that demanded fitness levels well in excess of those in traditional roles previously held by females. Recreational sport activities such as archery, badminton, golf, and tennis, and coed activities including volleyball and dance, were dropped from wartime secondary school and college programs. Activities stressed included aquatics, gymnastics, calisthenics, relays, tumbling, boxing, and wrestling. Obstacle courses with walls, ladders, pits, hurdles, and balance beams were installed on school athletic fields. Team sports, such as soccer, speedball, and touch football were played but with attention to especially quick tempo and increased intensity.[79] There was increased emphasis on physical education, with scaled-down versions of fitness activities, in elementary schools. Numerous physical educators with fitness specialization served as professional consultants to the armed forces in the development of programs to achieve high levels of physical fitness by servicemen in a short time.[82]

POST WORLD WAR II TO PRESENT. Since WW II, the United States has been relatively free from a total commitment to war, though the effects of the Cold War had a somewhat similar impact on physical education. This period has also been marked by increased federal attempts to promote equality of opportunity in various areas to its disadvantaged citizens. This resulted in the Title IX amendment to the Federal Education Act, passed in 1972, which mandated that there could be no discrimination on the basis of one's sex in any federally funded program. In the same context, the federal government also provided funding for the study of needs of handicapped individuals and the rapidly increased elderly population, as well as for the development of programs to meet those needs. Unlike the previous 40 years, there was no prolonged depression, which facilitated continued growth in economic prosperity for most citizens. This, together with additional increases in leisure time, resulted in further popularization of sports.[70] Substantial advances were made in scientific research in physical education, including the relationship of fitness and health in the adult population, which enabled the field to mature as a profession and to enter the developmental stage as an academic discipline.[79]

Continued advances in science and technology have not only increased leisure time since World War II, but many blue collar, common laborer jobs have disappeared, with an increase in professional and technical jobs. Individuals in the latter occupations have been shown to perceive the need for and participate in physically active recreation to a higher degree than do their blue collar counterparts.[21] Further, increased economic prosperity has meant that more individuals have more money to spend on active recreational pursuits. This has also helped facilitate substantial growth of interest in recreational lifetime participation sports, such as badminton, bowling, golf, swimming, and tennis. Physical education instruction in these activities increased sharply in the first 10 years following WW II, as the wartime emphasis on physical fitness receded. Somewhat later, especially in college, physical education courses in other lifetime sports, such as backpacking, cycling, flycasting, and skiing, were added. Siedentop[66] contends that instruction in these activities has been added primarily as a reflection of adult leisure trends and popular opinion, rather than careful analysis of their value in achieving well-identified educational objectives. Changes from instruction in team sports to other activities more popular at the particular time with students, has also accompanied reduction or loss of the requirement for physical education instruction in colleges and secondary schools. The latter occurred primarily during the late 1960s in response to students' request for fewer requirements and greater freedom of choice. In 1949, 92% of all secondary school children participated for an average of 132 minutes per week.[79] By 1980, only 36% of students in grades 5 to 12 had daily physical education, and less than 50% in grades 11 and 12 had any physical education.[49]

It should be recalled that sports in our society evolved outside of physical education in schools and colleges, with athletic programs only coming under faculty control in the late 1920s. Since WW II, the importance of sports in school and college physical education has increased, but not to the extent it has in our overall culture. Professional sports in the United States have grown exponentially since WW II, when only baseball and boxing commanded much attention. Subsequently, baseball, football, golf, and hockey have expanded in importance, while professional competition in basketball and tennis has been initiated and grown rapidly as well. Growth in the public's interest in sport has been facilitated by the media, especially television. Michener[45] cites a $200 million expenditure for sports coverage in 1975, with an additional 10% above usual growth expected in the 1976 Olympics year. Television payments to professional sports rose from 1961 to 1975 as follows: (1) baseball, from $3 million to $35 million; (2) football, from $4 million to $44 million; and (3) golf, from $150,000 to $5 million. More large stadia have been built, and sports spectatorism, when one includes those at live events and watching television, numbers many millions each day. Annual attendance at major spectator sports during 1979–1980 is summarized below:[70]

SPORT	ATTENDANCE
Horseracing	78,000,000
Baseball	65,000,000
Football (collegiate and professional)	50,000,000
Auto racing	48,000,000
Basketball	41,000,000

This modern American cultural fascination with sport as spectators is alarming to some, who describe it as the sports disease, "spectatoritis," and espouse concern because of its similarity to the behavior of Roman citizens in the waning years of the Empire ("It is a symptom of loss of national vigor when once hardy citizens are content merely to loaf and look"—[79]). The latter contention seems invalid, in that individual adult sports participation has contin-

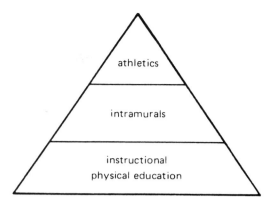

FIG. 1–8. Traditional symbolic relationship of physical education, intramurals, and athletics. (From Siedentop, D.: Physical Education: Introductory Analysis (3rd ed.). Dubuque, IA: Wm. C. Brown, 1980, p. 37.)

ued to increase.[74] Further, it has been estimated that Americans spend 10 times as much on participant sports as on spectator sports.[10]

The popularity of sports in our culture extends beyond the adult community, professional and intercollegiate competition, to interscholastic athletics and now, even to competitive sports for children generally conducted outside the schools. The latter has created enough concern amongst physicians, psychologists and physical educators to result in more appropriate competitive restrictions than originally existed.[28] Still, there are many physical educators who are vitally concerned about the profound influence of commercialized sports upon athletic programs in schools and colleges. The traditional relationship between secondary school instructional physical education, intramural sports, and athletics is depicted in Figure 1–8. The notion advanced is that instructional physical education is the base of a pyramid denoting primary emphasis of the overall program for the greatest number of individuals. For those more gifted, and/or interested, intramural sports competition represents an important intermediate level. The apex is intended to signify the few highly gifted individuals who desire intense competition with similar individuals in interscholastic/intercollegiate athletics. All too often, however, the funds and personnel provided for these programs are more accurately indicated by an inverted pyramid structure to that depicted in Figure 1–8. As Siedentop[66] correctly notes, physical educators have traditionally relegated athletics to a position that is inconsistent with that which it holds with the general public. This incongruity is such that many college athletic programs are no longer affiliated with their institution's physical education department. Further, interscholastic athletic programs usually draw far greater interest of parents and students, whether in urban areas or in small towns, than do the physical education or intramural sports programs. This usually means that disproportionate funding, personnel time and attention are routinely given to the few highly gifted student-athletes, rather than to the far more numerous other students who could benefit if increased resources were dedicated to physical education instruction and intramural sports programs. Even with the greatly enhanced popularity of athletic competition, now extending from youth to professional leagues, sports in America remains a much broader cultural phenomenon, in that such highly popular spectator sports as auto racing, boxing, dog racing, and horse racing do not properly fall within the educational domain.[70]

Individual developmentalism continued as the predominant educational philosophy influencing physical education programs.[79] Students were encouraged, especially in elementary and junior high school, to attempt a wide variety of activities to find one or more at which they could excel, or at least play well enough to enjoy. Accordingly, programs were expanded to include much more than the traditional team sports, including self-testing activities and lifetime sports. The focus of physical education programs moved more to the development of each student's potential. Movement education, which stressed the technique of individual problem solving and the need to establish basic movement competence at one's own pace as a basis for more advanced skills, was introduced in elementary school programs with great success during the 1960s. The

federal government provided funding to facilitate this effort of individual development for underprivileged children, the handicapped, and the mentally retarded.[79]

Adapted physical education increased rapidly following World War II, as physical rehabilitation of the wounded was found to facilitate vastly improved functional capacity. Physical education programs, particularly in the colleges, developed specially designed exercise and activity progressions for individuals with various physical handicaps. Federal grants helped in this effort, as well as for research, program development, and leadership training for those working with the mentally retarded. In 1975, the Federal Education of All Handicapped Children Act was passed to ensure that each individual would have an opportunity to develop his full potential and, wherever possible, in classes with non-handicapped students. This law increased adaptive physical education in colleges and schools. The Amateur Sports Act of 1978 charged the U.S. Olympic Committee with encouraging sports competition opportunity for the handicapped. The Committee of Sports for the Disabled arose from this charge, and amateur sports programs for individuals with various physical and mental handicaps have increased substantially[19] (Figure 1–9). A related phenomenon is the rapid increase in the use of physical activity as a therapeutic modality for individuals with a wide variety of disability or handicaps. This has resulted in expanded career opportunities in corrective therapy, dance therapy, occupational therapy, physical therapy, recreational therapy, and rehabilitative medicine.[39]

Individual developmentalism also facilitated the initial growth of interscholastic and intercollegiate athletic competition for girls and women in the late 1960s. While this effort, together with several national women's sports organizations' response to improve our women's performance in the Olympics, succeeded in partially countering the strong cultural bias against female participants in vigorous physical activity programs, it was again legislation (Title IX amendment to the Federal Education Act, 1972) that had by far the most profound

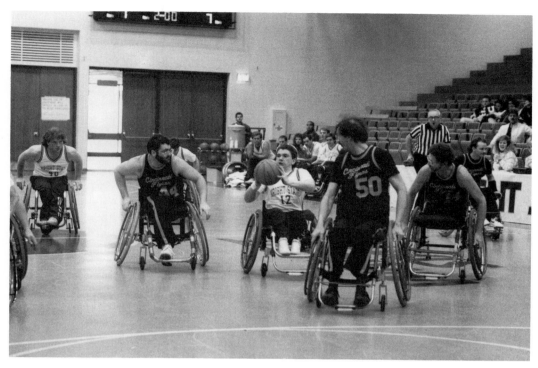

FIG. 1–9. Opportunities for athletic competition amongst persons with physical handicaps have expanded, including wheelchair divisions in marathon races and, in this photograph, a hotly contested basketball game. (Photograph courtesy of Wright State University, Ohio, adapted athletics program.)

effect. Title IX mandated that there can be no discrimination on the basis of sex in any federally funded education program. Interpreted broadly, this meant that an institution receiving any federal funds was required not to discriminate on the basis of sex in all of its programs. The impact on physical education has been less profound than for athletics, in that many schools were already providing comparatively equal facilities and equipment, personnel, and instructional time. The major change in many schools was reorganization of classes to a coeducational basis, though they could be separated on the basis of sex during participation in contact sports such as football and wrestling. Predominantly single-sex grouping could also occur in other activities if done on the basis of ability in order to facilitate more effective learning.

The impact of Title IX on interscholastic athletics for girls can perhaps best be ap-

preciated by comparison of the total number of participants: (1) 294,000 in 1970–71; (2) 1,600,000 in 1976–77, and (3) 1,747,000 in 1983–84.[24] In 1983–84 the number of female participants in interscholastic and intercollegiate athletics was about half that of males. Similar discrepancies still exist in the number of teams, support funding, and athletic scholarships. However, more nearly equal opportunity for practice and games, travel allowances, coaches' compensation, medical and training services, as well as equipment, has occurred.

Since the mid-1950s, there has been a near consistent concern with physical fitness in school and college physical education programs. It was initiated by the Kraus-Weber muscular fitness test comparison of American and European school children.[37] The fact that American children scored well below their European counterparts on most items was brought to President Eisenhower's attention, who established the President's Council on Youth Fitness in 1956. This action resulted in numerous national organizations encouraging attention to enhancement of youth fitness. In addition to encouraging more emphasis on fitness related activities in school and college physical education programs, the AAHPERD developed a 7-item youth fitness test which was administered to thousands of students in 1958, 1965, and 1975. For the first time, there was a strong demand for elementary school teachers of physical education. The scores of children on the AAHPERD fitness test in 1965 were near consistently better for both boys and girls in grades 5 through 12, with less dramatic improvement again observed in 1975.[54] President Kennedy advocated expansion of the fitness effort to include adults,[10] and this served to publicize widely the need for regular vigorous physical activity in our otherwise sedentary lifestyle. This action, together with several prominent medical doctors' strong advocacy of vigorous exercise to improve fitness and retard the development of chronic disease states,[15,38] spurred an unprecedented fitness boom. This interest has even extended to competition, especially popular in road running and swimming, in which several age ranges of master's level competition are used.[50]

The early performance oriented fitness tests and activity programs for school children were revised by AAHPERD[60] to reflect physical fitness components associated with health, including body composition and cardiorespiratory endurance. Between 1982 and 1984, the U.S. Public Health Office of Disease Prevention and Health Promotion, in cooperation with AAHPERD and several other national agencies, conducted the National Children and Youth Fitness Study. It surveyed both the school physical education program makeup and voluntary extracurricular physical activity participation in a nationwide sample of boys and girls, grades 5 through 12. Measurements of a 5-item health related fitness test, assessing body fatness, flexibility, abdominal strength, upper body strength, and cardiorespiratory endurance, were obtained.[60]

A primary impetus to the enhanced public awareness and interest in fitness, alluded to above, is that of a shift from curative and rehabilitative medicine to preventive medicine. This concept will be discussed in detail later, but in essence, preventive medicine seeks to identify effective strategies in reducing the effects of chronic disease that lead too often to severe illness or death well before 70 years of age. These strategies include participation in regular vigorous physical activity, as well as attention to optimal diet (in amount and types of foods), stress management, and abstention from smoking. Two reports from the U.S. Department of Health, Education, and Welfare[76,77] specify the potential of physical education's significant role in the adult population's achievement of health and well-being. More recent publications in the United States and Sweden attest to the medical community's increasing acceptance of the role of physical activity in public health and disease prevention.[2,52]

Physical education, as a profession, has assumed an umbrella role to several allied professions, which is reflected in the title of their premiere associative organization, the American Alliance for Health, Physical Education, Recreation, and Dance. In addition, interscholastic athletics has maintained an effective forum in this organization through the mid-1980s. Siedentop,[66] however, contends that though cooperation and interaction among these professions remains, each seems increasingly motivated to achieve a distinct entity. Perhaps this tendency is well conceived, in that this umbrella concept evolved when each was more closely oriented to the formal educational process in schools and colleges. While each of these professions retain this characteristic, they also have other unique service elements valued by society. For example, physical education is becoming increasingly important in the public health enhancement of all citizens, including adults who have completed formal education in schools and colleges.

A profound development in physical education since World War II is the increasingly important role of science and scholarly effort. This has been reflected in a more demanding academic major, which now entails study of a curriculum of basic sciences and liberal arts, in addition to theoretical and practical aspects of the application of this knowledge base. By 1969, there were 200 institutions of higher education conferring master's degrees in physical education and 50 that had doctoral degree programs.[79] This accelerated emphasis on the scientific basis of physical education was due, in part, to the widespread impetus on the life sciences provided by the U.S. space program. Also, it became apparent early that effective advances in space would necessitate detailed study of the effects of space flight on man and human physical performance. It became evident to the federal government and other agencies funding research, that the scientific study of human movement in all its dimensions was a fertile, relatively unexplored area for research. By 1966, 151 colleges/universities had physical education research facilities, including 58 for exercise physiology, 40 for fitness and motor functional measurement, 27 for motor learning, 24 for kinesiology, and 12 for growth and development.[79]

This accelerated research effort, made increasingly productive by computers and other technologic developments, resulted in a physical education knowledge explosion. By 1964, six areas of knowledge specialization were recognized: (1) sociology of sport and physical education; (2) biomechanics; (3) exercise physiology; (4) motor learning and sport psychology; (5) history and philosophy of physical education and sport; and (6) administrative theory.[88] Prior to this time, physical education major programs were almost totally oriented to general education philosophy and the training of teachers and coaches for professional careers as educators in the schools. A large portion of the curriculum was devoted to the acquisition of numerous sports and basic exercise skills and how to most effectively organize and teach this material to achieve desired educational goals. Elements of human movement studies, including exercise physiology, growth and development, kinesiology, motor learning, and sport psychology were in-

cluded, but were not a primary focus of the curriculum.

In 1964, Franklin Henry of the University of California, Berkeley, provided a theoretical framework for the study of physical education as an academic discipline, which he defined as "an organized body of knowledge collectively embraced in a formal course of study."[34] Henry contended that an academic discipline was theoretical and scholarly in content, rather than technical and professional. He also identified a unique developing scholarly field of knowledge basic to physical education, in which the focus of study was man as an individual engaged in motor performances of various types. He emphasized that this new academic discipline did not consist of the application of the study of related disciplines, including anatomy, physics, physiology, cultural anthropology, history, psychology, and sociology. Rather, it consisted of the study (as a discipline) of certain aspects of these traditional subject matter areas that are germane to the understanding of human movement. He stressed that scholars in other related disciplines generally had only peripheral interest in the study of man engaged in physical activity. It was only the academic discipline of physical education that had human movement as its central focus. Thus, physical education emerged as an academic discipline, as well as a previously well-recognized profession. Steinhaus has distinguished between an academic discipline and a profession as follows:

A discipline is a branch of learning . . . (whose) purpose is to extend in breadth and depth the content of their subject fields through study and research . . . A profession is the practice of an art that utilizes one or more disciplines in serving mankind.[73:69]

Since 1965, the undergraduate physical education major has become less professional course oriented, with increased emphasis on the academic discipline. In most cases, at least a 2-year liberal arts and basic science background is followed by a 2-year program of specialization. The bachelor's degree recipient might then elect to enter a teaching credential program, go on to physical therapy school, or to graduate school for advanced work in one of several subdiscipline areas. The rapid increase in knowledge has recently resulted in graduate students usually being required to elect a specialization from among biomechanics, exercise physiology, motor learning, history and philosophy of physical education, sport psychology, or sport sociology. Thus, their graduate training is becoming better characterized as that of a biomechanist, a sport psychologist, etc., rather than as a physical educator, per se.

Until the mid-1960s, with continued growth in school and college student enrollment, job prospects for a physical education graduate as a teacher and/or coach were good. However, by the early 1970s, enrollments leveled off or declined, and in the middle 1970s, economic conditions resulted in some education program cutbacks. Indeed, in 1975 colleges and universities were graduating 4 times more male and 3 times more female physical education majors than there were secondary school jobs.[39] This trend of reduced teaching positions available in physical education has continued through the late-1980s, but is projected to increase somewhat in the mid-1990s.[20] The change from a professional oriented curriculum to one with strong liberal arts and basic science preparation, together with the study of human movement from a broad perspective, has resulted in more versatile physical education graduates who have found an impressively wide range of alternate careers. A partial list, arranged in seven categories, is given in Table 1–1. Many of these alternate career options have arisen from the increased leisure time and increased financial resources for recreation enjoyed by much of the adult population, the enhanced popularity of sports in our culture, and the greater public awareness of fitness and health enhancement. In addition to the development of a large leisure and fitness industry in the private sector, industry and business corporations are providing "in house" recreational and health/fitness facilities and programs in increasing numbers.[35] There are also an increasing number of recreation programs in communities and the private sector. Other recent physical education graduates have initiated careers in sports administration, sports communication, and sports marketing. There are also an increasing number of graduates who are entering various allied health professions postgraduate programs to qualify for careers in these occupations.

PHILOSOPHIC FOUNDATIONS

Philosophy, as a discipline, can be defined as the pursuit of wisdom which involves inquiry into facts and principles of reality, and of human nature and conduct, utilizing logical reasoning rather than observation and experiment. The critique and analysis of fundamental beliefs, as they are conceptualized and formulated, are accomplished via structured processes of reasoning, taking as little as possible for granted. However, the term philosophy is also used to connote a basic theory or viewpoint, as in one's philosophy of physical education, or the system of values by which one lives, i.e., one's philosophy of life. Philosophy as a discipline will be examined first, in brief, followed by a more lengthy discussion of the philosophic bases of physical education.

Philosophy is characterized by an inquiring attitude that develops one's capacity to proceed past the immediate and familiar to underlying complexities. It represents an outgrowth of ordinary reflection, such as that we all engage in when we are confronted with great problems and try to determine their meaning and effect on our lives. But the philosopher goes through this process more seriously, more persistently, and more skillfully.[4]

There are six major areas of study in philosophy: metaphysics, epistemology, logic, axiology, ethics, and aesthetics.

1. Metaphysics is that area which systematically investigates the ultimate nature of reality. Utilizing a speculative, critical approach, questions related to all aspects of humanity and the universe are addressed.
2. Epistemology focuses on the nature and origin of knowledge. It deals with what kinds of knowledge exist and with the means of acquiring knowledge. Kinds of knowledge include authoritative (ob-

Table 1–1.   Alternate Career Opportunities for Physical Educators*

Equipment Design	*Sports Administration/Management*
footwear/other sports equipment designer	administrator (league, team, club, agency, clinic, health club, etc.)
therapy equipment designer	athletic director
Health/Medical/Rehabilitation/Therapy	athletic finance director
athletic trainer	business manager
biomechanist	facility director
cardiac rehabilitation specialist	military physical activity director
exercise physiologist	owner (team, club, camp, clinic, studio, wholesale or retail store or manufacturing)
exercise test technician	player representative
job analyst/disability evaluator/pre-employment testing specialist	recreation program director
medical specialties (wellness, sports medicine, orthopedic surgery, weight control)	*Sports Communication*
	broadcaster
	illustrator
pharmaceutical salesperson	information director
therapist (corrective, physical, occupational, recreation, dance, play)	journalist
	photographer
Performance	*Sports Marketing*
sports official	advertising
touring professional (pro teams, ice skater, dancer, etc.)	clothing salesperson
	club membership salesperson
Physical Activity Instruction	equipment salesperson
fitness leader (health club, community, corporate firm, weight control spa)	manufacturer's representative
	product advertising
geriatric/senior citizen activity leader	team or athletic program marketing director
infant/toddler development/activity leader	
private coach/consultant	
sport instructor (golf, skiing, tennis, etc.)	

*Modified from Clayton, R.D. and J.A. Clayton: Careers and professional preparation programs. JOPERD. *55(5)*:44–45, 1984; and Lambert, C.L.: What is physical education? JOPER. *51(5)*:26–27, 1980.

tained from experts), rational (acquired via reasoning and valid judgment), and empirical (that acquired through one's observations).
3. Logic deals with the principles of sound reasoning, and of the method and validity of deduction and induction. It describes the process to follow in thinking and in relating ideas into an appropriately structured sequence that produces valid conclusions.
4. Axiology is the study of the nature of values and value judgments. It is concerned with identification and description of values that exist, with their degree of permanency, and their relative importance.
5. Ethics, generally considered a subdivision of axiology, is the study of the general nature of morals and specific moral choices one should make in relationships with others. As such, it identifies and characterizes moral character, and provides a basis for development of an individual code of conduct.

6. Aesthetics is concerned with the study of theories of beauty and of its expression in the fine arts, such as dance, drama, music, painting, and sculpture. It is concerned not only with accurately describing beauty, but with the study of values in relation to the way artists express themselves.

Metaphysics and axiology, in general, form what is termed speculative philosophy, because they examine the postulation of first principles and the subsequent recognition of values. Epistemology and logic comprise what is usually called critical philosophy, in that they attempt to explain how knowledge is acquired and how thought is verified.[85]

PHILOSOPHY AND SCIENCE. Both philosophy and science arose from the human mind's large capacity to think. Until about the 17th century, all people systematically studying ideas regarding human existence were philosophers. Thus, the sciences arose from philosophy and, with the efficiency of the scientific method in producing reliable results useful to man, grew rapidly and broke away from philosophy. Some even envisioned that the true nature of things could now be determined analytically through accurate scientific measurement alone, and that philosophy should only concern itself with values.[85]

At present, philosophy and science have some common qualities, but also distinct differences. Both are interested in acquiring knowledge, and both use rigorous methods of study, though that for science is more clearly delineated.[4] Further, the scientific method entails direct observation and measurement, while philosophic analysis does not. The scientist's approach to a problem is limited, while the philosopher's is comprehensive. Finally, the scientist is interested in acquiring factual knowledge and establishing cause and effect (scientific law). On the other hand, the philosopher is concerned with understanding the very concepts of causality or scientific law themselves, and determining to what extent they are capable of analysis and clarification.[4]

PROMINENT PHILOSOPHICAL SCHOOLS OF THOUGHT. Historically, there has never been unanimous agreement among philosophers on how they viewed the nature of reality, truth, and values. Nonetheless, three leading Western philosophic schools of thought—idealism, realism, and pragmatism—emerged in the late 19th and early 20th centuries, and continued to have significant impact into the 1970s.[87] While each has had substantial influence on U.S. education, it has been an outgrowth of pragmatism, advocated by John Dewey, termed educational progressivism, that has been most influential.

Details of the impact of Dewey's ideas on education and on physical education have been presented earlier in this chapter. From a philosophic analysis perspective, they included implications for three fundamental issues: (1) the relationship among society, school, and the individual; (2) educational aims and objectives; and (3)

the process of education.[86] Changes were effected via a closer teacher-child relationship with a less rigid classroom atmosphere, accompanied by opportunity for self-directed study and use of the classroom (and field trips) as a laboratory for examining new ideas.[11]

Existentialism is a philosophic school that has emerged as a significant force only during the past century. It builds on, yet contrasts markedly with, many assertions of the traditional schools of idealism and realism regarding fundamental positions on reality, truth, and values. While more in agreement with pragmatism, it places even more emphasis on individual worth and freedom of choice in developing values. Self-determination, self-evaluation, and personal responsibility for consequences of value choices are stressed. Implications for education include providing an atmosphere promoting individual growth in the personal qualities identified above, with the teacher assisting in an impartial manner in the development of each individual's own values.[86]

PHILOSOPHY OF PHYSICAL EDUCATION AND SPORT

The nature and significance of physical education and sport has been largely ignored by philosophers.[81] In fact, systematic philosophic study by scholars in physical education and sport is of recent origin. When undertaken in a traditional manner, it can contribute to the comprehensive understanding of physical education and sport, interpreting data by means of general concepts that will assist in guiding better choices of professional goals and the methods to attain them.[87]

WHAT CAN BE GAINED FROM PHILOSOPHICAL RESEARCH IN PHYSICAL EDUCATION AND SPORT? In 1963, Van Dalen[78] wrote a brief essay addressing the essence of this question. He asserted that philosophy in physical education should strive to solve problems and controversies that lie beyond the help afforded by empirical science. It should examine, criticize, order, and interpret what is known in the field and structure a frame of reference from which we can gain a dependable sense of direction that would be lacking otherwise.

Davis and Miller[17] have identified five principal reasons for developing a philosophy of physical education. First, it can serve as a "common language" that facilitates more effective communication with other disciplines actively involved in the education enterprise. In this connection, it can move the profession beyond isolated concerns to expanded frames of reference. A third reason, is that it encourages careful examination of basic assumptions, including their source and validity. Stimulation of self-examination, which enables one to identify and critically examine his beliefs and convictions, is a fourth reason. Finally, these authors contend that developing a philosophy of physical education can crystalize professional purpose. Zeigler[87] contends that the systematic development of a philosophy of physical education would lead to greater consensus of purpose in the profession and place it in a much better position to deal with persistent problems.

DEVELOPMENT OF PHILOSOPHICAL INQUIRY IN PHYSICAL EDUCATION AND SPORT. Rivenes[57] asserts that until the late 1950s, philosophic study of physical education appeared to be largely limited to professionals expressing their point of view, rather than exemplifying the more rigorous, sustained, and disciplined reflection necessary for genuine philosophic inquiry. Indeed, in 1969, Ziegler[86] concluded that if a review of literature of the philosophy of physical education in which the structural analysis technique of philosophic research was used, the list of studies identified would be noticeably short. Zeigler[85–87] has utilized the rigorous philosophic approach in examining the most persistent problems facing the profession. Similarly, Davis and Miller[17] have presented an extensive treatment of the philosophic process in physical education.

In December 1972, a small group of philosophers interested in sport and a group of physical educators interested in philosophy formed the Philosophic Society for the Study of Sport. Since 1974, the society has published the *Journal of the Philosophy of Sport*. While some physical education departments have a specialist in philosophy on their faculty, as well as a few undergraduate and graduate courses, research productivity has not been closely comparable to that of the major subdisciplines in physical education. Further, Siedentop[66] concluded that most of the philosophic research in the 1970s was directed toward issues in the field of sport rather than physical education. Thus, the potential for significant contribution to the profession by philosophic research remains relatively untapped.[87]

IMPORTANCE OF DEVELOPING YOUR OWN PHILOSOPHY OF PHYSICAL EDUCATION. One who would teach, coach, or lead organized physical activity programs in a non-school setting, should understand that there is significant professional responsibility in developing the best structured presentation of well-selected movement experiences for an increasingly discerning clientele. This entails not only acquiring scientific knowledge, technical and pedagogic skills, but also examination of their effective integration via the philosophic process. Values of this effort include:

1. teaches one to question assumptions upon which current professional practices are based;
2. enables one to clarify aims and objectives of a structured physical activity program;
3. promotes clarification of one's beliefs and values, which profoundly influence one's behavior; and
4. enables one to use scientific knowledge and technical skills acquired in a more soundly based manner in his professional practice.

GUIDES TO DEVELOPING YOUR PHILOSOPHY OF PHYSICAL EDUCATION. One should understand that a person espousing a philosophy of physical education on an important issue might actually be stating an opinion or theory emanating from merely having jotted down a few notes. Actually, the latter represents only a rather feeble beginning. Each of you presently has acquired some information from your past experiences in physical education. This, together with your beliefs, values, and ideas that emanate from disciplined thought and synthesis, describes the essence of developing one's philosophy. Obviously, one's philosophy can become more profound as knowledge is increased and skill in the philosophic thinking process is developed. This knowledge base includes not only that from scientific data, but a basic understanding of the positions taken by the four primary schools of thought on reality, truth, and values. You should try to determine which positions you agree with, and incorporate them into your own basic philosophic position. Then, extend your reading and thinking to the field of physical education to determine which philosophic positions seems at odds with yours. Further reading and discussion with student peers and professors will provide help in advancing your philosophic growth.[17]

Logical induction and deduction are primary reasoning methods, while analysis and synthesis can be considered tools of philosophic inquiry. Clarke and Clarke[14] have outlined the steps involved by one who engages in philosophic inquiry:

1. Clearly identifies the problem area.
2. Collects available facts related to the problem.
3. Synthesizes and analyzes the facts, working them into patterns that identify relationships among them.
4. From these patterns, derives general principles that describe the relationships inherent in the principles.
5. States these principles in the form of hypotheses or tentative assumptions.

ROLE OF PHYSICAL EDUCATION PROGRAMS THROUGH 2000

One recurrent theme in the examination of the philosophic bases of physical education has been the potential of philosophic inquiry for clarifying programmatic aims and objectives. In this section, elements of the philosophic process appropriate to the task were utilized in preparing statements of the role of physical education during the remainder of the century in: (1) schools and colleges; and (2) in other societal locales.

ROLE OF PHYSICAL EDUCATION IN SCHOOLS AND HIGHER EDUCATION. The basic function of education in our society is to nurture the total development of young people in order that they might live enriched, abundant, and useful lives. Thus, education's charge extends well beyond the development of each student's intellectual potential and the acquisition of a large fund of liberal arts and technologic knowledge also inherent in the formal educational process. In this context, physical education can be defined as that process which, through the media of sports, dance, and exercise, strives to bring about physical, mental, social, and emotional development of the individual.[83] While a properly organized and directed physical education program does make significant contributions to the individual's social, mental, and emotional growth, these are shared goals of all aspects of education. However, physical education has a unique contribution to make in the physical development aspect of this total process.

The latter assertion is only valid with respect to the primary programmatic focus of physical education, as modern programs are grounded upon the biologic unity of mind and body. That is, one responds to any environmental input as a whole being, and not as a mind without a body, or vice versa. Nash elaborates:

The biological concept accepted today acknowledges an integration of all the capacities, traits, skills and powers of an individual into one personality which responds as a whole. Not only an individual's nervous system is an integrated whole, but also the entire organism is integrated. Each individual is a unit, a personality of many parts, functioning as a whole. No boy's mind by itself ever went to a football game, a classroom, a church or a jail. The total organism is equipped with a body, well or ill, a set of skills, a way of thinking, and emotionalized attitudes expressed in likes, dislikes, prejudices and principles.[47:264]

While the biologic unity of mind and body concept holds that the entire organism reacts to all stimuli encountered in its environment, it should be obvious that all stimuli do not have the same effect. This is easily appreciated by comparing the psychologic and physiologic responses to a 1-

hour calculus class to those from 1 hour of soccer warm-up drills and a practice game. Even the same activity, e.g., walking, can have substantially different effects when one hikes leisurely, as opposed to race-walking. Steinhaus, however, feels that there are few, if any, environments other than those of a physical education nature which permit, let alone encourage, the total organism to respond to a multiplicity of stimuli.[72]

While Steinhaus's perception of physical education providing rich potential for whole integrated organism response, there are many in the academic community who tend to categorize the physical education class as the time and place in the student's everyday curriculum for taking care of the body's needs by exercising (i.e., education of the physical). They assume that the student's mind is a virtual vacuum during physical activity. Further, there are many who consider the academic core subjects essential, and thus physical education, along with other "less important" curricular offerings, is decreased or eliminated upon cyclic occurrences of "back to basics" or shortage of funds. Dix, an educational administrator comments:

It is a very perverted education attitude to assume that children and young people in their growing stages need carefully planned arrangements for mathematics and for history more than they do for consistent opportunity and stimulation for physical activity. We have a hang-over of medieval contempt for the body, which is far less respectable in the modern age than was the pagan attitude of the Greeks. It is bad enough to have an increasing tendency for life occupations in a mature, complex society to become sedentary and physically malforming, without forcing young people in their growing period to cripple the magnificent heritage that the human physical organism still is. Apparently, only in time of war are we shocked to find widespread physical defects and a general lack of vital tone in the population. It is hard to find language strong enough to criticize so vicious a neglect.[22:87-88]

Until recently, most American physical educators have taught primarily sports skills and hoped that the beneficial by-products of these activities, together with occasional reminders of the values of continued participation in vigorous physical activity, would result in students' integrating these activities in their daily pattern of living following graduation. In fact, the recent upsurge in fitness among previously sedentary adults appears largely due to several years of heavy media exposure espousing the benefits of regular exercise in facilitating health enhancement. Logan and McKinney comment on the past failure of college physical educators in this regard, and offer suggestions to better achieve this important role in the future.

Students do need to be taught the *how-to* of skill, but this is not enough for our current, *thinking* student. He also needs to know the *why-of* participation in neuromuscular activities. He needs to know what the neuromuscular activity means to him in terms of his own physiologic, anatomic, psychological, and philosophic requirements. The combined *how-to* and *why-of* approaches to teaching physical education may help motivate the students to participate in an activity throughout their lifetime, because insight tends to facilitate foresight. Teachers should be concerned primarily with teaching activities so the students will be motivated to use the activities regularly throughout their lifetimes. The college physical education class should be a continuation of attention to physical fitness, not the end.[40:18]

Kraus and Raab[38] contend that school physical education programs have a vital role in attending to the physical fitness needs of youth and aiding in the prevention of hypokinetic disease. Following analysis of results from the 1985 President's Council on Physical Fitness and Sports' National School Fitness Survey, Reiff et al.[54] concluded that a great challenge for the 1990s and into the 21st century existed in the revitalization of school physical education programs. They recommended increased opportunities for students to develop fitness components, learn important concepts in exercise science, and experience fitness tests on a serial basis which would provide a profile of each youth's fitness, relationships to their peer age and sex group, and changes in their fitness achievement. Blair et al.[8] recommend that physical education programs at all levels should increase emphasis on exercise as it relates to health and well being. Further, principles of exercise prescription, physiologic effects (acute and chronic) of regular exercise, and health benefits and risks of physical activity should be taught in a carefully planned and sequenced curriculum. This breadth of perspective constitutes the collective intent of school physical education programs designed to produce the physically educated student of the 1990s.[42]

THE EXPANDED SOCIETAL ROLE FOR PHYSICAL EDUCATION. Until the 1970s, physical education's role was closely allied and essentially limited to the educational curricula of American schools and colleges. Indeed, in 1975, Terris stated that "physical fitness and physical education have no respected place in the American public health movement."[75] However, as mentioned earlier, there has been a substantial increase in adult physical activity participation in the decade following the mid-1970s. This phenomenon occurred largely outside the province of physical education, as the medical community, public health authorities, and the media communicated widely to the adult population the growing body of evidence that regular physical activity produces substantial physical and emotional benefits.[35,68] In 1979, the Public Health Service specified "physical fitness and exercise" as 1 of the 15 areas of greatest importance for improving the health of the public.[51]

For the first time, there is a large and still growing private physical education industry in the United States. Further, in addition to adults, children in the middle and upper classes have been receiving a good portion of their physical education from this source. Siedentop[66] considers it ironic that private physical education is growing at the same time when the public seems less willing to devote tax dollars to physical education in the schools. Blair et al.[8] contend that this is largely due to many school physical education programs continuing to maintain programs with a strong emphasis on instruction in traditional team sports. While this may still be the emphasis that physical education teachers and many students prefer, it is not consistent with the primary reasons of health and well-being given for participation in regular exercise by adults.

The collaborative promotion of physical activity participation in the United States population for public health enhancement was examined in 1985 by Iverson et al.[35] They also summarized the current status in medical, worksite, community, and school settings. Only a small portion of medical care settings offered physical activity programs, which were almost always associated with cardiac rehabilitation programs. Over 80% of the population sees a physician each year, with primary care physicians accounting for more than 50% of all patient encounters. Though the medical care encounter is considered an ideal situation to encourage patients to increase their physical activity level, surveys indicate that few physicians regularly discuss this with their patients. This seems particularly perplexing, in that most patients want physicians to be concerned with their health habits, including physical activity levels. Apparently, many physicians are concerned about their efficacy in counseling patients, and feel that lack of insurance reimbursement also curtails time available for nutritional and exercise counseling.[59] Another study suggests that there are important deficiencies in the final-year medical students' knowledge of exercise physiology and physical training.[84]

Iverson et al.[35] conclude that although the workplace is currently the focus of greatest interest by people who implement structured physical activity programs, there is little agreement in defining what constitutes the most appropriate program. Further, in 1985, only about 15% of employers in the United States provided worksite opportunities for formal exercise.[62] While worksite fitness programs have been shown to decrease absenteeism and increase productivity, there is still no conclusive proof that they reduce health care costs.[26,64] Nonetheless, there has been substantial growth in worksite fitness programs, as is indirectly reflected in an increased membership from 25 in 1974 to 3,000 in 1984 in the American Association of Fitness in Business.[30] Most worksite fitness programs exist in firms with 500 or more employees whose total work force constitutes less than 20% of the U.S. total. Thus, the challenge in future worksite fitness program growth will be in helping small firms meet their employees' health needs.[31]

The 1985 study by Iverson et al.[35] found that the greatest variety of physical activity programs were in community settings. They were offered by a number of non-profit private organizations, nonprofit public agencies, and for-profit organizations. While relatively little research has been done on community-based physical activity programs, it appears that when mass media are used as a primary mode of intervention, they clearly affect residents' interest and awareness in physical activity. However, whether they have a major effect on exercise behavioral changes in the short-term is not certain.[21]

It should be apparent that physical education in the United States is now in an era in which there is strong societal pressure to assume a vital collaborative role with other important societal elements in the enhancement of public health. This could be effected by modification of its programs in schools and colleges, as well as by extending its impact beyond these locales. Other important participants include the medical community and public health authorities, business and industry, private enterprise, the media, community organizations, and government.[35] The Public Health Service[77] has outlined specific objectives to be achieved by 1990, including:

1. At least 60% of youth, ages 10 to 17, should be participating daily in school physical education programs.
2. Greater than 90% of youth, ages 10 to 17, should be participating regularly in vigorous physical activities, particularly cardiorespiratory fitness programs that can be carried on into adulthood.
3. At least 60% of adults, ages 18 to 65, should be participating in vigorous physical activity at least 3 times per week for 20 minutes per session.
4. At least 50% of adults over 65 years should be engaging in appropriate physical activity, such as regular walking, swimming, or other aerobic activities.
5. At least 50% of primary care physicians should include a careful exercise history

as part of their initial examination of new patients.
6. At least 25% of companies and institutions with more than 500 employees should be offering employer-sponsored fitness programs.

Means of achieving these objectives include increased attention to providing information, improved physical activity programs, more facilities, as well as legislative, regulatory, and economic measures.[35] The more important specific measures advanced in the U.S. Public Health Service document[77:79-80] include:

1. Using television and radio public service announcements and print media to provide information on appropriate physical activity and its benefits.
2. The adoption of an exercise component by community service agencies, such as the American Red Cross and the American Heart Association.
3. Assuring that all programs and materials related to diet and weight loss have an active exercise component.
4. Encouraging health care providers, especially Health Maintenance Organizations (HMOs), community health centers and other organized settings, to prescribe appropriate exercise in weight loss regimens as a complementary treatment modality in the management of several chronic diseases, and to give patients 65 years and older and the handicapped more detailed information on appropriate physical activity together with warnings about starting up exercise too fast.
5. Providing physical fitness and exercise programs to school children, and ensuring that those programs emphasize activities for all children rather than just competitive sports for relatively few.
6. Providing physical fitness and exercise programs in colleges for students, faculty, and staff.
7. Providing worksite-based fitness programs which are linked to other health enhancement components and which have an active outreach effort.
8. Increasing the availability of existing facilities and promoting the development of new facilities by public, private and corporate entities (e.g., fitness trails, bike paths, parks, and pools).
9. Upgrading existing facilities, especially in inner city neighborhoods, and involving the population to be served at all levels of planning.

10. Developing and operating local, state and national park facilities which can be used for physical fitness activities in urban areas.
11. Increasing the number of school-mandated physical education programs that focus on health-related physical fitness.
12. Establishing state and local councils on health promotion and physical fitness.
13. Allowing expenditure of funds for fitness-related activities under federally funded programs guided by federal regulations.
14. Tax incentives for the private sector to offer physical fitness programs for employees.
15. Encouraging employers to permit employees to exercise on company time and/or giving employees flexible time for use of facilities.
16. Offering health and life insurance policies with reduced premiums for those who participate in regular vigorous physical activity.

Several important aspects of public health enhancement via regular exercise have been emphasized recently. Ramlow et al.[53] contend that if it were possible to take the 15% of the U.S. population who have physical activity limitations and raise their activity levels up to that of sedentary white collar workers, it might well have greater public health impact than attempting to transform an equivalent number of sedentary workers into regular joggers. Haskell et al.[32] state that health benefits attributable to physical activity are greater at lower levels, in that research shows greater improvement when moderately active individuals are compared to the least active, with much less effect apparent between the moderately active and very active. Dishman et al.[21] have advanced lower socioeconomic status as an apparent personal deterrent to initiating and adhering to a regular physical activity program. Each of these factors represent important components in organizing effective strategies for achieving public health goals in a more efficient manner.

In addition to programmatic modifications in schools and colleges discussed earlier, physical education must also continue to modify and expand its research and professional training curricula to meet the increased societal demand for public health enhancement via regular vigorous physical activity participation. This should not require major changes, as public health enhancement is not an entirely new objective, just a more powerful societal impetus than previously. Further, basic principles of organizing, administering, and leading appropriately selected physical activity programs tailored to the interests and needs of a particular group is not greatly different in the private sector from that in educational institutions. Finally, the focus of research and scholarly study remains human movement, though applied studies of fitness oriented programs to achieve primarily public health objectives will differ in specific content and scope from those addressing programmatic needs in school physical education and athletic performance contexts. Specific research recommendations for advancing knowledge relative to physical activity and public health have been addressed elsewhere.[32,46,51,67] These recommendations include areas in which physical education researchers are already actively involved, as well as others that could be upgraded, especially if participated in collaboratively with medical researchers.

Physical education has major contributions to make in modern American society, including the advancement of knowledge, basic and applied, in human movement encompassed in the modes of sport, dance, and exercise. Further, it has responsibilities for developing the best professional training curricula for preparing teachers, coaches, and physical activity program leadership personnel for community and private sector needs. Finally, it has responsibilities for structuring better programs in schools and colleges that attend to the optimum growth and development of the student's whole being, including a fitness component that enhances health and well-being. With regard to promoting the student's enrichment of life in terms of health and abundant living, physical education has responsibilities to:

1. Conduct research to discover the kinds and amounts of physical activity necessary to accomplish specific levels of health and fitness.
2. Provide activities which offer diversion

from anxiety and worry, and which afford wholesome relaxation during leisure hours.

3. Offer activities which counteract the effect of our modern technologic age on the strength, endurance, and flexibility weaknesses of our people.

4. Provide physical education programs for the masses, as well as the select few, to achieve the greatest good for the largest possible number of individuals.

5. Stress the importance of continued, regular physical activity participation after school years.

6. Assist in making the effects of physical training and sports participation well known to the general public.

CONCLUSION

In this chapter, it was stated that physical education in the United States has developed and expanded during the past quarter century in two principal ways: (1) it is increasingly an academic discipline (though it retains a strong professional context), with a growing body of knowledge whose central focus is human movement (i.e., man engaged in physical activity); and (2) via the dramatically enhanced societal awareness of the optimal health/fitness role of structured physical activity programs that now extend well beyond the traditional educational institution setting. Information related to these developments, and others of importance today, were examined from a broad perspective, viz., anthropologic, historic, and philosophic.

From an historic perspective, it was noted that organized physical activity programs evolved early in man's existence, but that their nature has varied widely to meet prevalent cultural aims emanating from the existent educational, political, religious, and economic conditions. A distinction between the roles of cultural and physical anthropology, as well as their interrelationship in human adjustment to the environment, was made. From this perspective, an argument supporting modern man's continued need for vigorous physical activity in our modern technologic—near activity void—society, was made. Finally, distinctions between the roles of science in the continued growth of the knowledge base in human movement and of the philosophic process in ferreting out elements of its comprehensive meaning in terms of benefit to modern man were made. In this context, aims and objectives for physical education in the advancement of basic knowledge in human movement, development of improved professional training curricula, and the provision of organized physical activity programs in educational institutions and other expanding societal settings, were detailed for the 1990s.

The first chapter, then, has set the stage for physical education as an academic discipline, with human movement as its focal point, and as a profession with an expanding societal impact. The next four chapters provide an overview of basic information from the four primary subdisciplines: (1) biomechanics, (2) exercise physiology, (3) motor learning and sport psychology, and (4) sport sociology. They include a basic theoretical overview of these subdisciplines, together with selected examples of applications to various aspects of physical education, exercise, and sport.

The last four chapters include basic information on (1) the interrelationships of physical activity, growth, and development, (2) exercise and aging, (3) the concepts of health, well-being, and fitness examined in the context of chronic, modern "life-style" disease, and (4) the relationship of exercise and chronic disease. Significant attention is given to applications of basic knowledge in terms of developmental and health maintenance and enhancements aspects.

SUMMARY

1. Physical education in the United States has, until recently, been considered almost exclusively as a profession providing programs in educational institutions, but is now also an academic discipline with a growing knowledge base whose focal point is human movement.

2. Growth as an academic discipline has caused some physical education depart-

ments to change their name—even to the extent of deleting it from their title, but no single term has emerged as a clear replacement.

3. From an evolutionary perspective, modern man's advanced technologically based culture has propelled him well ahead of his biologic adaptive capacity, such that substitute forms of vigorous physical activity are necessary to replace that inherent in man's normal everyday life until little more than 100 years ago.

4. Due primarily to increased leisure time, increased discretionary income, and an expanded societal awareness of the health/fitness benefits of exercise effected by federal public health support and expanded media exposure, organized physical activity programs are also available in numerous settings outside educational institutions.

5. Evidence indicates that organized physical activity programs developed early in man's existence, first being used to teach physical skills necessary for survival.

6. Subsequently, historic evidence of the role of organized physical activity programs reveals that various cultures have placed widely disparate value on the need for and purpose of physical education.

7. Early 19th century Western European physical education programs, particularly those in England, Germany, and Sweden, had an important impact on the early development of physical education and sport in the U.S.

8. Until about 1920, college physical education programs were usually devoid of sports, stressed primarily physical health and well-being, and were often directed by medical doctors.

9. Sport developed outside the formal educational sphere, but was incorporated as the primary component of physical education programs in schools and colleges by 1930, primarily as a result of the education progressivism movement stimulated by the ideas of John Dewey.

10. During WW II, there was renewed emphasis on the physical fitness objective to enhance young males' preparedness for military service and females' readiness for occupational roles that demanded fitness levels well beyond that of traditional roles.

11. Since WW II, the federal government has provided a substantial societal impact on physical education. This included presidential concern for enhanced fitness levels for youth and adults, followed by legislation to promote equality of opportunity for persons with handicaps, and federal agency support for exercise as an effective means of intervention in public health problems.

12. Sport has assumed an increasingly influential role in the United States, which has resulted in increased physical activity levels for many individuals, but has also produced an enhanced commercialization of athletic programs in educational institutions, particularly at the college level.

13. Scientific inquiry in various realms of human movement has grown rapidly, providing much useful information for application in effecting enhanced performance and improved health/fitness.

14. Philosophic inquiry in physical education and sport strives to resolve comprehensive problems and controversies that lie beyond the realm of empirical science.

15. As an example, elements of the philosophic process were utilized to develop statements of aims and objectives for physical education in the 1990s.

16. Physical education's role in schools and colleges was held to include increased emphasis on teaching activities more likely to be used into one's advanced years. Further, principles of exercise prescription, physiologic effects of exercise, and health benefits and risks of physical activities should be taught in a carefully planned and sequenced curriculum.

17. It was also stated that physical education should take a more assertive role in research, training of leadership personnel, and in organized physical activity program development in societal settings outside educational institutions.

REFERENCES

1. Astrand, P.-O.: Why exercise? An evolutionary approach. Acta Med. Scand. Suppl. *711*:241–242, 1986.
2. Astrand, P.-O., and G. Grimby (editors): Physical

activity in health and disease. Acta Med. Scand. Suppl. *711*:1–244, 1986.

3. Bates, M.: Man in Nature. (2nd ed.) Englewood Cliffs, N.J.: Prentice-Hall, 1964.

4. Beck, L.W., and R.L. Holmes: Philosophic Inquiry: An Introduction to Philosophy. (2nd ed.) Englewood Cliffs, N.J.: Prentice-Hall, 1968.

5. Bennett, B.L.: Dudley Allen Sargent: the man and his philosophy. JOPERD. *55*(9):61–64, 1984.

6. Berryman, J.W.: The tradition of the six things non-natural: exercise and medicine from Hippocrates through ante-bellum America. In Exercise and Sport Sciences Reviews. Vol. 17., edited by K.B. Pandolf, Baltimore: Williams & Wilkins, 1989, pp. 515–559.

7. Blair, S.N., D.R. Jacobs, and K.E. Powell: Relationships between exercise or physical activity and other health behaviors. Public Health Rep. *100*:172–180, 1985.

8. Blair, S.N., R.T. Mulder, and H.W. Kohl: Reaction to secular trends in adult physical activity: exercise boom or bust? Res. Quart. Exer. Sport. *58*:106–110, 1987.

9. Bortz, W.M.: Disuse and aging. JAMA. *248*:1203–1208, 1982.

10. Boyle, R.H.: The new wave in sports. Sports Illustrated. 21:41, (21 December 1964).

11. Bucher, C.A., and D.A. Wuest: Foundations of Physical Education and Sport. (10th ed.) St. Louis: Times Mirror/Mosby, 1987.

12. Cassidy, R.: The cultural definition of physical education. Quest. IV:11, April, 1965.

13. Cheffers, J., and T. Evaul: Introduction to Physical Education: Concepts of Human Movement. Englewood Cliffs, N.J.: Prentice-Hall, 1978.

14. Clarke, D.H., and H.H. Clarke: Research Processes in Physical Education. (2nd ed.) Englewood Cliffs, N.J.: Prentice-Hall, 1984.

15. Cooper, K.H.: The New Aerobics. New York: Bantam, 1970.

16. Davies, G.: Wellington and His Army. Oxford: Basil Blackwell, 1954.

17. Davis, E.C., and D.M. Miller: The Philosophic Process in Physical Education. (2nd ed.) Philadelphia: Lea & Febiger, 1967.

18. deGrazia, S.: Of Time, Work, and Leisure. New York: Twentieth Century Fund, 1962.

19. de Pauw, K.P.: Commitment and challenges: sport opportunities for athletes with disabilities. JOPERD. *55*(2):34–43, 1984.

20. Dewar's Guide to Career Development. New York: Research & Forecasts, 1983.

21. Dishman, R.K., J.F. Sallis, and D.R. Orenstein: The determinants of physical activity and exercise. Public Health Rep. *100*:158–171, 1985.

22. Dix, L.: A Charter for Progressive Education. New York: Teacher's College, Columbia University, 1939.

23. Dobzhansky, T.: Mankind Evolving: The Evolution of the Human Species. New Haven: Yale University Press, 1962.

24. Eitzen, D.S., and G.H. Sage: Sociology of North American Sport. (3rd ed.) Dubuque, Iowa: William C. Brown, 1986.

25. Ellis, M.J.: Warning: the pendulum has swung far enough. JOPERD. *59*(3):75–78, 1988.

26. Fitness Research: It's a game of numbers. Athletic Business. November 1985, pp. 14–25.

27. Fraleigh, W.P.: Unresolved tensions in college physical education—constructive and destructive. Quest. *37*:135–144, 1985.

28. Godshall, R.W.: Junior league football: risks versus benefits. J. Sports Med. *3*:139–166, 1975.

29. Goldman, L., and E.F. Cook: The decline in ischemic heart disease mortality rates: an analysis of the comparative effects of medical interventions and changes in lifestyle. Ann. Intern. Med. *101*:825–836, 1984.

30. Gray, H.J.: The role of business in health promotion: a brief overview. Prev. Med. *12*:654–657, 1983.

31. Hargadine, H.K.: Health promotion programs: limited funds no stumbling block. Occupat. Health and Safety. *54*:69–74, 1985.

32. Haskell, W.L., H.J. Montoye, and D. Orenstein: Physical activity and exercise to achieve health-related physical fitness components. Public Health Rep. *100*:202–212, 1985.

33. Heath, G.W., J.M. Hagberg, A.E. Ehsani, and J.O. Holloszy: A physiological comparison of young and older endurance athletes. J. Appl. Physiol. *51*:634–640, 1981.

34. Henry, F.M.: Physical education—An academic discipline. National College Physical Education Association for Men. Proceedings. 1964, pp. 6–9.

35. Iverson, D.C., J.E. Fielding, R.S Crow, and G.M. Christenson: The promotion of physical activity in the United States population: the status of programs in medical, worksite, community, and school settings. Public Health Rep. *100*:212–224, 1985.

36. Janz, K.F., S.L. Cottle, C.R. Mahaffey, and D.A. Phillips: Current name trends in physical education. JOPERD. *60*(5):85–92, 1989.

37. Kraus, H., and R.P. Hirschland: Minimum muscular fitness tests in school children. Res. Quart. *25*:178–188, 1954.

38. Kraus, H., and W. Raab: Hypokinetic Disease. Springfield: Charles C Thomas, 1960.

39. Lambert, C.L.: What can I do besides teach? JOPER. *51*(9):74–76, 1980.

40. Logan, G.A., and W.C. McKinney: The service program: a challenge to the intellect. National College Physical Education Association for Men. Proceedings. 1963, pp. 17–21.

41. Malina, R.M.: Physical activity in early and modern populations: an evolutionary view. In Physical Activity in Early and Modern Populations: Amer.

Acad. of P.E. Papers No. 21. Edited by R.M. Malina and H.M. Eckert, Champaign, Ill.: Human Kinetics, 1988, pp. 1–12.

42. Marsh, R.L.: Physically educated: what it will mean for tomorrow's high school student. JOPER. *49*(1):49–50, 1978.

43. Mead, M.: Growing Up In New Guinea. New York: Mentor, 1958.

44. Metheny, E.: Movement and Meaning. New York: McGraw-Hill, 1968.

45. Michener, J.A.: Sports in America. New York: Random House, 1976.

46. Morris, J.N.: Exercise and public health. Acta Med. Scand. Suppl. *711*:243–244, 1986.

47. Nash, J.B.: Physical Education—Its Interpretation and Objectives. Dubuque, Iowa: William C. Brown, 1963.

48. Nixon, J.E., and A.E. Jewitt: An Introduction to Physical Education. (9th ed.) Philadelphia: Saunders, 1980.

49. Office of Disease Prevention and Health Promotion, Public Health Service. Summary of findings from national children and youth fitness study. JOPERD. *56*(1):2–90, 1985.

50. Pollock, M.L., and T.T. Gushiken: Aerobic capacity and the aged athlete. In The Elite Athlete. Edited by N.K. Butts, T.T. Gushiken, and B. Zairns. New York: Spectrum, 1985, pp. 267–274.

51. Powell, K.E., and R.S. Paffenbarger: Workshop on epidemiologic and public health aspects of physical activity and exercise: a summary. Public Health Rep. *100*:118–126, 1985.

52. Public Health Aspects of Physical Activity and Exercise. Public Health Rep. *100*:113–252, 1985.

53. Ramlow, J., A. Kriska, and R. Laporte: Physical activity in the population: the epidemiologic spectrum. Res. Quart. Exer. Sport. *58*:111–113, 1987.

54. Reiff, G.G., et al.: The President's Council on Physical Fitness and Sports 1985: National School Population Fitness Survey. HHS—Office of the Assistant Secretary for Health, Research Project 282–84–0086, The University of Michigan, Ann Arbor, 1986.

55. Report of Inter-Society Commission for Heart Disease Resources. Circulation. *70*:153A–205A, 1984.

56. Rice, E.A., J. Hutchinson, and M. Lee: A Brief History of Physical Education. (5th ed.) New York: Ronald Press, 1969.

57. Rivenes, R.S. (editor): Foundations of Physical Education: A Scientific Approach. Boston: Houghton-Mifflin, 1978.

58. Robinson, J., and G. Godbery: Work and leisure in America: how we spend our time. JOPER. *49*(8):38–40, 1978.

59. Rosen, M.A., D.N. Lodgsdon, and M.M. Demak: Prevention and health promotion in primary care: baseline results on physicians from the INSURE project on lifecycle preventive health services. Prev. Med. *13*:535–548, 1984.

60. Ross, J.G., and G.G. Gilbert: The national children and youth fitness study. A summary of findings. JOPERD. *56*(1):45–50, 1985.

61. Sage, G.H.: The quest for identity in college physical education. Quest. *36*:115–121, 1984.

62. Shephard, D.S., and L.A. Pearlman: Healthy habits that pay off. Business and Health. March, 1985, pp. 37–41.

63. Shephard, R.J.: Fitness boom or bust—A Canadian perspective. Res. Quart. Exer. Sport. *59*:265–269, 1988.

64. Shephard, R.J.: Practical issues in employee fitness programming. Physician and Sportsmed. *12*(6):161–166, 1984.

65. Siedentop, D.: Developing Skills in Physical Education. Boston: Houghton-Mifflin, 1976.

66. Siedentop, D.: Physical Education: Introductory Analysis. (3rd ed.) Dubuque, Iowa: Wm. C. Brown, 1980.

67. Siscovick, D.S., R.E. Laporte, and J.M. Newman: The disease-specific benefits and risks of physical activity and exercise. Public Health Rep. *100*:180–188, 1985.

68. Skinner, J.S.: The fitness industry. In Physical Activity in Early and Modern Populations. Amer. Acad. of P.E. Papers No. 21. Edited by R.M. Malina and H.M. Eckert. Champaign, Ill.: Human Kinetics, 1988, pp. 67–72.

69. Smith E.L., and C. Gilligan: Physical activity prescription for the older adult. Physician and Sportsmed. *11*(8):91–101, 1983.

70. Snyder, E.E., and E.A. Spreitzer: Social Aspects of Sport (2nd ed.). Englewood Cliffs, N.J.: Prentice Hall, 1983.

71. Sorokin, P.A.: Society, Culture and Personality. New York: Harper & Bros., 1947.

72. Steinhaus, A.H.: Significant experiences—A challenge to physical education. The Physical Educator. *19*:5–11, March 1962.

73. Steinhaus, A.H.: The disciplines underlying a profession. Quest. *IX*:68–72, 1967.

74. Stephens, T.: Secular trends in adult physical activity: exercise boom or bust. Res. Quart. Exer. Sport. *58*:94–105, 1987.

75. Terris, M.: Approaches to an epidemiology of health. Am. J. Public Health. *65*:1037–1045, 1975.

76. U.S. Department of Health, Education, and Welfare. Healthy People: The Surgeon General's Report on Health Promotion and Disease Prevention. Washington, D.C.: U.S. Government Printing Office, 1979.

77. U.S. Department of Health and Human Services. Promoting Health/Preventing Disease: Objectives for the Nation. Washington, D.C.: U.S. Government Printing Office, 1980.

78. Van Dalen, D.B.: Philosophy: an initial consideration in quest. Quest. *1*:19–21, 1963.

79. Van Dalen, D.B., and B.L. Bennett: A World History of Physical Education: Cultural, Philosoph-

ical, Comparative. (2nd ed.) Englewood Cliffs, N.J.: Prentice Hall, 1971.

80. Weiss, M.L., and A.E. Mann: Human Biology and Behavior: An Anthropological Perspective. (4th ed.) Boston: Little Brown, 1985.
81. Weiss, P.: Sport: A Philosophic Inquiry. Carbondale, Ill.: Southern Illinois University Press, 1969.
82. Weston, A.: The Making of American Physical Education. New York: Appleton- Century-Crofts, 1962.
83. Williams, J.F.: The Principles of Physical Education. (8th ed.) Philadelphia: Saunders, 1964.
84. Young, A., J.A. Gray, and J.R. Ennis: Exercise medicine: the knowledge and beliefs of final-year medical students in the United Kingdom. Medical Educ. 17:369–373, 1983.
85. Zeigler, E.F.: Philosophic Foundations for Physical, Health, and Recreation Education. Englewood Cliffs, N.J.: Prentice-Hall, 1964.
86. Zeigler, E.F.: Problems in the History and Philosophy of Physical Education and Sport. Englewood Cliffs, N.J.: Prentice-Hall, 1968.
87. Zeigler, E.F.: Physical Education and Sport Philosophy. Englewood Cliffs, N.J.: Prentice-Hall, 1977.
88. Zeigler, E.F., and K.J. McCristal: A history of the Big Ten body-of-knowledge project in physical education. Quest. IX:79–84, December 1967.

BIBLIOGRAPHY

1. Dobzhansky, T.: Mankind Evolving: The Evolution of the Human Species. New Haven, Conn.: Yale Univ. Press, 1962.
2. Kraus, H., and W. Raab: Hypokinetic Disease. Springfield, Charles C Thomas, 1961.
3. Rice, E.A., J.L. Hutchinson, and M. Lee: A Brief History of Physical Education. (5th ed.) New York: Ronald Press, 1969.
4. Van Dalen, D.B., and B.L. Bennett: A World History of Physical Education. (2nd ed.) Englewood Cliffs, N.J.: Prentice-Hall, 1971.
5. Weiss, M.L., and A.E. Mann: Human Biology and Behavior: An Anthropological Perspective. (4th ed.) Boston: Little, Brown, 1985.
6. Weston, A.: The Making of American Physical Education. New York: Appleton-Century-Crofts, 1962.

2 BIOMECHANICS OF HUMAN MOVEMENT

INTRODUCTION

Biomechanics is the science concerned with the interrelationship "of the biologic and material properties of the skeletal, articular, and neuromuscular systems and of the laws and principles set forth in mechanical physics."[20:1] It arose from the subdiscipline kinesiology (literally defined as the scientific study of movement) which, until the mid-1960s, entailed the study of (1) the structure and function of the skeletal and neuromuscular systems, and (2) mechanical aspects. However, with the rapid advancement of knowledge of mechanical principles applicable to human movement, this area of study became the most significant part of kinesiology, thus resulting in increased usage of the term biomechanics. Further, at about the same time, some physical educators began to use the term kinesiology to encompass all scientific areas of study relating to human movement, including exercise physiology, psychologic and sociologic aspects, as well as biomechanics.[1]

Biomechanics is concerned with both internal and external factors that affect not only movement of one's body, but also the movement of implements or other equipment used in exercise, sport, or other physical activity. Applications of biomechanics in human movement are readily seen in: (1) athletics, where performance technique can be better analyzed and corrected, and injury incidence reduced; (2) physical education, in which fundamental movement patterns such as walking, running, jumping, throwing, and striking, can be more effectively taught; (3) medicine, in prostheses design and in the physical therapist's attempts to reestablish normal movement patterns in stroke patients; and (4) in industry, where the worker-equipment interface is designed to maximize work efficiency. There is current debate as to whether an athlete's knowledge of biomechanic principles facilitates performance, but general agreement that those who teach others to move efficiently, viz., coaches, physical education teachers, and physical therapists, must be able to observe the learner's movement patterns, determine errors, and provide appropriate information to improve performance. To accomplish these tasks efficiently, a sound working knowledge of biomechanics is necessary.[20]

As depicted in Figure 2–1, mechanics is that branch of physical science which deals with the physical laws and principles relating to objects at rest or in motion, and when combined with the interrelated effects of musculoskeletal and neurophysiologic factors inherent in goal oriented human movement, becomes **biomechanics.** Mechanics consists of two aspects: (1) statics, in which forces acting on an object are balanced and thus, in equilibrium; and (2) dynamics, in which motion of an object is brought about by unbalanced forces. There are two branches of dynamics: (1) kinematics, which deals with descriptive analysis of motion without consideration of forces causing motion; and (2) kinetics, which deals with the interrelationship of forces causing motion.

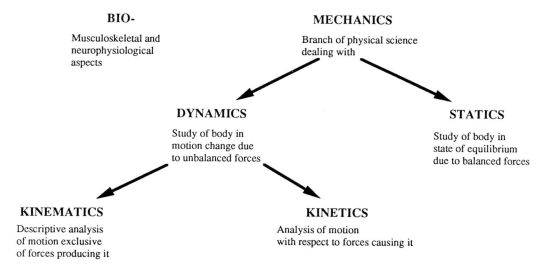

FIG. 2–1. Components of biomechanics.

MUSCULOSKELETAL AND NEUROPHYSIOLOGIC ASPECTS OF HUMAN MOVEMENT

Before examining the mechanics of human movement and selected applications to exercise, sport, and basic movement tasks, it is necessary to review the basic structure and function of the skeletal, muscular, and nervous systems. This is because effective movement is dependent on coordinated integration of these systems. That is, appropriate neural stimulation activates muscular contraction that generates force which, together with the skeletal system's bones and articulating joints, serve as elements of anatomic levers that function in accord with the laws of mechanics. Further, knowledge of fundamental musculoskeletal relationships facilitates understanding of gravitational and other external forces on muscle actions, which has important implications for performance, exercise prescription, and prevention of injury.

THE SKELETAL SYSTEM

BONES. The human skeleton is made up of the axial skeleton (consisting of the skull vertebral column, and thorax), which con-

tains 80 bones, and the appendicular skeleton (consisting of the upper and lower extremities), which contains 126 bones. Figure 2–2 identifies the bones primarily involved in human movement.

FUNCTION. The skeletal system serves five major functions:

1. It provides the rigid supporting framework of the body.
2. Bones, through their shape or location, provide protection for vital organs.
3. Bones make up a lever system upon which attached muscles act to effect movement.
4. The internal portion of long and flat bones serves as the manufacturing area of red and white blood cells, as well as blood platelets which are essential for clotting.
5. Bone serves as a calcium storehouse.

STRUCTURE. There are two types of bone tissue: a solid compact type, and a spongy cancellous tissue. The amount of each varies throughout life, with bone becoming less flexible and more brittle with age. Bone is usually a hard outer layer of compact tissue with cancellous bone as the core. For example, long bones consist of a shaft of compact bone surrounding an internal cavity which contains the marrow. Compact tissue gives bone its strength, while the cancellous portion allows for the distribution of forces over its interwoven network,

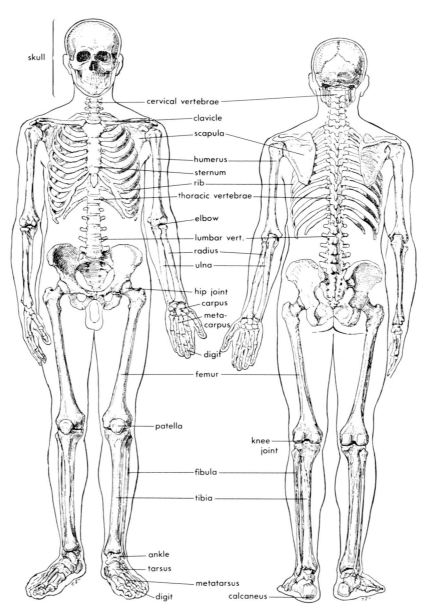

FIG. 2–2. Selected aspects of the skeletal system. (Modified from Crouch. J.E.: Essential Human Anatomy: A Text-Atlas. Philadelphia: Lea & Febiger, 1982, p. 78.)

thus lessening the effect of impact. The hardness of bone is due to mineral salts, of which calcium carbonate and calcium phosphate constitute the major portion.

CLASSIFICATION OF BONES. Bones may be divided into four classes according to their shape—long, short, flat, and irregular. Long bones are located in the arms and legs, and are characterized by long slender shafts with broad bumpy ends. They usually serve as levers in the body, facilitating movement. Short bones are found in the wrist and ankle, and are often cubical in shape with equal width and length. These bones are important where strength is concerned more than mobility. Flat bones, including the ribs, the shoulder blade (scapula) and the larger bones of the skull, generally serve a protective function. Irregular bones are of varied shapes, and include the vertebrae, which play a role in protection, support, and leverage in movement.

JOINTS. A joint is a junction, or articulation, between two or more bones. Some bones articulate at immovable joints characterized by stability (e.g., sutures of the skull),

others at joints permitting slight movements (e.g., intervertebral disks of the spinal column), and still others articulate at a variety of movable joints (diarthrodial). The latter are of particular interest due to their importance in motor skill and movement analysis.

The diarthrodial (synovial) joint is so structured that the opposed ends of the bones have a thin cartilagenous covering over their articulating surfaces and are separated by a membranous covered cavity. This arrangement permits great freedom of movement. Support is furnished by the counteracting pull of muscles and tendons across the joint, by widening of the bony surfaces at the joint, by adjacent fascia, and by strong accessory ligaments which resist movements in undesired directions.

There are six types of synovial joints of which two are of primary concern, viz., (a) the hinge and (b) the ball and socket (Fig. 2–3). A hinge joint permits movement about a single axis of motion, such as flexion and extension of the lower arm at the elbow joint. A ball and socket joint is triaxial and provides the greatest freedom of movement. It consists of the head of a long

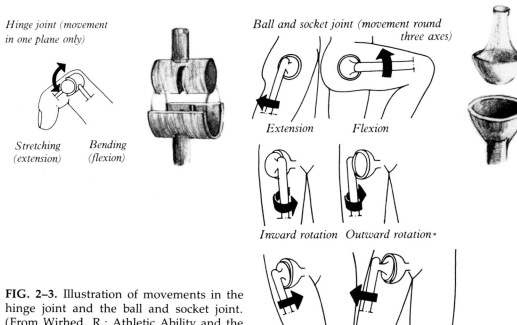

Hinge joint (movement in one plane only)

Stretching (extension) *Bending (flexion)*

Ball and socket joint (movement round three axes)

Extension *Flexion*

Inward rotation *Outward rotation*

Adduction *Abduction*

FIG. 2–3. Illustration of movements in the hinge joint and the ball and socket joint. (From Wirhed, R.: Athletic Ability and the Anatomy of Motion. London: Wolfe Medical, 1984, p. 13.)

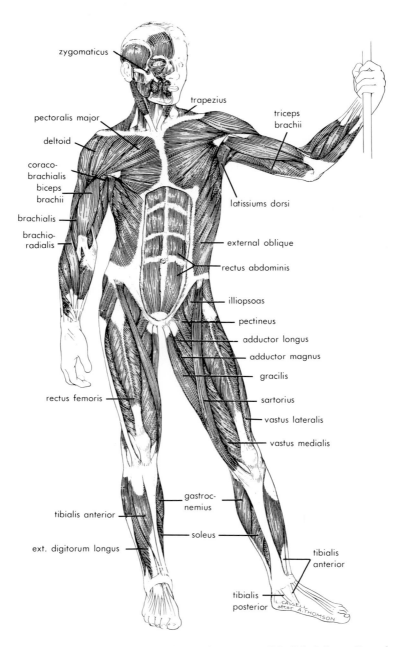

FIG. 2–4. Selected aspects of the skeletal muscle system. (Modified from Crouch, J.E.: Essential Human Anatomy: A Text-Atlas. Philadelphia: Lea & Febiger, 1982, pp. 150–151.)

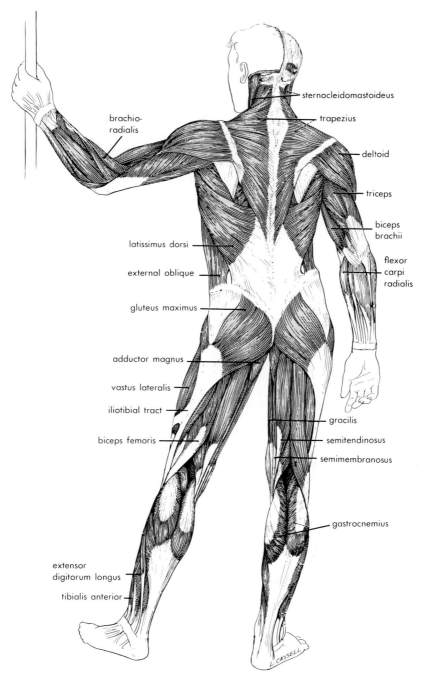

sternocleidomastoideus

trapezius

deltoid

triceps

biceps
brachii

flexor
carpi
radialis

brachio-
radialis

latissimus dorsi

external oblique

gluteus maximus

adductor magnus

vastus lateralis

iliotibial tract

biceps femoris

gracilis

semitendinosus

semimembranosus

gastrocnemius

extensor
digitorum longus

tibialis anterior

L. CASSELL

FIG. 2–4 *continued.*

bone inserted into a cup-like cavity, e.g., the shoulder or hip joint. This type of joint allows flexion, extension, abduction, adduction, circumduction, and rotation.

In spite of the biologic adaptations for support and stability, highly movable joints are extremely susceptible to injuries to the articulated bones, to their ligaments, and to adjoining structures. The most common injury to joints is called a sprain. Sprains occur when the joint is forced past the point of ligamentous restriction of its range of motion. The result is a rupture of one or more ligaments about the joint.[29] Dislocated shoulders, "trick" knees, sprained wrists or ankles, and "whip-lash" neck injuries are amongst the most common examples of sprains.

THE MUSCULAR SYSTEM

There are three types of muscle tissue in the body: skeletal, smooth, and cardiac. Smooth muscle is sometimes referred to as involuntary because it is not responsive to an act of will. It also differs from skeletal muscle in that its fibrous arrangement is nonstriated. Examples of this type of muscle are found in the blood vessels and the inner walls of the digestive system and other vital organs. Cardiac muscle, which forms the muscular wall of the heart, is striated but involuntary. A unique characteristic of cardiac muscle is its autorhythmicity, i.e., it contracts in a rhythmic and automatic fashion initiated from a signal originating in the heart itself.

SKELETAL MUSCLE. Major skeletal muscles affecting body movement are depicted in Figure 2–4. Skeletal muscle is sometimes called voluntary muscle, in that it effects movements initiated by will. The muscle is enclosed on the outside in a connective tissue covering which fuses with the tendon. The tendon consists of non-contractile fibrous tissue attaching the fleshy muscle body at both ends to bone. Within each muscle are the individual fibers grouped into bundles, which are covered by a sheath. This bundle arrangement yields the shape and size of each individual muscle.

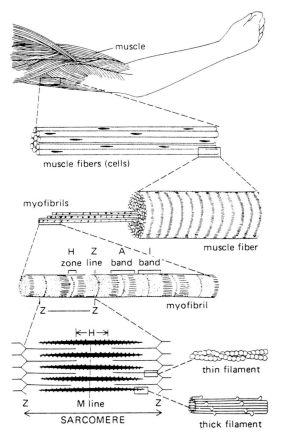

FIG. 2–5. Components of skeletal muscle. (From Vander, A.J., et al: Human Physiology. 3rd ed. New York: McGraw-Hill, 1980, p. 212.)

Basic structural aspects of a skeletal muscle are illustrated in Figure 2–5. The individual muscle fibers making up the muscle bundle are the basic structural unit of the muscle, i.e., the muscle cells. These cells are long and slender, varying in length from 1 to 50 millimeters. Each muscle fiber consists of a mass of protoplasm, called the sarcoplasm, which is surrounded by a thin tough elastic sheath or sarcolemma. Embedded in the sarcoplasm of each cell are long filaments or column-like structures known as myofibrils. The myofibrils are the contractile elements of skeletal muscle and are subdivided into sarcomeres which serve as the functional unit of the myofibril. A myofibril filament contains two different proteins in parallel with the muscle fiber; actin is thin and continuous with the full length of the muscle cell, while the myosin protein is thick and short, and is found in the middle of sarcomeres.

The contractile process is best explained by what is known as the sliding filament theory,[40] in which a neural impulse induces a biochemical change producing an interaction between the actin and myosin. The actin appears to slide past the myosin in an interlacing pattern that forms cross-bridges between the two proteins resulting in contraction.

Skeletal Muscle Form. The structure of skeletal muscle is reflected in the number, arrangement, and length of its fibers. These structural differences allow for variation in primary function. The more powerful muscles have a large number of fibers which are relatively short and are attached to the bone by extensive use of tendinous fibers. Conversely, less powerful muscles with greater range of movement have a smaller number of fibers that are relatively longer.

The arrangement in which the fibers run parallel along the length of a muscle is termed fusiform (Fig. 2–6). When the points of attachment of a fusiform muscle are widely separated, a long tendon of insertion is provided. An example of this type of muscle fiber arrangement is the sartorius, the long strap-like muscle that winds from the hip down and across the inside of the thigh and attaches to the inside of the knee.

The penniform type of fiber arrangement is observed when power is of prime importance. In the unipenniform arrangement (Fig. 2–6), the fibers are parallel to one another and diagonal to the central tendon of the muscle. An example is the vastus medialis muscle. In other modifications of the same arrangement—bipenniform, which is a feather-like structure (rectus femoris; Fig. 2–6) and multipenniform (deltoid; Fig. 2–6)—still greater power per area of muscle mass can be achieved.

The force a muscle is able to generate is proportional to its physiologic cross-sectional area (Fig. 2–7), which gives a better estimation of force than simple cross-sectional area, since it considers the sum of the cross sections of all the individual fibers.[24] The physiologic cross-sectional area is calculated by multiplying the average thickness of the muscle by the sum of the lengths of peripendicular lines through all the fibers. In general, the more powerful muscle groups, as stated above, are of penniform arrangement and, although more

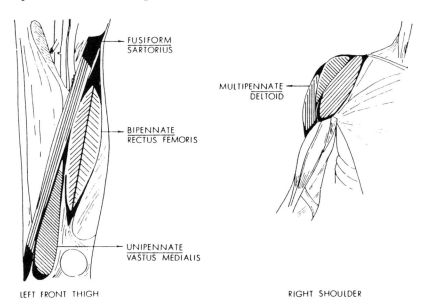

FUSIFORM
SARTORIUS

MULTIPENNATE
DELTOID

BIPENNATE
RECTUS FEMORIS

UNIPENNATE
VASTUS MEDIALIS

LEFT FRONT THIGH

RIGHT SHOULDER

FIG. 2–6. Skeletal muscle fiber arrangements. (From Adams, W.C., et al.: Foundations of Physical Activity. Champaign, Ill.: Stipes, 1968, p. 25.)

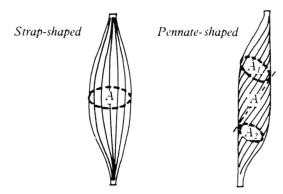

Strap-shaped   *Pennate-shaped*

FIG. 2–7. Physiologic cross-sectional area (A) of fusiform (left) versus unipenniform (right) muscles. In the fusiform arrangement, the physiological cross-sectional area is simply equal to the geometrical cross-sectional area since this transects all of the muscle fibers. In the penniform arrangement, A1 and A2 must be added together to determine A, since a simple geometrical cross-sectional cut would not transect all fibers. (From Wirhed, R.: Athletic Ability and the Anatomy of Motion. London: Wolfe Medical, 1984, p. 17.)

force can be generated, this is at the expense of range of motion.

In addition to the arrangement of muscle fibers, other factors are also important in muscle force production, including:

1. disuse, which causes muscle atrophy and less muscular strength;
2. leverage position, or the angle of pull of the muscle;
3. velocity of the muscular contraction;
4. distance over which the force is being generated; and
5. physiologic factors, especially metabolic fatigue products.

Types of Muscular Contraction. Skeletal muscle is capable of either developing tension (contracting) or relaxing (elasticity). Although the word contraction literally means shortening, not all types of muscular contraction involve shortening of the muscle fibers. There are three basic types of muscular contraction: isotonic (including both concentric and eccentric); isokinetic; and isometric.

1. Concentric contraction (shortening) occurs when one end of the muscle remains stationary while the other shortens and

pulls the bone, thus resulting in movement. Movement occurs because the force developed in the contracting muscle is greater than the resistance it is contracting against.
2. Eccentric contraction (lengthening) is the gradual releasing of a contracted (shortened) muscle. This is effectively illustrated when one lowers a weight slowly while "giving in to" an external force, which is greater than the force being exerted by the contracted muscle. In effect, the muscle is working against the force of gravity to control the speed of the downward motion. The muscle does not actually stretch; rather, it merely returns to its resting length or, in other words, lengthens from its shortened position.
3. Both concentric and eccentric contractions are isotonic, as the tension within the muscle during movement remains relatively constant. A more recent type of muscular training regimen results in a constant speed of movement, i.e., isokinetic contraction, while the resistance to be overcome is accommodated accordingly.
4. Isometric (static) contraction takes place when the force developed by a muscle against an external force, or against a muscle working in the opposite direction, is equivalent. During isometric contraction, tension in the muscle is increased but the length of the muscle remains the same. Though no mechanical work is done in an isometric contraction, the muscle undergoes the complete metabolic contractile process.

Modern muscle function testing devices can assess force production during isometric, isokinetic, and isotonic contractions (Fig. 2–8).

Roles in Which Muscles Act. The fact that muscles are attached to bones across a joint allows their contractile force to be effective in performing movement. However, not all skeletal muscle contractions actually effect movement. In nearly all body movements, certain muscles steady or support a body part, while others stabilize a bone to which another muscle is attached, or neutralize the undesired actions of a muscle which might cause any one of several movements.

A mover, or agonist, muscle contraction role is exemplified when it directly produces a movement. In many movements,

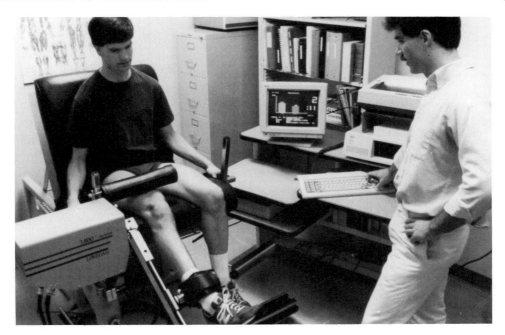

FIG. 2–8. Use of a modern muscle function testing device, shown here with computer driven graphic display, to assess isometric strength. This device can also be used to measure isotonic and isokinetic force production, and has been used in efforts to enhance athletic performance, as well as in rehabilitation following injury.

however, there are several movers utilized. The ones responsible for the greatest portion of the movement are called principal movers. Those of less importance, or which contract only under particular circumstances, are termed assistant movers. For example, the supinator muscle is the principal mover in supination of the forearm, while the biceps brachii is an assistant mover in this action.

Stabilizers contract statically to steady, support, or anchor a bone or other part of the body. This fixation may be made against the pull of gravity or against the effect of momentum and recoil in certain vigorous movements. A neutralizer muscle also contracts statically to prevent extraneous, undesired movements of the mover muscles. For example, if a mover muscle can both flex and abduct a body part, a neutralizer muscle contracts to prevent abduction during flexion.

An antagonist muscle is one that produces a joint action opposite that of another muscle. For example, in elbow flexion, the flexors are the movers and the extensors are the antagonists. Conversely, in elbow extension, the extensors are the movers and the flexors are the antagonists.

Muscle Team Work. A muscle seldom, if ever, acts alone. Even simple movement is based upon some static or dynamic posture which necessitates a number of stabilizer and neutralizer contractions in addition to those of the mover muscles and their antagonists. Hence, movements generally require the combined contraction of several muscles to produce an efficient, coordinated effect.

Movement that is initiated by vigorous contraction of the prime movers and simultaneous relaxation of the antagonists is referred to as ballistic. When the moving limb reaches a high velocity during a ballistic movement, the movers relax and the developed momentum completes the action. Momentum of the moving part may be checked by the passive resistance of the ligaments of the joint, by opposing muscle groups contracting near the end of the movement, or by striking an external object. The movement of limbs effecting throwing, kicking, and striking illustrates the ballistic type of movement.

THE NERVOUS SYSTEM

The nervous system is the body's primary adaptive and adjusting mechanism, through which stimuli are received, interpreted, and subsequent responses made. The nervous system can be divided into two parts: the central nervous system (CNS), which consists of the brain and spinal cord, and the peripheral nervous system (PNS), which includes all the nerves outside the CNS. The major parts of the brain include the cerebrum, thalamus, and cerebellum. The cerebrum is the highest integration center of the nervous system and contains sites for psychic functions, such as sensation, perception, memory, judgment, and volition. Most sensory information goes to the cerebrum through the thalamus which plays an important role in complex reflex movements. The cerebellum is intimately involved with cerebral neural outflow in the coordination and refinement of motor skills. The spinal cord contains the many important neural pathways carrying impulses to and from the brain, and is also involved in reflex activity. The PNS is the connection between the CNS and the muscle, skin, and viscera of the body. It communicates via thousands of nerves with various characteristics. A diagrammatic representation of the integration of the CNS and PNS is depicted in Figure 2–9.

While structurally the nervous system can be divided into the CNS and PNS, functionally it consists of the somatic and autonomic systems (Table 2–1). The somatic system is involved with reception and conduction of nervous impulses and ultimately the activity of skeletal muscle. The autonomic nervous system regulates the involuntary visceral structures of the body (e.g., the heart and stomach). This regulation is accomplished by a system of double innervation from the parasympathetic and sympathetic divisions. These divisions are antagonistic to each other (e.g., the sympathetic division increases heart rate, while the parasympathetic decreases

Table 2–1.   Subdivisions of the Nervous System*

Anatomic Divisions
  Central Nervous System
  A. Brain
  B. Spinal Cord
  Peripheral Nervous System

Functional Divisions
  Somatic Nervous System
  A. Cranial Nerves
  B. Spinal Nerves
  Autonomic Nervous System
  A. Sympathetic Nerves
  B. Parasympathetic Nerves

*From Wilmore, J.H. and D.L. Costill: Training for Sport and Activity. 3rd ed. Dubuque, Iowa: Wm. C. Brown, 1988, p. 83.

it). In general, the sympathetic division acts to prepare the body to meet emergency "fight or flight" situations, while the parasympathetic acts to conserve or preserve the basic body functions, e.g., digestion. However, the internal environment or condition of the internal viscera at any given time reflects a balance of stimulation of both the parasympathetic and sympathetic nerves.

The basic structural and functional unit of the nervous system is the nerve cell, or neuron (Fig. 2–10). Efferent neurons are those that transmit impulses from the brain or spinal cord to the muscles. They are called motor neurons since movement results from the impulses they transmit. A motor neuron (Fig. 2–10A) is composed of a cell body, its dendrite processes and a single axon process. The dendrite processes, which branch out short distances from the cell body, receive the neural impulses which are then carried to the cell body from the CNS. The axon process usually protrudes from the opposite side of the cell body, is quite long, and carries impulses from the cell body on to the nerve endings in the muscle. The axons of some neurons are encased in a fatty layer called a myelin sheath (Fig. 2–10B) which permits faster transmission of impulses. Afferent neurons (Fig. 2–10C) are those that transmit impulses or "messages" from the periphery, or environment, to the spinal cord or brain. They are also called sensory neurons because the impulses for the sensa-

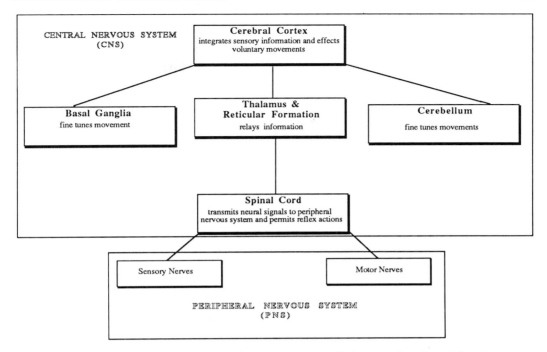

FIG. 2–9. Diagrammatic representation of the integration of the central and peripheral nervous systems.

tions of touch, sight, hearing, and pain are transmitted over them.

The CNS is constantly kept aware of muscle condition through stimuli produced from sensory receptors located in muscles, tendons, ligaments, and joints. These neural impulses enable the higher brain centers to integrate the various movements necessary for skilled performance. Nervous stimulation for voluntary muscle contraction orginates from the motor area of the cerebral cortex. With practice, many of the adjustments that modify the strength, duration, and range of muscular movement become involuntary. Pain, pressure, or irritation sensations, which come from the surface of the body or from sensory organs, initiate simple spinal reflexes.

To effect movement, the nerve impulse travels from the higher brain centers down the spinal cord and then, by way of a motor neuron, propagates itself to the myoneural junction. The impulse conduction involves changes in the electrical nature of the nerve membrane. The impulse does not flow through the nerve as water through a pipe, but more like a row of bowling pins, each falling in rapid succession after the first one is struck, and then popping up again.

At the myoneural junction the impulse stimulates the production of a chemical substance, called acetylcholine. This substance is thought to aid in transmitting the impulse across the gap between the nerve ending and the motor end plate A new self-propagating impulse, which is created at the motor end plate, is then received by the muscle membrane (sarcolemma) and transmitted through the membrane to the contractile substance within the muscle cells. The stimulus subsequently innervates a series of chemical reactions that release energy for contraction.

THE NEUROMUSCULAR SYSTEM

A motor nerve supplying a muscle is composed of many nerve fibers, each originating from a separate nerve cell in the spinal cord. Within the muscle the nerve fiber splits into numerous branches, with each branch ending at the motor end plate

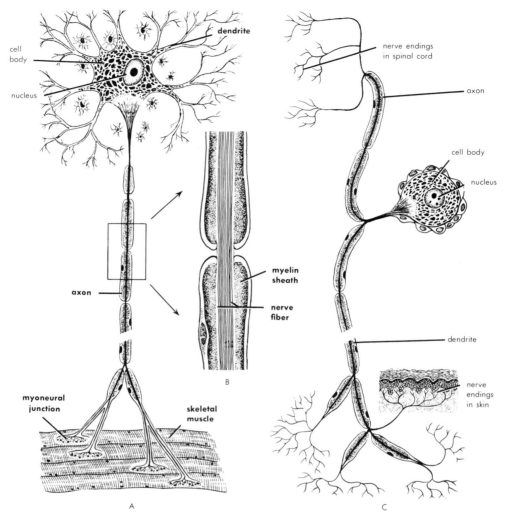

FIG. 2–10. Types of neurons. A. Efferent (motor) neuron. B. Enlarged portion of axon showing myelin sheath. C. Afferent (sensory) neuron. (Modified from Crouch, J.E.: Essential Human Anatomy: A Text-Atlas. Philadelphia: Lea & Febiger, 1982, p. 211.)

closely adjacent to a single muscle fiber. A single motor nerve cell in the spinal cord, together with its nerve fiber and the group of muscle fibers supplied by its branches, form a *motor unit* (Fig. 2–10A).

The neuromuscular stimulus-response mechanism can best be understood in terms of the motor unit—that is, a single motor neuron and the muscle fibers that its axon supplies.[24] Nervous stimulation received by the motor unit must be of sufficient intensity and duration to elicit a minimal response. When a motor unit re-

ceives this threshold stimulation, all of its muscle fibers contract according to the "all-or-none" law; i.e., the muscle fibers of a single motor unit contract completely or not at all.

The operation of the entire muscle, however, does not conform to the "all-or-none" law. Instead a graded mechanism, which regulates the amount of force needed to overcome resistance, is utilized. Only the number of muscle fibers necessary for the performance are activated. For example, the force required to lift a 50-pound weight is obviously greater than that needed to lift a book, and thus requires activation of more motor units. During prolonged work motor units actually take turns, and only during work requiring maximal effort do all units operate at the same time. It is also possible to increase the amount of strength developed by increasing the frequency of motor unit firing, which is often the case in maximal work when all the motor units have been employed. Successive stimulation at a high frequency results in a cumulative effect increasing the total tension of the muscle. Thus, the strength of contraction is determined by both the number of motor units within the muscle that have been stimulated and the frequency at which they have been stimulated.

The number of muscle fibers contained in a given motor unit is dependent on the muscle's function. Muscles performing fine, delicate movements have a low innervation ratio of neurons to muscle fibers, i.e., one nerve fiber to five or fewer muscle fibers. On the other hand, muscles involved with heavy work or gross movements have a high innervation ratio of as many as 150 or more fibers per motor unit. A vivid illustration of an error in judgment during the operation of the graded mechanism is afforded when one lifts an empty box which was presumed to be heavily loaded. Having lifted such heavy boxes previously, one's nervous system is set to "fire" the supposed required number of motor units. When the empty box is lifted, much more force is generated than is actually required. Unless the grading mechanism can quickly adjust by inhibiting the unnecessary motor units, the body's balance will be noticeably disturbed, even to the extent of causing the individual to fall.

KINESTHESIA. The nervous system provides one with an awareness of the position and movement of the body and its parts in space without full visual or other conscious awareness.[36] This ability, or feeling, is termed kinesthesia, and is the apparent result of proprioception, which is the mechanism of sensory input about body position and movement, and of the position and tension within the muscles and joints.

The vestibular proprioceptors, found in the inner ear, transmit information to the brain concerning linear and rotational acceleration and deceleration, positional information, and equilibrium to maintain balance. Other important types of kinesthetic proprioceptors, each of which provide sensory information without necessitating visual awareness, include muscle spindles, golgi tendon organs, and Ruffini endings.

Muscle spindles are sensitive to length and tension changes in the muscle fibers. When the muscle fiber is stretched, the spindle is also stretched, activating it and sending impulses which eventually effect contraction of fibers antagonistic to the stretch. Golgi tendon organs respond to high tension, whether due to active or passive shortening of the muscle. They serve as a protective mechanism and send signals to the CNS to inhibit contraction and relax the muscle involved. Ruffini endings, found in joint capsules, are important in both static and dynamic conditions.

MECHANICS AND HUMAN MOVEMENT

The basic elements of biomechanics have been identified in Figure 2–1, including previously discussed musculoskeletal and neurophysiologic aspects. Coordinated integration of the skeletal, articular, and neuromuscular systems produces effective human movement in accord with the laws of mechanics. Thus, a more complete understanding of the internal and external factors affecting goal oriented movement can be obtained by knowledge of the basic elements of mechanics.

MOTION

Motion can be defined as the act or process of changing position with respect to some reference point. In general, there are three basic kinds of motion—translatory, rotary, and combinations of the two. Translatory motion occurs when an object moves from one location to another, with all its parts traveling in the same direction,

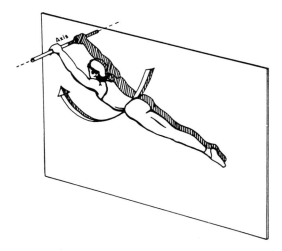

FIG. 2–11. An example of rotary (angular) motion. (From Hay, J.G.: The Biomechanics of Sports Techniques. 2nd ed. Englewood Cliffs, N.J.: Prentice-Hall, 1978, p. 5.)

the same distance, and with the same speed. Translatory motion can occur in a straight line, or in a curvilinear pattern, but occurs infrequently in human physical performance, since various body parts change their relative positions during movement. Rotary, or angular, motion occurs when one portion of an object is stationary and the rest of the object moves about this given point, termed the axis. As the object moves about this circular path, all parts are traveling through the same angle in the same direction, and in the same amount of time. An example of rotary motion is illustrated by the gymnast's performance of a giant swing on a horizontal bar (Fig. 2–11). More typical in human physical performance is a combination of translatory and rotary motion, termed general motion,[12] as illustrated in the 1½ somersault dive depicted in Figure 2–12.

KINEMATICS

Kinematics is that aspect of mechanics concerned with descriptive analysis of motion without concern for the forces causing it. Basic considerations include displacement, velocity, speed, and acceleration.

The distance an object travels is the length of the course it has taken to reach its destination. The distance covered differs from displacement, which is the length of a straight line drawn from the starting position to the ending position (i.e., straight as the crow flies). For example, if a person jogs one lap of a track, his displacement will be zero because he starts and stops at the same place, yet the distance traveled is the circumference of the track.

The distance an object travels in a certain amount of time represents its speed. This is an average over the entire period and does not consider the variations in speed over the total distance. Further, speed is distinguished from velocity, in that speed is distance divided by time and thus, considers only the rate at which an object is traveling (a scalar quantity). Velocity, however, usually has two components—horizontal (X) and vertical (Y)—which are re-

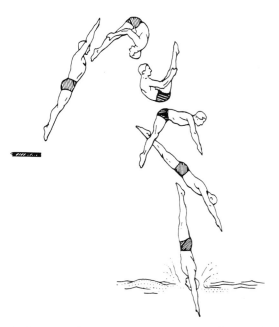

FIG. 2–12. Kinematic representation of general motion in the forward one and one half somersault dive—a combination of rotary motion and translatory motion of the body as it moves through a curvilinear path of flight. (From: Jensen, C.R., C.W. Schultz, and B.L. Bangerter: Applied Kinesiology and Biomechanics. 3rd ed. New York: McGraw-Hill, 1983, p. 209.)

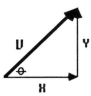

FIG. 2–13. Components of a velocity vector. Unlike speed, velocity also has direction, indicated by the angle theta.

solved to find the resultant velocity (v) (Fig. 2–13).

Acceleration, another vector quantity dealing with motion, is defined as the rate of change in velocity with respect to time (t) (i.e., v ÷ t). Assuming movement along a straight line, acceleration refers to an increase in the rate of speed. A decrease in velocity is termed deceleration. Like velocity, acceleration is rarely constant in human performance, and if one changes the other must also.

In human performance, one's body, as well as objects that one propels, are subject to physical laws appropriate to projectile motion. In air free space (which neglects air resistance), the horizontal component of an object in flight remains constant. The parabolic path transcribed by the object (i.e., curvilinear motion) is due to the gravitational effects that pull the object back to earth. The horizontal range of the object is then primarily dependent on the speed, angle, and height of release. The speed of release largely defines the horizontal component, whereas the angle of release affects the relative size of horizontal and vertical components. An increased angle of release will result in a decreased horizontal velocity, while a decreased angle yields a decreased vertical velocity. Thus, the optimum angle of release depends on both the speed and height of release. When the vertical and horizontal components of velocity are equal, the optimum angle of release is 45 degrees, regardless of the velocity (provided that the point of landing is at the same height as that of the release). In reality, air resistance exerts a profound effect on the path of projectile motion in many aspects of human performance. The amount depends on several factors to be discussed subsequently.

As with linear motion, rotary (angular) motion can be analyzed descriptively without respect to the forces causing it. This can occur in a crude manner, such as the description of the diver's 1½ revolutions about a horizontal axis parallel to the diving board, as exemplified in Figure 2–12. However, rotary motion equivalencies to linear motion calculations for distance, displacement, speed, velocity, and acceleration only involve incorporation of an angular/radius relationship, viz., a radian, which equals 57.3 degrees (2 π radians = 360°). A particularly important consideration, though, is that the velocity of an implement at the point of contact (or release) is equal to the product of its angular velocity and the radius of rotation (Fig. 2–14).

KINETICS

As previously mentioned, kinetics is that aspect of dynamics concerned with analysis of motion with respect to the *forces* producing it. For motion to occur, a net force must be exerted on the object. Such a force alters motion, and therefore can set

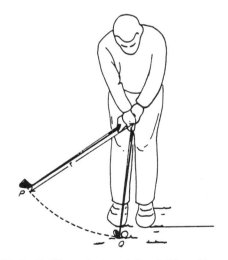

FIG. 2–14. The velocity of the clubhead is equal to the product of its angular velocity and the radius of rotation. (From: Hay, J.G.: The Biomechanics of Sports Techniques. 2nd ed. Englewood Cliffs, N.J.: Prentice-Hall, 1978, p. 53.)

an object into motion, slow it down, speed it up, or even cause a change in direction. Thus, force is a vector quantity possessing both magnitude and direction. A force also has a given point of application which plays a role in its effect.

With respect to human physical performance, forces are usually categorized as internal or external. External forces include gravity, air resistance, and friction via contact with the ground or other objects. Internal forces develop within the body due to the action of muscles across the joints of articulating bones. As mentioned earlier, muscle force depends on the type of muscular architecture. The direction of force exerted by any one muscle is influenced by the muscle's insertion angle and how it is related to the pulling axis of the long bone which constantly changes with movement.

NEWTON'S LAWS OF MOTION. In the 17th century, Newton advanced a profound integrative understanding of forces affecting objects in motion with his three laws addressing inertia, acceleration, and reaction. The mass of an object can also be considered as a measure of its inertia, which represents its resistance to change. That is, if an object is at rest, it will remain at rest—or if it is in motion, it will continue in motion at a constant velocity—unless it is acted upon by an external force great enough to change its state. Once in straight-line motion, the tendency is to maintain it, but this varies as is evidenced in the example of baserunning where a player swings wide to make the turns or slides into the bag to avoid over running it.

The sliding example also illustrates Newton's second law of motion, which deals with the change in velocity of an object (positive or negative—in this case, the latter) produced by applying force. The magnitude of this change will be proportional to the force applied, inversely proportional to the mass, and in the direction of the applied force. Thus, with mass constant, the force applied to decelerate or accelerate is directly proportional to the change in velocity. On the other hand, if two sprinters differing notably in mass accelerate from the start together and cover the same

distance in the same time, the heavier sprinter will have developed more force. In equation form, Newton's second law is: $F = m \cdot a$, where F is force, m is mass, and a is acceleration.

Newton's third law of motion states that for every action, there is an equal and opposite reaction, i.e., for every force exerted, there is an equal and opposite force. Thus, single forces cannot occur; i.e., forces work in opposing pairs. The equivalent opposing forces are equal to each object's mass times its acceleration. Both objects can be perceived to move, as in the case of an individual stepping from a canoe onto a dock. However, when the mass of the opposing object is large, movement of that object will not be perceived, e.g., when a jumper "takes off" from the earth, only the movement of the jumper is observed.

FORCES THAT MODIFY MOTION. *Gravitation* is an external force acting on all objects. The concept of weight of a body depends on the gravitational force acting on it. Mass, a term often used synonymously with weight, is an intrinsic property of a substance. The amount of matter in a body determines its mass, and this value stays the same no matter where the body is. Thus, an object has a constant mass, whether on the earth or on the moon, while the gravitational change affects weight. On the earth's surface, changes in gravitational effects on performance are predictable, but not large. For example, because the earth is not a perfect sphere (being somewhat flattened at the poles), the effect of gravity on a given mass is less at the equator than at the poles. Kirkpatrick[16] has calculated that a shot put performance of 57 ft. and 1 in. in Oslo, Norway (~60° latitude) would be improved by 2 in. at the equator. This positive effect would also occur in the discus, hammer, and javelin throws, while the long jumper's distance would be improved by about ¾ in.

Friction is the force that arises when one object moves across the surface of the other and the roughness of the two surfaces bond as they pass. Friction can never be completely eliminated and always opposes the direction of movement, thus acting to slow the object down. When a force is applied to a stationary object, friction will inhibit motion until a threshold level is reached. At this threshold level, the force has become great enough to overcome the frictional force and movement results. Because of its slowing effect on rapid movement, friction is usually considered a consistent deterrent to human performance. However, there are numerous situations where an increase in friction is advantageous to performance; e.g., when one exchanges rubber sole shoes for a pair with cleats when running on a grass surface made slippery by rainy weather.

Momentum is the product of an object's mass times its velocity. Thus, the greater the momentum of an object, the greater the effect it can produce upon impact with another object. If two objects have the same velocity, but one's mass is substantially larger, it will have a greater momentum and cause a greater impact. In a collision situation, momentum is conserved. That is, the momentum gained by one object is lost by the other object, with the momentum of the whole system remaining constant.

Momentum can be transferred within the body from segment to segment, as well as from one object to another. For example, in walking, momentum is transferred from the upper leg to the lower leg during the forward swing. At a certain point in a given stride the upper leg stops, but the lower leg continues forward as the leg extends. This is due to the transfer of momentum and results in less muscular effort needed for knee extension as the lower leg swings comfortably into place for the foot to make contact with the surface.

Transferring momentum and imparting it to another object is exemplified in hitting a baseball. The batter's stride forward, trunk rotation, arm movement, and wrist rotation all contribute to developing speed to be transferred to the end of the bat. In fact, the speed of the bat at the time of contact with the ball can be conceptualized as a resultant of the summation of internal forces developed with transfer of momentum. Success in athletics and other motor skill activities depends on the ability to efficiently transfer momentum through sequential body movements, an ability that increases with the skilled performer.

When two bodies collide they exert a force on each other when in contact. This force (f) over a given period of time (t) is termed *impulse* (i.e., f·t). Through application of Newton's second law, it can be shown that impulse is equal to the change of momentum that is produced. Thus, to change the speed of a body or object, not only is the force that is applied important, but also the time it is applied. When landing from a height or catching a hard thrown ball, the idea is to decrease the effective force by increasing the time of its application. This can be done by flexing the arms from their initially fully extended position when catching the ball and, when jumping from a height, by landing with the feet and legs extended, followed by flexion of the ankles, knees, and hips.

Impact occurs when two objects collide. Success in many sports depends on the outcome or result of impacts taking place, e.g., the ball rebounding off the walls and floor in racquetball, or in soccer, the striker's attempt to impart particular direction and speed when heading or kicking the ball for a goal. Rebound after impact is influenced by several factors, including elasticity, angle of incidence, angle of reflection, and the presence or absence of rotation, i.e., spin.

1. Elasticity is the property of an object that allows it to restore its shape after compression. It can be measured by the coefficient of restitution (elasticity), which is equal to the square root of the bounce height divided by the drop height. Since a tennis ball dropped from a given height does not bounce as high as a golf ball, it has less elasticity.
2. The angle of incidence is that of the velocity vector relative to the surface at the point of contact.
3. The angle of reflection represents the velocity vector upon rebound relative to the point of contact, and is dependent upon friction and the object's elasticity and spin.
4. Rotation (spin) of an object impacting another object at the same angle of incidence and velocity will affect both its angle of reflection and rebound velocity. Backspin

causes the ball to rise at a lower angle with slower velocity, while topspin increases the angle of reflection and velocity with which the ball rises.

WORK. Work is used in everyday language to describe any situation in which muscular effort is exerted, even when there is no movement, i.e., isometric contraction. However, with respect to mechanics, work is equal to the force applied to a body times the distance through which the body moves, i.e., $W = F \cdot d$, where W is work, f is force, and d is distance. A force acting in the same direction as the object is moving results in positive work done. If the object is moving in the opposite direction than the force is acting, then negative work is being done.

Whereas work is independent of time, *power* is the rate at which work is done and is expressed in equation form as: $P = W \div t$, where P is power, W is work, and t is time. *Energy* is the capacity to do work. It can exist in many forms, including chemical, heat, and mechanical. Mechanical energy, or that which a body in motion possesses, can be classified as either kinetic or potential. Kinetic energy is that demonstrated by a body by virtue of its motion, and increases with speed; when velocity is zero, kinetic energy is zero. Since the total amount of energy possessed by a body remains constant, potential energy is the inverse of kinetic energy. When one initiates a dive from a springboard, potential energy is greatest when the peak height is reached. If there were no horizontal velocity, the potential energy would be equal to the diver's weight times the height above the water.

FORCES IN EQUILIBRIUM. As stated earlier, *statics* is that aspect of mechanics in which forces acting on an object are in equilibrium; for example, when an object is at rest, it is in a state of static equilibrium. Concepts associated with static equilibrium include center of gravity, stability, and balance.

The *center of gravity*, also known as the center of mass, is a theoretical point of an object at which its entire weight at rest can be balanced. The force of gravity acts perpendicularly through the center of mass to the ground. In symmetrically shaped objects (such as a cube or sphere) of constant composition, the center of gravity lies in the exact center of the object. In the standing position, with the arms hanging at the sides, the center of gravity of the average adult male is at a point about 57% of his total height from the floor; for the average young adult female, it is at 55% of her height. These values would be higher if one were to raise his arms in the normal standing position, and lower if one bends at the knees.

Stability represents a body's resistance to losing balance or the maintenance of equilibrium. It depends upon three factors, viz., the height of the center of gravity of the object, its base of support and its weight. Stability is decreased as the center of gravity is elevated. Conversely, the lower the center of gravity, the more stable a body becomes. The base of support of a body is the area encompassed by connecting all the points in contact with the ground. If the base of support is increased, stability is also increased because the line drawn perpendicular to the surface from the center of gravity is now farther from the outside edge of the base of support.

In any position except the recumbent, muscles are called upon to resist the pull of gravity on the body. In the normal standing position, the center of gravity is high and the base of support is small. Greater stability can be obtained through flexing the knees slightly, bending the trunk forward, and lowering the arms (Fig. 2–15 A and B), but will be reduced if the center of gravity is moved toward the edge of the base (Fig. 2–15C). A heavier object of similar size as a lighter one will have greater inertia and thus greater stability. The heavier object's inertia, i.e., resistance to change, will increase the force required to dislodge the object by causing movement of the body's center of gravity outside its base of support.

Balance during movement, termed *dynamic balance*, is achieved by a continuous interaction of the forces moving the body in the desired direction and speed. In essence, dynamic balance is achieved via a smooth transition of the body's center of

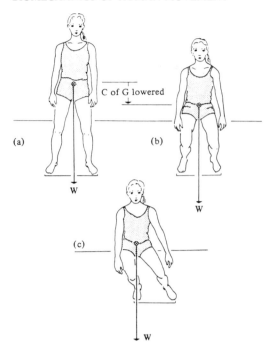

(a)

(b) C of G lowered

W

W

(c)

W

FIG. 2–15. A and B, Greater stability is obtained by lowering the center of gravity. C, Moving the center of gravity closer to the edge of the base of support results in instability. (From Kreighbaum, E., and K.M. Barthels: Biomechanics. A Qualitative Approach For Studying Human Movement. Minneapolis, Minn.: Burgess, 1981, p. 255.)

gravity from one base of support to the next. It should be realized, however, that an individual may be properly balanced for accomplishment of an athletic movement task at a given instant, yet exhibit poor stability characteristics. An example of this situation is illustrated in Figure 2–16, in which the centripetal force is "balanced" by leaning in the opposite direction with the line drawn perpendicular from the body's center of gravity falling well outside the small base of support.

ANGULAR KINETICS. As with linear motion, angular motion (also known as rotary motion) can be analyzed with respect to forces causing it. In general, the quantities used to describe and analyze rotary motion are similar to those for linear motion. Indeed, Newton's three laws of motion have been adapted to angular form.[12]

Torque is the magnitude of twist around a center of rotation and, in angular motion, is analogous to force in linear motion. It is equivalent to the product of the perpendicular component of force applied to the lever arm times the distance from the center of rotation to the line of application of the force. This concept is graphically depicted in Figure 2–17.

In linear motion, an object's mass is its sole measure of inertia, i.e., a greater mass yields a greater resistance to change. With angular motion, the resistance depends not only on mass, but on the distribution of mass about the axis which the body is rotating. This angular motion resistance to change is called *moment of inertia*, and is defined by the equation: $I = m \cdot r^2$, where I is the moment of inertia, m is the mass, and r is the distance of the mass from the center of rotation. Thus, the closer the mass is to the axis of rotation, the easier it is to initiate rotary movement. This concept supplies the logic for choking up on the bat to make it easier (less force needed) to initiate the swing.

Angular velocity can be defined as the angle through which the object turns in a given time period. The product of angular velocity and the moment of inertia is equal to the *angular momentum*, and, like linear momentum, is conserved, in that once established it tends to remain constant until outside forces change it (analogue of Newton's first law of motion). However, during movement one can alter the body's shape and configuration, and thus the distribution of mass and its moment of inertia. By changing the moment of inertia of body positions during spins and rotations, the turning rate, or angular velocity, can be increased or decreased while the total angular momentum remains unchanged throughout. This is how the ice skater is able to spin so fast (i.e., increased angular velocity) by bringing the arms in closer to the axis of rotation (decreased moment of inertia). The diver also utilizes this concept (Fig. 2–18)—in the tuck position there is an increased angular velocity, but as soon as the extended, pike configuration is assumed for entry, the rotation (angular velocity) slows, yet the angular momentum

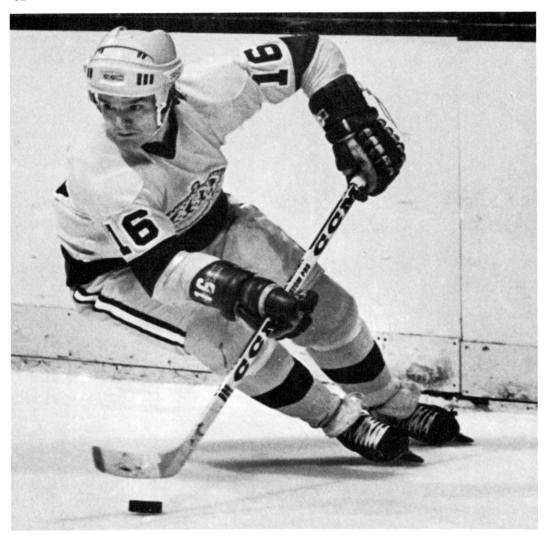

FIG. 2–16. Professional hockey player exhibiting poor stability characteristics in order to counterbalance centripetal force. (From Rasch, P.J.: Kinesiology and Applied Anatomy. 7th ed. Philadelphia: Lea & Febiger, 1989, p. 80.)

of the whole body remains essentially constant throughout the dive.

The work accomplished in rotary motion is dependent in part on the *mechanical advantage* of the *lever* system(s) employed. A lever may be thought of as a rigid bar that turns about an axis through application of an external force. In the human body the bones act as rigid bars, the joints as fulcra (or axes), and the contraction of muscles supplies the force to effect movement of the bones (levers).

As previously noted, torque in angular motion is analogous to force in linear motion. The angular analogue of Newton's third law can be stated as: "for every torque that is exerted by a body on another, there is an equal and opposite torque exerted by the second on the first."[12:152] The most common illustration of this law of angular motion in human physical performance occurs when one applies torque to one part of the body by muscular contraction, thus causing that part to rotate. The equal and op-

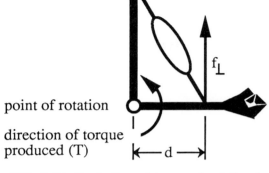

point of rotation

direction of torque
produced (T)

FIG. 2–17. Production of torque about the elbow joint. $T = f_\perp \cdot d$, where T = torque, $f_\perp$ = perpendicular component of muscular force, and d = distance from point of rotation to point of force application to the lever arm.

posite reaction to this applied torque causes some other part of the body to rotate in the opposite direction, as illustrated in the legs action and arms reaction on the long jumper in Figure 2–19.

Generally, the purpose of a lever is to gain mechanical advantage so that application of a relatively small force over a long distance will result in a larger force over a smaller distance. Mechanical advantage (MA) may be defined as the ratio of the length of the effort arm over the length of the resistance arm, i.e., the distance between effort application (E) and the fulcrum (F), divided by the distance from the resistance (R) to the fulcrum, or in equation form: $MA = EF/RF$. Thus, one gains mechanical advantage by increasing the length of the effort arm and/or decreasing the length of the resistance arm (Fig. 2–20).

In human movement, the muscles moving the bones are usually attached near the joints (which serve as fulcra) and resistance is applied at the end of the bones. This leads to a small effort arm (EF) and a relatively large resistance arm (RF), thus leaving man at a disadvantage in accomplishing power movements. However, this same mechanical arrangement facilitates speed movements against relatively light resistance, as a given muscular force will generate the greatest speed of movement at the end of the lever (Fig. 2–20).

Some individuals have muscle insertions

farther than the normal distance from joints, thus giving them the mechanical advantage for more powerful movements. This is usually less than 15%; thus, the principal gain in work production is accomplished by increasing the effort applied, e.g., through increasing muscle strength.

Tall individuals, because of long body levers, are generally at a disadvantage in activities requiring power. Further, unless they possess reasonably strong muscles, they are not able to take advantage of the speed which long levers are capable of generating against light resistance.

It should be recognized that a muscle can exert its greatest force only when it is perpendicular to the bone on which it has its insertion, since at this angle, the entire force of the muscle acts to rotate the bony lever around its axis.

FLUID DYNAMICS. In human physical performance, movements of one's body, as well as those of objects kicked, thrown, or caught, take place in a fluid environment. In some, such as badminton, cycling, golf, and tennis, the surrounding air (especially in the form of wind), can have a profound effect on performance. In other activities, such as basketball, gymnastics, and handball, however, the effects of the fluid environment on performance are negligible. In rowing and swimming, however, the effects of the fluid environment (water) substantially affect performance.

Aerodynamics is that subdivision of fluid dynamics concerned with the forces that affect moving bodies in space. External forces which can directly affect an object or body in flight are air resistance and gravity, as well as other environmental factors such as humidity, atmospheric pressure, and temperature. Other factors which have a significant effect on an object's flight include projectile motion principles mentioned previously, such as velocity of the object and its angle of projection when it becomes airborne, density of the air, wind direction and speed, shape of the object, texture of the object's surface, and rotation of the object (spin). Even a track sprinter's performance is notably affected by a tailwind of 2 m/s in a 200 m race (0.35 sec faster than in still air) at sea level; a 2 m/s head-

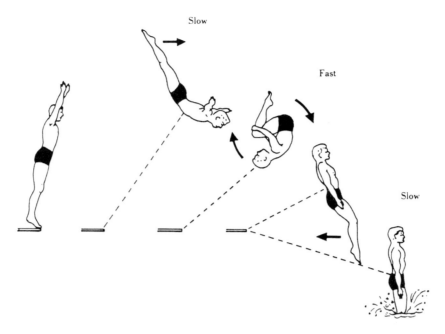

FIG. 2–18. Conservation of angular momentum. Alterations in the moment of inertia cause reciprocal changes in angular velocity, thus maintaining a constant overall angular momentum. (From: Jensen, C.R., G.W. Schultz, and B.L. Bangerter: Applied Kinesiology and Biomechanics. 3rd ed. New York: McGraw-Hill, 1983, p. 217.)

wind would result in a 0.43 sec slower time. Further, since air density is significantly reduced at altitude, a 200 m race can be run 0.32 sec faster at 7,500 ft elevation than at sea level in still air.[9]

There are two different drag effects which can alter substantially one's performance when air resistance is encountered. These drag forces act in the opposite direction to movement of the object, thus decreasing velocity of the object. *Form drag* is related to the object's shape or form. By altering the body's shape, the surface area exposed to air resistance forces can be decreased and thus, the form drag effect is decreased. Such action is of substantial value in cycling, speed skating, and downhill skiing.[8,21] *Surface drag* is caused by the characteristics of the surface of the object that affect the development of friction and air turbulence, which can, in turn, affect speed of movement and time in the air. The smooth surface of the bottom of a pair of skis and the dimples in a golf ball are both designed in such a manner as to reduce surface drag and enhance performance.

Lift is the force which develops perpendicular to the direction of movement, or in other words, at right angles to the drag force. These two forces, drag and lift, acting perpendicular to each other, produce a net or resultant propulsive force, whether the object in motion is in air or in water.

Hydrodynamics is the branch of fluid dynamics dealing with the movement of a body or object through water and the external forces which affect this movement. Gravitational effects no longer play as significant a role when a body is submerged in water. Instead, water resistance must now be overcome and the effects of buoyancy must be dealt with.

Buoyancy is an upward pressure exerted by the water on the object. If this force is greater than the weight, the object will float; if less, it will sink. The buoyancy of the human body is primarily dependent on a person's body composition (a person with a greater percentage of fat will float more easily). One's buoyancy can be increased by increasing volume without adding appreciable weight. One way to accom-

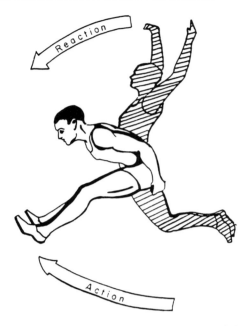

FIG. 2–19. Illustration of Newton's third law applied to angular motion. (From Hay, J.G.: The Biomechanics of Sports Techniques. 2nd ed. Englewood Cliffs, N.J.: Prentice-Hall, 1978, p. 153.)

plish this is to take a deep inspiration and inflate the lungs, which will increase the volume of the body but not its weight. An inflated life jacket has essentially the same effect.

Movement in water, as in air, produces a drag force or resistance in the opposite direction of motion. As in air, this drag force depends on form and surface characteristics, as well as the velocity of the object. Swimmers, for example, often shave their body hair and wear "skintight" suits when competing to decrease the amount of surface drag produced and thus, enhance performance. Figure 2–21 illustrates the application and direction of external forces acting on a breast-stroke swimmer: buoyancy (B), weight (W), and drag (D). Drag would be reduced if the swimmer floated higher in the water and maintained a more streamlined body configuration, i.e., less downward flexion of the arms and legs.[27]

ENHANCEMENT OF SPORTS AND EXERCISE PERFORMANCE VIA BIOMECHANICAL ANALYSIS TECHNIQUES

In the previous section, illustrations of the applicability of fundamental laws and principles of mechanics to performance of motor skills in various sports was examined. Contini[4] has termed this area of emphasis, general biomechanics; applied biomechanics is concerned with the more practical problems of analyzing motion to improve performance and prevent injury. Examples of improved sports performance via biomechanical analysis are increasingly abundant. In 1976, Nelson[30] cited numerous research studies providing evidence that prevalent coaching techniques regarding the time of force application and the optimal angle of projecting implements, as well as that for the athlete in diving and jumps, were at odds with that observed in biomechanical analysis of championship performers. Subsequently, Dillman[8] provided a summary of an extensive biomechanical analysis of cross-country skiing training techniques, and of downhill skiing air resistance effects, which led to improved performances. Kyle[21] has reported a greater than 10% reduction in air resistance effects on bicycling performance by the use of streamlined clothing, including shoes, canopied shaped helmet, and a one-piece skintight suit. Further reductions in air resistance measured in a wind tunnel have been achieved by streamlining components of the bicycle, including wheel spokes.[6,11] Considerable biomechanical research has been done on running shoes with respect to the relationship of their weight and amount of energy cost, their cushioning effects to absorb ground contact forces, and other design features to reduce musculoskeletal strain.[21] In comparing the running efficiency (i.e., energy cost), ground reaction forces, and rear foot motion characteristics of running shoes from four major companies, Williams, et al.[42] observed "trade-offs in terms of lighter shoes resulting in reduced energy cost, but at the expense of characteristics that would be expected to increase the likelihood of injury to the foot and knees."

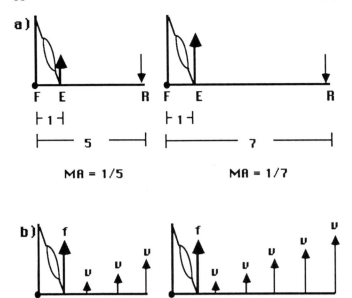

FIG. 2–20. A, Comparison of mechanical advantage. Given all other parameters equal, an individual with a shorter lever arm would have to exert less muscular force to overcome a given downward resistance applied at the end of the arm. B, Comparison of velocity of movement at given distances from the point of rotation, assuming muscular forces equal and an equal, light resistance. Despite a lesser mechanical advantage, the long limbed individual is able to create greater velocity at the lever's end, which becomes important in transferring momentum from the arm to an object being thrown.

An increasingly wide variety of mechanical and electrical devices are being utilized to measure specific skeletal and neuromuscular interactions with mechanical factors affecting human movement. The equipment utilized in a particular situation depends on the primary objectives of the study and the availability of appropriate equipment. Research biomechanists utilize increasingly sophisticated equipment, both to advance fundamental knowledge in the field and to conduct state-of-the-art analyses of athletic performances to discover effective means of improvement.

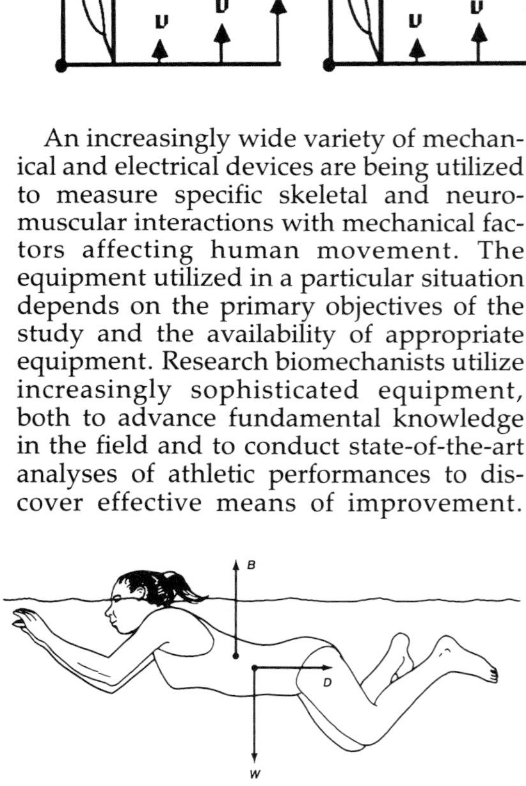

FIG. 2–21. External forces acting on a breaststroke swimmer: buoyancy (B), weight (W), and drag (D). The more streamlined the body configuration is with respect to the flow, the less will be the drag. (From Luttgens, K., and K.F. Wells: Kinesiology. Scientific Basis of Human Motion. 7th ed. Philadelphia: Saunders, 1982, p. 340.)

However, many who work with the direct application of biomechanics to enhance physical performance, such as teachers or coaches at the high school or college level, will usually be limited in equipment available to facilitate their efforts.

QUALITATIVE BIOMECHANICAL ANALYSIS TECHNIQUES

One who has a sound working knowledge of biomechanics and human physical performance can often make helpful suggestions to correct errors in a performer's movement pattern, even without equipment. Northrip et al.[32] stress the necessity of the teacher or coach training himself to see what is actually taking place, as opposed to what he thinks is occurring in the observed performance. To facilitate the effective teaching of motor skills and enhanced physical performance, Luttgens and Wells[24] have isolated five components of an effective biomechanic analysis system: (1) identification of the primary purpose of the skill with respect to accuracy, speed, form, distance, etc; (2) classification of the skill in terms of giving impetus to one's own body or to external objects, and receiving impetus; (3) anatomic analysis, including examination of skeletal-joint action, muscle participation, and neuromuscular considerations; (4) mechanical analysis that identifies the most appropriate form for successful performance; and (5) a succint prescription for improvement of performance.

For the teacher or coach, the big advantage in utilizing cinematography or videotaping for motion analysis lies in the available permanent record afforded and the ability to use slow motion and stop-action playback features. In this manner, the performance can be reviewed in more detail at various speeds, with particularly critical sequences viewed frame by frame. Obviously, this provides the potential for an objective and more careful biomechanic analysis. Videotape is particularly valuable in practice situations, as the near instant playback permits the performer to view the performance while errors are identified and corrections provided. Subsequently, the tape can be erased or if a permanent record is desired, it can be transferred to a 16mm film before reusing.

QUANTITATIVE BIOMECHANICAL ANALYSIS TECHNIQUES

Because of the difficulty in accurately measuring forces (i.e., kinetics) produced and encountered during sports performance, the most frequently researched parameter by biomechanists has been the relationship between space and time (i.e., kinematics).[32] Because motion can be viewed as a series of isolated positions linked in space and time, and since position is location in space, motion is the change that occurs from one position to another over time.

Cinematography has been the most widely used technique to study spatiotemporal relationships during human movement. Use of high-speed cameras with film speeds of up to 500 frames per second, coupled with a stop motion film analyzer, easily provide sufficient data points for analyzing the fastest human movements. This procedure usually entails careful placement of markers on body landmarks, such as that shown on the runner in Figure 2–22, so that measurements of segment displacements can be

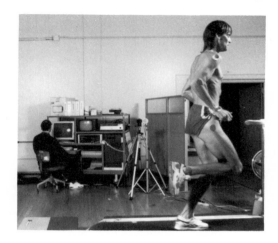

FIG. 2–22. Markers on body landmarks of this runner permit measurement of segment displacement in the analysis of rapid human movement.

made from graphic representations obtained by hand tracings from frame images (one by one) or, as depicted in Figure 2–23, by computer analysis. From these data, calculations of speed, range, angle, and sequence of body segments can be made. Figure 2–24 depicts sequential elements of the coupled cinematographic data acquisition system (top) and a sequential stick-diagram of lower body segment trajectories during a walking stride. A trained observer can analyze specific positions of body landmarks or segments at critical points of a movement and distinguish incorrect from correct movement patterns observed in skilled performers.[24] An example, utilizing a computer supported cinematography system, is Mann and Herman's study[25] of the 1984 Olympic Games 200 meters sprint finals. They found that the 1st and 2nd place finishers differed significantly from the 8th place finisher in numerous important lower limb kinematic responses which were associated with shortened ground support time, greater stride rate, and higher horizontal velocity.

Stroboscopy is a single frame photographic technique in which the camera shutter remains open throughout the movement while multiple images are obtained from accurately timed light flashes against a darkened background. This re-

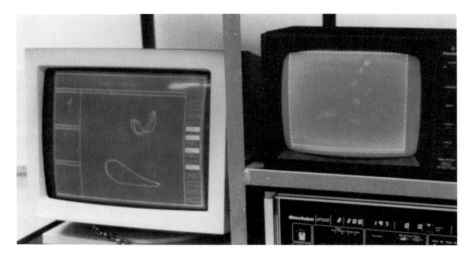

FIG. 2–23. Computer assisted graphic display of a cinematographic analysis of the ankle motion (lower portion, left screen) and wrist motion (upper portion, left screen) with each stride in the runner depicted in the previous figure.

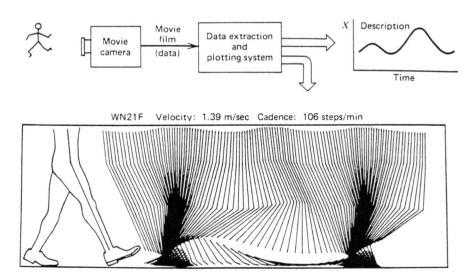

FIG. 2–24. Stick figure diagram of lower body segment movement generated by cinematographic data extraction and plotting system. (From Winter, D.A.: Biomechanics of Human Movement. New York: Wiley & Sons, 1979, p. 4.)

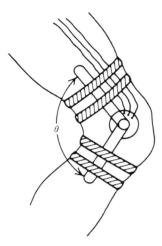

FIG. 2–25. Electrical potentiometer located at the knee joint for measurement of angular change. (From Winter, D.A.: Biomechanics of Human Movement. New York: Wiley & Sons, 1979, p. 12.)

sults in a continuous image of the path of the moving body, body parts, and any implement being used at selected time-constant points. Thus, this single photograph serves as primary data for measurements of position as a function of time for any part of the image. This technique has proved useful in the study of movement patterns involved in the golf swing, tennis serve, dance leap, basketball jump shot, and softball throw.[26] The movement paths evidenced by novices can be compared to skilled performers to determine appropriate corrections for effecting improved performance, or studied for changes noted following instruction and practice.[41]

Electrogoniometry utilizes an electrical potentiometer attached at the center of rotation to indicate the angular change of the two arms of a goniometer attached to limb segments across a joint (Fig. 2–25). Continuous recording of electrical current change caused by changes in joint angle can be obtained. This permits assessment of ranges of motion at various joints, as well as determination of joint angles at given points of a total motion pattern. Angular velocity and acceleration can also be determined. While early models were somewhat cumbersome, modern equipment uses solid state devices to make the

detection equipment smaller and lighter.[32] Knutzen et al.[17] have utilized this technique to demonstrate range of motion differences permitted by knee braces utilized during slow running rehabilitation therapy following surgical repair from knee injury.

Electromyography (EMG) is a technique utilized to measure the type and magnitude of muscle-action potentials that are produced during muscular contractions. The electrical discharge is measured by electrodes attached to the skin over the muscle(s) involved in the movement. Needle electrodes embedded in the muscle are used for studying the deeper underlying muscles. In either case, electrical activity is received, amplified, and integrated for analysis. These electrical potentials describe the neural input to the muscles as a function of time during movement. This provides information as to when a muscle begins to contract, with what force, and when it ceases contraction during a movement. Further, electrodes can be arranged so that the interplay of muscles within a group, as well as antagonistic muscle action, can be studied. Lagasse[22] contends that champion athletes demonstrate a specific temporal and sequential order of muscle activation in the execution of their specific skill. Further, temporal and sequential order of muscle activation, which can be assessed by EMG, has been shown to be modified by practice. He also recommends measurement of antagonistic muscle activity, since practice has been found to inhibit undesired activity from the antagonistic muscles during performance.[15,31] Lagasse[22] also recommends utilizing the EMG to study power athletes' ability to rapidly contract a muscle in reaching a desired level of muscular tension.

Force platforms employ strain gauge transducers to measure the relative force exerted upon a spring-loaded flat surface. Via utilization of multiple strain gauges and subsequent mathematic calculations, measurement of the force imparted by the foot, hand or other body part in the vertical and two horizontal directions, and about three axes is accomplished, thus permitting analysis of linear forces and torques.[34] Panzer et al.[33] used force platforms to measure lower extremity joint loads experienced by elite gymnasts during landing following a double back somersault. Comparison of these data with those obtained during computer simulation enabled these authors to suggest specific methods of landing training for injury prevention and skill improvement.

Telemetry has facilitated significant advances in biomechanics research because it permits electrical signals from devices used to monitor movement without the encumbrance of wires to electrical receivers. Further, miniaturization of detection and broadcasting equipment has reduced the weight and size significantly. Thus, any mechanical or physiologic event that can be converted to an electrical signal can be amplified, recorded, and analyzed. de Koning et al.[18] have utilized telemetered EMG data to study the relationship between muscle action and movement pattern in ice speed skating in an effort to improve transformation of rotational velocity into horizontal velocity.

Computers. Perhaps the most significant advance in biomechanics research has been the utilization of high-speed computers. Previously, hand tabulation and reduction of recorded data entailing substantial mathematic calculations limited the amount of cinematographic and force measurement data that could be analyzed. Now, analysis of high-speed cinematographic data from multiple trials of a performance by an individual, and comparison to other individuals, is possible with the use of motion analyzer and computer interfacing.

Computers can also be programmed to present graphic displays of analyses. These can range from simple X-Y plots to sequential graphic representations of the entire movement. A graphic comparison of an individual's performance can be made to that of an ideal performance previously stored. This procedure can facilitate the detection of errors in performance, and can lead to the development of appropriate strategies for improvement, particularly if done in real time. An example of immediate computer generated feedback facilitating changes in movement patterns that could improve performance is the study by Sanderson and Cavanagh.[37] These investigators were able to show competitive cyclists that they were not pulling up on the toe-clips of the foot opposite the one pushing down on the pedal. Instead, they were actually pushing down slightly and thus, working against the positive force generated by the other limb. By watching the force pattern in real-time on the computer screen, they were able to correct this fault rapidly.

Another principal advance in biomechanics research has been the utilization of computers to generate simulations of ideal performance. Numerous mathematic models have been developed that simulate human movement patterns in sports performance.[28] Following validation against experimental conditions, they provide a powerful means of varying one or more key parameters under controlled conditions to determine the effect on performance. Ramey[34] utilized equations of rigid body dynamics to show that the three major styles of flight in the long jump were equally effective, given the proper angular momentum at takeoff.

APPLICATIONS OF BIOMECHANICS TO SELECTED DAILY LIVING ACTIVITIES

Numerous examples of exercise and sports applications have been presented in the preceding biomechanics discussion. Principles of biomechanics, however, are applicable to all human movement, including ordinary daily living activities and occupational tasks. Technologic advances have generally reduced the vigorous physical activity necessary in our modern day life, but man still uses his/her body for locomotion and handling of objects, and there are still many occupations which require manual materials handling. While many of these tasks do not entail intensive effort, movements may be repeated often or performed for prolonged periods of time. If these activities are performed improperly, they can lead to undue musculoskeletal strain, fatigue, and injury. Injury due to improper handling techniques is quite prevalent in our labor force and results in significant costs for sick leave, worker's compensation, and rehabilitation.[38] Many companies now offer or require back care or materials handling classes for their employees. Further, physical therapists often become involved in retraining employees or restructuring their work tasks in order to incorporate biomechanically safe materials handling techniques. When tasks are performed in accord with fundamental principles of basic body mechanics, incidence of strain and injury are reduced, fatigue is lessened, and movement is more efficient and aesthetic.[24,36]

MAN'S UPRIGHT POSTURE

Evolution has brought about many structural adaptations to the human's upright posture.[36,40] However, there is still inherent instability in the structure of man's axial skeleton which appears to be associated with some of today's most common health problems. First, the spine is a series of vertebrae stacked on top of each other, not a single rigid bone. These vertebrae are stacked not in a straight line, but rather in a slight zigzag shape due to the curves of the spine. This stack is then topped with a heavy skull and supported by a pelvis which can rock back and forth. These characteristics all lead to instability in the erect position. Other factors augment this problem. For example, man's center of gravity is relatively high, and the base of support formed by the feet is relatively small. Furthermore, the heavy viscera in the abdomen tend to exert a forward and downward pull on the trunk, thus increasing the curvature in the lumbar region of the spine.

POSTURE ASSESSMENT. For many years physical educators attempted to evaluate the erect standing posture and to correct postural faults, especially in school-age children. However, individual variation in structure, body composition, and age make objective evaluation difficult. Also, the body is not actually static in the standing position; it oscillates over a small range within the base of support, as the trunk flexors and extensors are alternately activated. Thus, a single measurement would

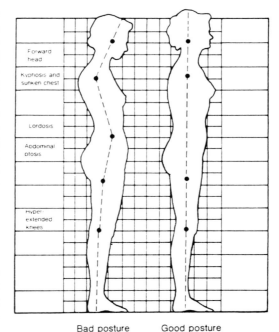

Bad posture　　Good posture

FIG. 2–26. Comparison of good and bad posture. (From Corbin, C., et al: Concepts in Physical Education. Dubuque, Iowa: Wm. C. Brown, 1981, p. 99.)

be an inaccurate assessment of erect posture. Though there is no one correct model of erect posture for the entire population, numerous general guidelines have been advanced. As depicted in Figure 2–26, the spinal curves should be minimal and the major body segments in near vertical alignment.

MAINTENANCE OF POSTURE. Erect posture is maintained by muscles working to stabilize the joints by acting in opposition to each other, to gravity, or to other external forces. The groups of muscles most frequently employed are those used to maintain the erect position of the body against the force of gravity. The abdominal muscles tend to pull up on the anterior part of the pelvis, thus minimizing excessive curvature in the lumbar region of the spine (or "pelvic tilt"). They also produce pressure inside the abdomen, which creates a torque about the spine to counterbalance the forward pull as one lifts an object or bends forward. The long spinal muscles act in op-

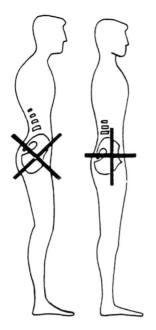

FIG. 2–27. Improper (a) and proper (b) angle of pelvic tilt. (From Adams, W.C., et al.: Foundations of Physical Activity. Champaign, Ill.: Stipes, 1968, p. 116.)

position to the abdominal muscles, and the quadriceps and hamstrings groups also act in opposition on the pelvis, thus affecting the extent of "pelvic tilt."

ADVERSE EFFECTS OF POSTURAL MISALIGNMENT. Persistent imbalances in posture have been associated with certain chronic health problems, including headache, susceptibility to back injury, painful menstruation, joint strain, and ligament stretch.[23] The most important problem, however, is low back pain, suffered by approximately 75% of the adult population at some time in their life in most industrialized nations. Nearly 15% of these populations experience back pain *every year*.[39] Several other factors are associated with low back pain, such as obesity, improper lifting, and hypokinetics. However, muscular imbalances and improper pelvic tilt appear to be primary causes.[19,36] The weak abdominal muscles fail to provide the upward pull on the front of the pelvis (Fig. 2–27), thus resulting in the lumbar curve becoming exaggerated (lordosis). This excessive lordosis causes a shift in position of the lumbar ver-

tebrae relative to one another. With this change in position, the vertebral articular processes can press against one another, creating excessive pressure on nerve roots and pain in the lower portion of the back.[3,36]

In order to prevent or rehabilitate problems associated with poor posture, one is best advised to seek strategies to eliminate the cause(s). Strengthening the appropriate muscles is one of the most important preventive and rehabilitative measures. However, in developing a therapeutic approach to posture correction, one must realize the limitations of postural evaluation techniques, and be especially attendant to individual structural variation.[24]

WALKING

Walking is man's most universal and frequently employed locomotor activity. A well-coordinated walking gait necessitates properly functioning reflexes, normal flexibility of the joints, and achievement of appropriate stability in the weight-bearing phases. Though walking appears to be a relatively simple activity, biomechanical analysis reveals it to be an effective illustration of the exceedingly complex synchronization of neuromuscular and joint movements common to all skilled motor performance.

Walking entails alternate, rhythmical propulsive force from the legs and a co-ordinated loss and recovery of balance with each step. The foot strike is heel first, and the knee and foot should be aligned straight ahead in all phases of the gait. Minimum lateral motion occurs when the feet strike such that their inner borders describe a single straight line. Actions of the upper body should be coordinated to facilitate smooth transition from the supporting phase to the swing phase of the gait.

Effective forward propulsion in walking (i.e., without slipping) necessitates counterpressure and friction of the contact surface greater than that of the horizontal force developed through muscular contraction. If one desires to walk faster than his normal rate, or walks into a strong wind, the body should be inclined farther forward.

The muscular action and movement mechanics involved in walking have been carefully studied by numerous research workers, yet there is little agreement as to what constitutes a "proper" walking gait. Individual variations in walking gait have been ascribed to habits developed in childhood, differences in body mass, in leg length, in joint restrictions, in distribution of body weight, and in modifications caused by sickness or injury.[2]

CLIMBING AND DESCENDING STAIRS

Muscular strain and energy expenditure can be minimized in ascending stairs by inclining the body slightly forward (primarily from the feet, rather than from the hips), placing the entire sole of the foot on the stair tread, and by raising the body via extension of the knee joint.[5] By keeping the center of gravity forward, the resistance arm of the thigh lever is reduced and energy expenditure is reduced. Even so, ascending stairs at a normal rate (i.e., about two steps per second) requires about 5 times more energy than descending stairs at the same rate.[14]

Descending stairs safely requires that the body be kept more erect to keep the center of gravity near the center of the base of support. When landing on the foot, the extensor muscles of the hip, knee, and ankle joints perform eccentric ("lengthening") contraction. This is negative work, as gravity does the work and the muscles resist it to facilitate a controlled rate of descent. Hurrying and leaning too far forward compromise effective balance due to the line of gravity coming too close to the anterior margin of the base of support.

SITTING AND RISING FROM A SEATED POSITION

The movements of being seated and rising from a seated position are, for most people, the most common examples of changing body levels. The basic biomechanic problem in sitting down and in ris-

ing is that of supporting the body while the center of gravity is moving. To keep the body's center of gravity within the base of support during these movements, one foot should be placed slightly to the rear of the front edge of the chair and the trunk inclined forward. In sitting, the body is lowered gradually and eased into the chair by bending the knees in eccentric contraction of the knee extensors to control the effects of gravity. In rising from a chair, it may be necessary first to move the center of gravity near the edge of the chair seat. The standing erect position is reached by concentric contraction of the knee extensors, with the weight gradually shifted from the rear to the forward foot.

SQUATTING

When squatting with a heavy weight, it is best to spread the feet about shoulder width apart and to extend one foot slightly forward. The heels should maintain contact with the floor for better stability. It is not advisable to perform a full knee bend, especially when handling heavy weights, since damage may be done to the ligaments of the knee by overstretching them.[24] With this in mind, half knee bends (i.e., 90 degree angle between upper and lower leg) are recommended. Care should also be taken to avoid loss of balance and twisting of the knee joint, which can result in tearing of the medial cartilage.[13]

LIFTING HEAVY OBJECTS

Since neither the spine or spinal muscles are effectively designed for lifting heavy weights, it is not surprising that the incidence of back injury attributed to lifting is high.[3,38] Figure 2–28 illustrates the increased bending moment on the lumbar spine by assuming a forward-bending position. When attempts to lift heavy objects are made in this position, compressive forces can be great enough to result in slipped, or herniated disks. Use of basic mechanic principles, however, can increase economy of effort and reduce back strain. Basic to effective lifting is keeping

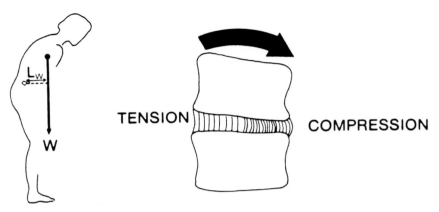

TENSION   COMPRESSION

FIG. 2–28. Lumbar vertebral force development. Forward bending produces a forward torque (moment) on the body via action of the upper body weight (W) on the lever arm, Lw. This results in an increase in pressure on the front of the lumbar vertebral disc, and tension on the rear portion. (From Nordin, M., and V.H. Frankel: Basic Biomechanics of the Musculoskeletal System. 2nd ed. Philadelphia: Lea & Febiger, 1989, p. 193.)

the resistance arm of the lever used for lifting as short as possible, and the angle at which the gravitational force applies to the lever as small as possible.[24] Effective balance is achieved by keeping the feet flat on the floor about shoulder width apart. Preparatory to lifting, the object is grasped with the knees flexed and the back kept as straight as possible (Fig. 2–29). Lifting is accomplished by straightening of the legs via forceful contraction of the powerful knee extensor muscles, and *not* by pulling with the arms and back. The object should be kept close to the body's line of gravity during the lifting motion. This will bring the resistance (R) closer to the fulcrum (F), reducing the distance between R and F and thus, increasing the mechanical advantage. When lifting a suitcase or load with both hands at the side of the body, the foot far-

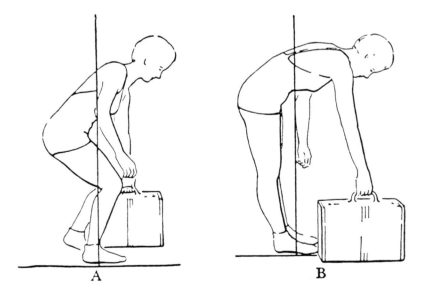

A   B

FIG. 2–29. Lifting a suitcase: A) correctly, and B) incorrectly. (From Luttgens, K., and K.F. Wells: Kinesiology: Scientific Basis of Human Motion. 7th ed. Philadelphia: Saunders, 1982, p. 519.)

ther from the load is placed forward in order to give better stability during the lifting motion (Fig. 2–29).

CARRYING HEAVY OBJECTS

The most common cause of injury in carrying loads is loss of balance resulting in momentary inadequately compensated muscular strain.[36] Maintenance of balance, as well as more efficient leverage, are achieved by carrying the object close to the midline of the body near the body's center of gravity. When carrying a heavy unilateral load (e.g., a suitcase), compensatory movements, such as lifting the other arm and inclining the trunk to the opposite side, are required to help keep the center of gravity of the body and suitcase over the body's base of support. Since the strain on the opposite hip is greater when the load is carried on one side than if double the weight is carried bilaterally,[10] the load should be alternated from one side of the body to the other. Heavier loads can be carried longer distances with less muscular strain and energy cost if they can be effectively balanced on the head or shoulders.[7]

PUSHING AND PULLING HEAVY OBJECTS
(Fig. 2–30)

Though the shape and weight of the object to be moved, as well as surface friction and amount of control needed in moving are primary considerations sometimes in conflict, it is generally best to slide rather than carry, and to push rather than pull a heavy object. The basic problem in sliding a heavy object is the efficient application of force to move the object without undue strain and risk of injury, and to conserve the mover's energy. Rasch[36] has advanced four principles for effecting an efficient pushing technique.

1. The feet are placed a comfortable distance apart, with one foot near to the object to be pushed and the other extended to the rear.
2. The spine is kept straight and the hips are kept low.
3. The hands are placed at or near the level of the object's center of gravity.

4. The object is moved by contracting the extensors of the hip, knee, and ankle and straightening the legs, not by extending the arms.

Force should be applied in the desired direction at a point near the center of gravity to maximize the horizontal component. If there is significant friction to overcome, force is applied below the center of gravity in order to counterbalance the downward force due to friction with an upward component of applied force. Once the object is in motion, it is best not to stop until one tires. At this point, it may be advisable to alternate the primary muscles used by changing from facing the object to a position with one's back facing the object. Starting again will require application of a large initial force to overcome inertia.

An efficient pulling action necessitates application of similar mechanical principles as those for pushing. As illustrated in Figure 2–30, the body is inclined away from the object and positioned in a manner to maximize horizontal force application consistent with the frictional force encountered. If the object has a low center of gravity, lengthening the handle or rope attached to the object will permit reduction of the upward (vertical) lift component.

WORKING WITH LONG HANDLED IMPLEMENTS

Working with implements such as a hoe, rake, or mop, involves the movements of pushing, pulling and occasional lifting. The basic characteristic of this type of work is maintenance of a fixed posture for a considerable period of time, which can result in tension and fatigue. This can be partially alleviated by varying the worker's position to one with his side aligned to the work task. Additional reach is obtained by bending the knee of the lead leg and inclining the trunk toward the work site. As the stroking motion is completed, the knee and trunk are straightened. This method results in an alternate contraction and relaxation of primary muscle groups used, and consequently reduces the tension from static contraction of back muscles normally associated with such work tasks.

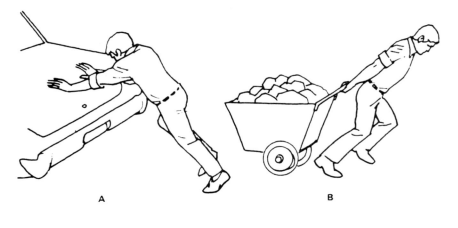

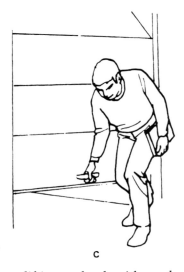

FIG. 2–30. Correct methods of A, pushing, B, pulling, and C, lifting objects. (From Luttgens, K., and K.F. Wells: Kinesiology: Scientific Basis of Human Motion. 7th ed. Philadelphia: Saunders, 1982, p. 508.)

When lifting a load with a shovel or snow spade, one should slide the lower hand well down the shaft near the resistance in order to lengthen the effort arm (EF) and increase mechanical advantage. This is of particular importance because of the invariably long resistance arm (RF), with the resistance taken at the end of the lever opposite the effort application. Efficiency of movement and reduction of muscular fatigue, strain, and risk of injury can be accomplished by keeping the back relatively straight, inclining the body forward from the trunk, and bending the knees. In this manner, upward lifting movement is done primarily by coordinated action of the knee and hip extensors which reduces lower back muscle strain.

SUMMARY

1. Biomechanics is the science concerned with the interrelationship of the biologic properties of the skeletal, articular, and neuromuscular systems and of the laws and principles of mechanics.

2. Biomechanics is concerned with both internal and external factors that affect movement of one's body, as well as the movement of implements or other equipment used in exercise, sport, or other physical activity. Applications of biomechanics are seen in medicine, industry, and the military, as well as in physical education and athletics.

3. Bones of the skeletal system that articulate at a joint serve as anatomic levers

effecting movement upon application of force generated by skeletal muscle contraction.

4. Primary functions of skeletal muscle are affected by number, arrangement, length, and type of fibers. Some muscles are more powerful, while others permit greater endurance or range of movement.

5. Even relatively simple movements, e.g., walking, involve the action of numerous muscles in one or more of several roles to produce an efficient effort.

6. The somatic nervous system is involved with reception (afferent) and conduction (efferent) of neural impulses and ultimately, with the activity of skeletal muscle.

7. The basic functional structure of the neuromuscular system is the motor unit, which consists of a single motor nerve cell, together with its nerve fiber and the group of muscle fibers supplied by its branches. The strength of muscle contraction is dependent on how many motor units are activated by the central nervous system.

8. Dynamics is the aspect of mechanics in which motion of an object is brought about by unbalanced forces. There are two branches of dynamics: (a) kinematics, which deals with descriptive analysis of motion without consideration of forces causing motion; and (b) kinetics, which deals with the interrelationship of forces causing motion.

9. Kinematics includes the measurement of displacement, velocity, speed and acceleration in both linear and rotary (angular) motion about an axis.

10. Newton's three laws of motion addressing the concepts of inertia, acceleration, and action-reaction, provide an integrative understanding of forces affecting objects in motion, and are the cornerstone of kinetics.

11. Forces that modify motion include gravity, friction, momentum, impulse, and impact.

12. Statics is that aspect of mechanics, in which forces acting on an object are in equilibrium. Center of gravity and stability are concepts basic to static balance.

13. Torque, moment of inertia, angular velocity, and angular momentum provide analogues of Newton's three laws applicable to rotary motion. The work accomplished in rotary motion is dependent on the mechanical advantage of the lever system(s) employed.

14. In human physical performance, movements of one's body, as well as those of objects kicked, thrown, or caught, take place in a fluid environment, and are subject to the net propulsive force of drag and lift.

15. An increasingly wide variety of mechanical and electrical devices are being utilized to measure specific skeletal and neuromuscular interactions with mechanical factors affecting human movement.

16. The development of high-speed computers has provided the most important impetus for advances in biomechanics research. Some of this research has been successfully applied to effect improvements in performance and prevention of exercise and sports related injuries.

17. Principles of biomechanics are also applicable to movement entailed in daily living activities and many occupational tasks which, if employed properly, lead to reduced incidence of strain and injury, more efficient movement, and less fatigue.

REFERENCES

1. Atwater, A.E.: Kinesiology/biomechanics: perspectives and trends. Res. Quart. 51:193–218, 1980.
2. Basmajian, J.V.: Muscles Alive. 4th Ed. Baltimore: Williams & Wilkins, 1979.
3. Cailliet, R.: Low Back Pain Syndrome. Philadelphia: F.A. Davis, 1981.
4. Contini, R.: Preface. Human Factors. 5:423–425, 1963.
5. Cooper, J.M., M. Adrian, and R.B. Glassow: Kinesiology. (5th ed) St. Louis: Mosby, 1982.
6. Dal Monte, A., L.M. Leonardi, C. Menchinelli, and C. Marini: A new bicycle design based on biomechanics and advanced technology. Int. J. Sport Biomech. 3:287–292, 1987.
7. Datta, S.R., and N.L. Ramanathan: Ergonomic comparison of seven modes of carrying loads on the horizontal plane. Ergonomics. 14:269–278, 1971.
8. Dillman, C.J.: Applied biomechanics research for the United States ski team. JOPERD. 53(1):27–29, 1982.
9. Frohlich, C.: Effect of wind and altitude on record

performances in foot races, pole vault, and long jump. Am. J. Physics. 53:726–730, 1985.

10. Greene, E., and A. Bilger (Editors): Winter's Protective Body Mechanics. New York: Springer, 1973.

11. Gross, A.C., C.R. Kyle, and D.J. Malewicki: The aerodynamics of human powered land vehicles. Sci. Amer. 249(2):142–152, 1983.

12. Hay, J.G.: The Biomechanics of Sports Techniques. 2nd ed. Englewood Cliffs, N.J.: Prentice-Hall, 1978.

13. Helfert, A.J.: Mechanism of derangements of the medial semilunar cartilage and their management. J. Bone Joint Surg. 41-B:299–336, 1959.

14. Hesser, C.M.: Energy cost of alternating positive and negative work. Acta Physiol. Scand. 63:84–93, 1965.

15. Kamon, E., and J. Gormley: Muscular activity pattern for skilled performance and during learning of horizontal bar exercise. Ergonomics. 11:345–357, 1968.

16. Kirkpatrick, P.H.: Unscientific measurement in athletics. Sci. Amer. 156(4):226–228, 1937.

17. Knutzen, K.M., B.T. Bates, and J. Hammill: Electrogoniometry of post-surgical knee-bracing in running. Am. J. Phys. Med. 62(4):172–181, 1983.

18. Koning, J.J. de, R.W. de Boer, G. de Groot, and G.J. Ingen Schenau: Muscle coordination in speed skating. In International Series on Biomechanics, Vol 7-B. Edited by G. de Groot, A.P. Hollander, P.A. Huijing and G.J. Ingen Schenau. Amsterdam: The Netherlands Free Press, 1988, pp. 878–882.

19. Kraus, H., and W. Raab: Hypokinetic Disease. Springfield: Charles C Thomas, 1960.

20. Kreighbaum, E., and K.M. Barthels: Biomechanics: A Qualitative Approach for Studying Human Movement. Minneapolis: Burgess, 1981.

21. Kyle, C.R.: Athletic clothing. Sci. Amer. 254(3):104–110, 1986.

22. Lagasse, P.: Neuromuscular considerations. In Standardized Biomechanical Testing in Sport. Edited by D.A. Dainty and R.W. Norman. Champaign, Ill.: Human Kinetics, 1987, pp. 59–71.

23. Lindsey, R., B.J. Jones, and A.V. Whitley: Body Mechanics. Dubuque, Iowa: Brown, 1968.

24. Luttgens, K., and K.F. Wells: Kinesiology: Scientific Basis of Human Motion. 7th ed. Philadelphia: Saunders, 1982.

25. Mann, R., and J. Herman: Kinematic analysis of Olympic sprint performance: men's 200 meters. Int. J. Sport Biomech. 1:151–162, 1985.

26. Merriman, J.S.: Stroboscopic photography as a research instrument. Res. Quart. 46:256–261, 1975.

27. Miller, D.I.: Biomechanics of swimming. In Exercise and Sport Sciences Reviews. Vol. 3. Edited by J.H. Wilmore and J.F. Keogh. New York: Academic, 1975, pp. 219–248.

28. Miller, D.I.: Modeling in biomechanics: an overview. Med. Sci. Sports. 11:115–122, 1979.

29. Morehouse, L.E., and P.J. Rasch: Sports Medicine for Trainers. 2nd ed. Philadelphia: Saunders, 1963.

30. Nelson, R.C.: Contribution of biomechanics to improve human performance. In Beyond Research—Solution to Human Problems. Amer. Acad. of P.E. Papers No 10. Edited by M.B. Scott. Iowa City, Iowa: Amer. Acad. of P.E., 1976, pp. 6–11.

31. Normand, M.C., P.P. Lagasse, C.A. Rouillard, and L.E. Tremblay: Modifications occurring in motor programs during learning of a complex task in man. Brain Research. 241:87–93, 1982.

32. Northrip, J.W., G.A. Logan, and W.C. McKinney: Introduction to Biomechanic Analysis of Sport. 2nd ed. Dubuque, Iowa: W.C. Brown, 1979.

33. Panzer, V.P., G.A. Wood, B.T. Bates, and B.R. Mason: Lower extremity loads in landings in elite gymnasts. In International Series on Biomechanics, Vol. 7-B. Edited by G. de Groot, A.P. Hollander, P.A. Huijing, and G.J. Ingen Schenau Amsterdam: The Netherlands Free Press, 1988, pp. 727–735.

34. Ramey, M.R.: Significance of angular momentum in long jumping. Res. Quart. 44:448–497, 1973.

35. Ramey, M.R.: Force plate designs and applications. In Exercise and Sport Sciences Reviews. Edited by J.H. Wilmore and J.F. Keogh. New York: Academic, 1975, pp. 303–319.

36. Rasch, P.J.: Kinesiology and Applied Anatomy. 7th ed. Philadelphia: Lea & Febiger, 1989.

37. Sanderson, D.J., and P.R. Cavanagh: An investigation of the use of automated feedback to modify the application of forces to the pedals during cycling. Med. Sci. Sports Exer. 18(2 Suppl.): S63, 1986.

38. Shephard, R.J.: Economic Benefits of Enhanced Fitness. Champaign, Ill.: Human Kinetics, 1986.

39. Steinberg, G.G.: Epidemiology of low back pain. In Chronic Low Back Pain. Edited by M. Stanton-Hicks and R.A. Boas. New York: Raven Press, 1982.

40. Vander, A.J., J.H. Sherman, and D.S. Luciano: Human Physiology: The Mechanics of Body Function. 3rd ed. New York: McGraw-Hill, 1980.

41. Vorro, J.R.: Stroboscopic study of motion changes that accompany modifications and improvements in a throwing performance. Res. Quart. 44:216–225, 1973.

42. Williams, K.R., R. Snow, C. Agruss, J. Litschert, and W. Austin: Differences in running biomechanics and running economy associated with different types of running shoes. Proceed. Amer. Soc. Biomech. 1989, pp. 184–185.

BIBLIOGRAPHY

1. Cailliet, R.: Low Back Pain Syndrome. 3rd ed. Philadelphia: F.A. Davis, 1981.

2. Crouch, J.E.: Functional Human Anatomy. 4th ed. Philadelphia: Lea & Febiger, 1985.

3. Dyson, G.H.G.: The Mechanics of Athletics. 3rd ed. London: University of London Press, 1964.
4. Hay, J.G.: The Biomechanics of Sports Techniques. 2nd ed. Englewood Cliffs, N.J.: Prentice-Hall, 1978.
5. Jensen, C.R., G.W. Schultz, and B.L. Bangerter: Applied Kinesiology and Biomechanics. 3rd ed. New York: McGraw-Hill, 1983.
6. Luttgens, K., and K.F. Wells: Kinesiology: Scientific Basis of Human Motion. 7th ed. Philadelphia: W.B. Saunders, 1982.
7. Marion, J.B.: General Physics with Bioscience Essays. New York: John Wiley, 1979.
8. Rasch, P.J.: Kinesiology and Applied Anatomy. 7th ed. Philadelphia: Lea & Febiger, 1989.
9. Wirhed, R.: Athletic Ability and the Anatomy of Motion. London: Wolfe Medical Publications, 1984.

3

EXERCISE PHYSIOLOGY

INTRODUCTION

Physiology is the branch of biologic science which deals with the functions and vital processes that characterize living organisms, especially the controlled physiochemical processes inherent in maintaining a near constant internal environment in the face of changes in the external environment.[59] In humans, as with other higher level animals, physiochemical processes are tightly controlled in order to maintain a near constant internal environment. This state of homeostasis, as identified by Cannon,[19] is achieved through a complex integration of physiologic systems. In effect, homeostasis necessitates that the body's vital physiologic processes be effectively responsive to external environmental challenges, including changes in the internal milieu induced by disease, exercise, and nutritional status.

Exercise physiology is a subfield of physiology concerned with the study of functional responses to a single bout of exercise (acute) and to repeated exercise sessions (chronic, or training effects). Though we usually think of exercise physiology as applied, its roots stem from the preeminent investigations of pioneer 20th century physiologists such as August Krogh, A.V. Hill, and D.B. Dill, who effectively demonstrated the basic physiologic responses of primary organ systems to the perturbations of exercise and accompanying environmental stressors.

The development of exercise physiology over the past 50 years has paralleled increased economic and other societal concerns related to athletic and occupational performance, as well as the now evident relationship of one's lifetime activity habitus to general health and fitness. Much of this development occurred within college and university physical education departments, though significant contributions have also been made in laboratories located in other university departments, in medical schools, and in military and private sector settings. Their principal research focus ranges from cellular to whole body systems responses and adaptations.

From previous discussion, it should be recalled that the initiation of effective movement is not possible without skeletal system support and muscular contraction via appropriate neural input. Further, since intense exercise may increase muscle cell metabolism by as much as 50-fold above that at rest, the circulatory and respiratory systems, mediated by endocrine and neural input, must assume an essential supportive role in sustaining exercise. In the initial portion of the remainder of the chapter, exercise metabolism and the requisite cardiorespiratory system support are examined.

EXERCISE METABOLISM

ENERGY SUPPLY PROCESSES FOR MUSCULAR WORK

Some fundamental aspects of the physiology of muscular contraction were presented in the previous chapter. Here, our focus is on how energy needs are met by the transformation of potential energy in chemical bonds to mechanical energy for work. Muscular contraction can only proceed via the breakdown of adenosine triphosphate (ATP), which is an energy rich molecule in short supply in the human body. ATP is the body's basic energy currency and thus, must be replenished for muscular contraction to continue. Fortunately, this can occur via anaerobic metabolism (without the presence of oxygen) as well as through aerobic metabolism (in the presence of oxygen).

As indicated in Figure 3–1, for ATP to be resynthesized, it is dependent on enzymatically induced breakdown of another cellular high energy compound, phosphocreatine (PC). PC is also in short supply and its resynthesis is dependent on a third chemical reaction, the breakdown of muscle glycogen or glucose via glycolysis, which involves at least 10 steps catalyzed by specific enzymes. However, when oxygen is not present, the end result is only two ATP molecules reconstituted per molecule of glucose, while the resultant pyruvic acid and hydrogen atoms combine to form lactic acid which, when production substantially exceeds removal, can inhibit performance. Also shown in Figure 3–1, it is only in the presence of oxygen (i.e., aerobic phase) that lactic acid can be reconverted to pyruvic acid and used as an energy source, or to resynthesize glycogen. Thus, while anaerobic metabolism is vital to the achievement of short-term maximum performance and, indeed, is necessary to initiate even moderate work, it is only in the presence of adequate oxygen supply (aerobic metabolism) that physical exertion can continue for appreciable periods of time.

A particularly important point depicted in Figure 3–1 is that the first three steps are common to both anaerobic and aerobic metabolism. That is, sustained (aerobic) performance proceeds in chemical transformation essentially as does anaerobic until the step at which pyruvic acid is formed. In the presence of sufficient oxygen, pyruvic acid diffuses into the muscles' mitochondria, and is irreversibly converted to acetyl CoA (a form of acetic acid), which subsequently enters the Krebs cycle as citric acid. Numerous hydrogen atoms are generated and then oxidized via electron transport-oxidative phosphorylation, with the whole process yielding 38 ATP molecules per molecule of glucose. The oxidation of the complex carbon glucose molecule also yields carbon dioxide and water. If the oxygen supply or level of enzymes in the citric acid cycle or respiratory chain becomes insufficient, substantial reduction in ATP production results.

Figure 3–2 shows that degradated forms of fat and protein, as well as carbohydrate, eventually enter the Krebs cycle. In the case of fat, most of which is stored in fat cells, it is initially hydrolyzed into glycerol and free fatty acids (FFA). The FFA enter the circulation and are carried to the muscle

I.   Anaerobic Phase (no oxygen required)

    1. ATP————————► ADP + P + energy for muscle contraction
    2. PC —————————► P + C + energy for resynthesis of ATP
    3. Glycogen ————► Glucose ————►Pyruvic acid + H$^+$ ——►Lactic
        acid + energy for resynthesis of PC.

II.   4. 1/5 of the lactic acid———►Pyruvic acid————► (Krebs cycle) +
        oxygen (O_2) —————►Water (H_2O) + carbon dioxide (CO_2)
        + energy for resynthesis of remaining lactic acid back to glycogen.

FIG. 3–1. Elementary chemical schematic of processes related to muscle contraction. (Modified from Karpovich, P.V.: Physiology of Muscular Activity. 5th ed. Philadelphia: Saunders, 1959, p. 21, and de Vries, H.A.: Physiology of Exercise for Physical Education and Athletics. 4th ed. Dubuque, Iowa: Wm. C. Brown, 1986, p. 33.)

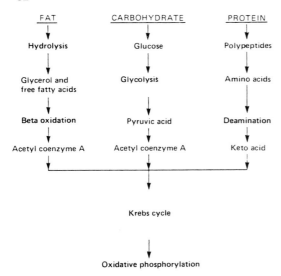

FIG. 3–2. Derivation of energy from the metabolism of the three basic foodstuffs by way of the final common path: the Krebs cycle and oxidative phosphorylation. (From de Vries, H.A.: Physiology of Exercise for Physical Education and Athletics. 4th ed. Dubuque, Iowa: William C. Brown, 1986, p. 37.)

mitochondria where, via beta oxidation, they are transformed to acetyl CoA. The resultant citric acid continues into the Krebs cycle in the presence of oxygen to formulate ATP molecules in the same manner as that described previously for glucose. Although a single fatty acid molecule yields 130 molecules of ATP, it provides only 5½ ATP molecules per molecule of oxygen consumed, while the complete breakdown of glucose yields approximately 6½ ATP molecules. Thus, to reconstitute ATP, fat requires that about 15% more oxygen be delivered via the blood during its combustion than when glucose is metabolized. It is important to realize the FFA metabolism cannot proceed without a continuing, adequate presence of oxygen to accept hydrogen atoms for beta oxidation to occur.

Also indicated in Figure 3–2, protein in the form of deaminated amino acids, can be catabolized to furnish energy substrate directly via the Krebs cycle, or via the muscle alanine-glucose cycle involving gluconeogenesis in the liver. In well nourished individuals, as much as 10 to 15% of total

energy has been attributed to protein metabolism during prolonged exercise.[34]

OXYGEN REQUIREMENT FOR MUSCULAR WORK

Some basic life processes, such as brain and heart function, are dependent upon a continuously adequate oxygen supply (i.e., oxygen supply equals oxygen demand). In the immediately preceding discussion, it was emphasized that skeletal muscle contraction can proceed anaerobically for a limited time, but that a near completely adequate oxygen supply is necessary to sustain muscular work beyond several minutes. Further, it was implied earlier that metabolism of high energy phosphates and glycogen via glycolysis would ultimately necessitate oxygen to restore normal cellular metabolite levels.

At rest, the oxygen available to the tissues is sufficient to insure continuous aerobic metabolism. Thus, the oxygen consumption (uptake) is equivalent to that required for resting metabolism. During exercise, however, there are two distinct demands that exceed the capacity of the cardiorespiratory system to provide a continuously adequate oxygen supply to the skeletal muscle. The first, identified as oxygen deficit in the upper panel of Figure 3–3, reflects the transition period between the initiation of exercise at a constant, submaximal workload in which cardiorespiratory adjustments lag behind before the oxygen uptake reaches a steady rate after several minutes.

Upon cessation of submaximal exercise, oxygen uptake falls to near resting levels within 10 minutes. The oxygen consumed in excess of resting values during recovery is termed oxygen debt. In moderate exercise, oxygen debt reflects primarily the extra energy needed to replenish the stores of ATP and CP. Thus, the total oxygen requirement of a given submaximal bout of exercise is equal to the oxygen consumption during exercise plus the oxygen debt.

As shown in the lower panel of Figure 3–3, the energy demand of severe, near exhausting exercise can exceed one's max-

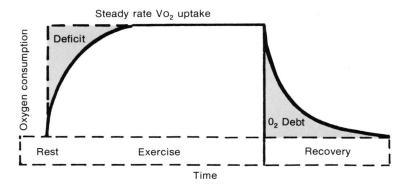

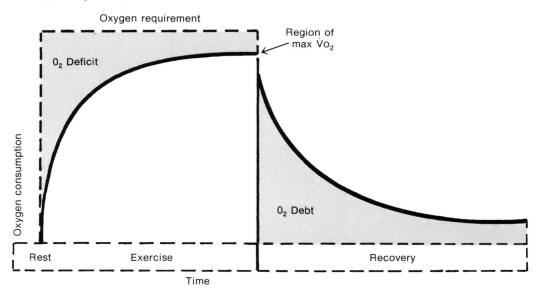

FIG. 3–3. Oxygen consumption during and in recovery from light to moderate steady-rate exercise (A), and heavy exercise that exceeds $\dot{V}_{O_{2max}}$ and results in an increased oxygen debt (B). (From McArdle, W.D. et al.: Exercise Physiology: Energy, Nutrition, and Human Performance. 2nd ed. Philadelphia: Lea & Febiger, 1986, p. 112.)

imal oxygen uptake (aerobic) capacity. This extra energy demand necessitates substantial, sustained anaerobic metabolism, and a more prolonged recovery. In such conditions, the rate of lactic acid production rises well above the removal rate, and blood lactate levels rise. The larger oxygen debt only partially reflects the need for oxygen to reconvert lactic acid to glycogen, as strenuous exercise also leads to postexercise energy demands of the circulatory, respiratory, hormonal, and thermoregulatory systems, which can take as long as 24 hours to return to normal resting levels.[15]

ENERGY REQUIREMENT OF
PHYSICAL ACTIVITY

In humans, as with other animals, the major byproduct of energy metabolism is heat, which is usually expressed in kilocalories (a kilocalorie is the amount of heat required to raise 1 kilogram of water 1°C). The energetics of muscle contraction was discussed earlier with reference to stored chemical energy transformation to accomplish work in both anaerobic and aerobic conditions, but without consideration of metabolic heat production.

One's metabolic heat production can be measured directly by determining the temperature change of a known volume of circulating water within a heavily insulated copper container. However, such facilities are expensive and confining. The principle of indirect calorimetry, in which oxygen consumption is measured to estimate metabolic heat production, was validated during rest and exercise by Atwater, Benedict and Cathcart in the early 1900s via simultaneous measurement of both oxygen consumption and metabolic heat production in a respiration calorimeter.[7] The oxygen caloric equivalent was found to be approximately 1 liter of oxygen consumed per 5 kilocalories (kcal) of metabolic heat production, but to vary according to the proportion of carbohydrate and fat being metabolized. It was also determined that the latter could be rather accurately estimated by measurement of carbon dioxide production (lower per unit of oxygen in fat metabolism, but the same when carbohy-

drate only was being metabolized). This ratio of metabolic gas exchange, i.e., the volume of carbon dioxide production to oxygen consumption, is termed the respiratory quotient (RQ), and can be accurately assessed during rest and in aerobic exercise by indirect calorimetry. However, during and immediately following strenuous exercise, blood buffering of anaerobically induced lactic acid creates extra carbon dioxide production and a higher respiratory exchange ratio.[74]

Estimates of energy requirements for most human physical activity entailed in daily living, household and occupational tasks, exercise, and athletics have been determined via indirect calorimetry (i.e., measurement of oxygen consumption and carbon dioxide production). This is of practical importance, as there is a near 15-fold difference between the minimum and maximum energy expenditure values given in Table 3–1 which, depending on the duration of activity, can have profound effects on balancing daily caloric expenditure with that from food intake. Somewhat surprising are the relatively low energy expenditure values for sports activity. This is because the values given do not represent just the momentary intensive spurts of activity inherent in these activities, but the average energy expended during a simulated contest which includes periods of standing and walking. For example, the value given for tennis was determined with an accompanying videotape analysis that revealed the following time spent in 30 minutes of match play: (1) standing, 31%; (2) walking, 35%; (3) swinging at the ball, 20%; and (4) running, 14%.

Values given for walking, running, bicycling, and swimming increase with speed in a near rectilinear manner. Since they entail continuous, rhythmic activity of much of the large skeletal muscle mass, most individuals can maintain a substantially higher energy expenditure for prolonged periods than the average expenditure entailed in "stop and start" recreational sports. It should be noted that the values given in Table 3–1 are for a young adult 70 kg "reference" man. Since most physical activities entail weight bearing, energy expenditure values given in

Table 3–1.   Energy Cost of Selected Activities for a 70 kg Person*

Activity	Caloric Cost (kcal/min)
Lying at ease	1.3
Sitting, reading	1.6
Standing at ease	2.0
Bowling	3.5
Walking (zero grade), 3 mph	4.5
Golf	4.8
Bicycle riding (touring position), 10 mph	5.0
Walking, 4 mph	6.1
Bicycle riding, 12½ mph	6.3
Swimming crawl stroke, 1.34 mph	7.0
Tennis	7.1
Skiing downhill, hard snow	7.6
Badminton	7.8
Handball	8.4
Bicycle riding, 15 mph	9.6
Swimming crawl stroke, 1.79 mph	9.8
Squash	10.7
Jogging, 6 mph	11.6
Swimming crawl stroke, 2.24 mph	12.5
Running, 7½ mph	14.3
Bicycle riding, 17½ mph	14.4
Skiing, cross country, hard snow, moderate speed	14.5
Running, 8½ mph	16.3
Swimming crawl stroke, 2.68 mph	16.5
Running, 10 mph	18.9

*Above values are adjusted to a 70 kg (154 lbs) man from data presented in: (1) Banister, E.W. and S.R. Brown: The relative energy requirements of physical activity. In Exercise Physiology. Edited by H.B. Falls. New York: Academic Press, 1968, pp. 267–322; (2) Consolazio, C.R., R.E. Johnson, and L.J. Pecora: Physiological Measurements of Metabolic Functions in Man. New York: McGraw-Hill, 1963, pp. 328–332; (3) Holmer, I.: Oxygen uptake during swimming in men. J. Appl Physiol. 33:502–509, 1972; (4) Passmore, R. and J.V.G.A. Durnin: Human energy expenditure. Physiol. Rev. 35:801–840, 1955; and (5) from data collected at the Human Performance Laboratory, University of California, Davis.

Table 3–1 would be proportionally less, or greater, depending on one's body weight.

Numerous other factors can affect one's energy expenditure in physical activity, including air resistance, extremes of environmental temperature, and the performer's skill level. The latter is of little consequence in walking, but trained runners may use 10% less energy than their nontrained counterparts at slower running speeds,[56] while an elite swimmer may require only ⅔ to ¾ of the energy used at the same recreational swimming speeds by poorly skilled swimmers.[54] Another factor affecting one's energy expenditure in dual sports competition is the skill level of one's competition. It appears that one participates more strenuously if their competition is of near equal skill, rather than distinctly better or poorer.[6]

Indirect calorimetry laboratory equipment needed to measure oxygen consumption is expensive and the expired air collection devices can be inhibiting to normal performance in some physical activities. Fortunately, with the advent of biotelemetry, measurement of heart rate with a "package" weighing no more than a few ounces is possible during virtually all physical activity. However, to estimate energy expenditure from heart rate, it is necessary to "calibrate" each individual's heart rate-oxygen consumption relationship over a wide range in an activity similar to that for which actual oxygen consumption measurement would be inhibiting. Further, numerous factors such as environmental heat stress and emotional state can substantially elevate the heart rate at a given oxygen consumption (energy expenditure).

CARDIORESPIRATORY SUPPORT OF EXERCISE METABOLISM

THE RESPIRATORY SYSTEM

As discussed earlier, the body requires an increased oxygen supply during exercise. The respiratory system functions to bring oxygen into the blood for use at the tissues, and is also responsible for disposal of carbon dioxide into the environment and aiding in the control of blood acidity.

Figure 3–4 depicts the basic anatomy of the respiratory system. Air passes through the nose and mouth, and then through the *conducting airways*, which include the larynx, trachea, and bronchi. The latter consist of left and right divisions which branch successively into smaller airways called bronchioles. Air then passes into the respiratory zone to respiratory bronchioles,

which lead into the smallest division, the alveolus.

The functional unit of respiration in the lung is the *alveolus* (pl., alveoli), a small pouch which facilitates diffusion of gases (oxygen and carbon dioxide) to and from the blood in the pulmonary capillaries with which the alveoli are closely associated. Oxygen diffuses from the alveolus into the blood to be carried to the body tissues. Carbon dioxide diffuses from the blood into the alveolus, then up through the conducting airways, through the mouth and nose, to the environment (Fig. 3–4).

The respiratory musculature consists of the diaphragm and intercostal muscles. Contraction of these muscles leads to an increase in the size of the chest cavity and creates a pressure gradient such that air is drawn into the lungs. Passive elastic recoil of these muscles results in expiration, especially during exercise, but they can also be used in forced expiration.

In order to understand the role of the respiratory system in exercise, some basic functional terms associated with the system must be clarified:

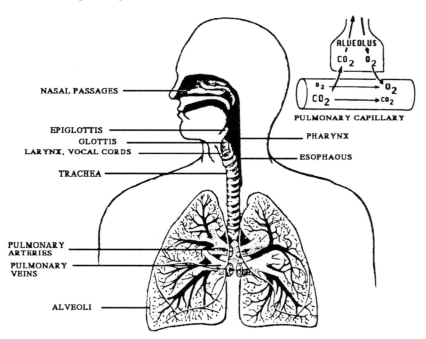

FIG. 3–4. Diagram of the external respiratory system, showing the respiratory passages and function of the alveolus to oxygenate the blood and to remove carbon dioxide. (From Guyton, A.C.: Physiology of the Human Body. 5th Ed. Philadelphia: Saunders, 1979, p. 8.)

1. *Ventilation:* movement of air into and out of the pulmonary system via mouth and nose (i.e., breathing).
2. *Respiration:* actual exchange of gases across cell membranes. Respiration occurs both at the lungs (externally) and in the body tissues (internally).
   a. *External Respiration:* exchange of oxygen and carbon dioxide between the alveoli and lung capillaries; oxygen enters the blood, while carbon dioxide enters the alveolus.
   b. *Internal Respiration:* gas exchange between body tissue capillaries and the cells of these tissues; oxygen enters the cells, while carbon dioxide enters the blood for transport to the lungs.
3. *Diffusion (pressure) Gradient:* If the pressure of a given gas is greater in one area than another, it will move from the area of high pressure to the area of low pressure.
4. *Pulmonary Minute Volume:* amount of air breathed per minute ($\dot{V}_E$), which is calculated as the product of frequency of breaths (f_B = breaths/minute) times the tidal volume (V_T = liters of air moved into the lungs per breath).
5. *Ventilation-perfusion Ratio:* the pairing of respiratory system and circulation, such that an increase in ventilation is matched by an increase in blood flow in the lung capillary system for effective oxygen pickup.

THE CARDIOVASCULAR SYSTEM

During sustained exercise, continually adequate oxygen supply and carbon dioxide removal are vital. The respiratory system provides the contact with the environment, while the cardiovascular system functions to transport the gases from one place to another in the body (i.e., from lungs to tissues, or cell to cell). The cardiovascular system also transports nutrients and hormones to cells and carries metabolic wastes to the appropriate organs for excretion.

The three main structural divisions of the cardiovascular system are the *heart, blood, and vessels of transportation.* The heart consists of four chambers including two atria and two ventricles. The atria are thin-walled and serve as reservoirs for blood before it enters the ventricles. The ventri-cles, on the other hand, have thick muscular walls which contract forcefully to pump blood to the lungs and body tissues. The course of blood flow in the heart is directed by one-way valves. The blood supply to the heart itself is delivered through the coronary arteries; the heart muscle cells receive no nourishment from blood within the chambers.

Blood serves as a fluid medium for nutrient and gas transport. Structurally, blood is divided into plasma (fluid) and formed elements. Plasma consists of water and solutes, including inorganic ions and protein molecules. The *hematocrit* is the percentage of the total blood volume which is made up of formed elements: red and white blood cells, and platelets. Red blood cells are important here because they contain a protein called *hemoglobin* which enables them to transport oxygen and carbon dioxide. The average size adult male has a blood volume of 5½ liters.[103]

The vessels, along with the heart, maintain a complex pressure gradient system for the regulation of blood flow. The high pressure side of the vascular system begins with the *aorta,* a large diameter vessel with thick elastic walls which exits from the left ventricle in the heart. The aorta branches successively into smaller and smaller *arteries,* which also have thick elastic walls, but decrease in internal diameter as they branch. The small arteries then branch into *arterioles,* which still have elastic walls but are extremely small in diameter, i.e., approximately 0.2 mm, or just greater than the size of a strand of hair. This tiny diameter coupled with thick, strong walls creates high resistance to the flow of blood, but the diameter can be altered by the contraction or relaxation of the smooth muscles in the walls. In this manner, the amount of blood flow to a given tissue can be regulated. The arterioles eventually branch into *capillaries* which are associated with the tissue cells, such that gas exchange takes place at this level.

At the other end of the capillaries, the *venous* system begins, with smaller vessels leading into progressively larger vessels and finally back to the right atrium of the heart. First, the capillaries empty into *venules,* which are larger, relatively inelastic, and have more fibrous walls than the capillaries. These lead into thin-walled *veins,* which have some smooth muscle in their walls. Veins are referred to as compliant vessels, meaning that a large change in the volume of blood inside the vessels will produce only a small change in pressure. The venous system is thus the low pressure side of the cardiovascular system. Venous flow is primarily determined by contraction of the skeletal muscles surrounding the veins which acts as an external pump. However, it is also affected by posture, gravity, and environmental temperature.

Figure 3–5 illustrates the course of blood flow through the cardiovascular system. The *systemic* circulation begins at the left atrium and ends as the blood is emptied into the right atrium. The *pulmonary* circulation begins at the right atrium and ends with the blood emptying into the left atrium. When the blood leaves the pulmonary capillaries and returns to the left atrium via the pulmonary veins, it is *oxygenated,* meaning sufficient oxygen is present for tissue metabolism. Once the blood passes through the tissue capillaries, it becomes "*deoxygenated,*" since much of the oxygen has been extracted for respiration in the tissue cells. In cellular respiration, carbon dioxide is given off as a waste product which diffuses into the capillaries and is carried in deoxygenated blood, through the right side of the heart, to the lungs to be blown off.

As with the respiratory system, there are some essential terms to understand before discussion of cardiovascular function in exercise. Some average resting values for a 70 kg young adult male are included in parentheses for later comparison to exercise values.

1. *Heart Rate:* number of heart beats per minute (70 beats/min.).
2. *Stroke Volume:* volume of blood pumped by one heart beat (70 ml).
3. *Cardiac Output:* rate of blood flow from the heart, calculated as the product of heart rate times stroke volume (70 bpm × 70 ml ≃ 5 liters/minute).
4. *Cardiac Cycle:*
   a. Systole: period during which blood is pumped from the ventricles.
   b. Diastole: period when the ventricles

are being filled with blood from the atria.
5. *Systolic* blood pressure is the maximal value, and *diastolic* blood pressure is the minimal value obtained during systole and diastole, respectively.
6. *Vasoconstriction:* decrease in diameter of blood vessels resulting from contraction of smooth muscle in the walls.
7. *Vasodilation:* increase in diameter of blood vessels due to relaxation of the muscles in the walls.
8. a-v_{O_2} *Difference:* (arteriovenous oxygen difference) The difference between oxygen content of the blood on the arterial and venous sides of the capillaries. (A measure of the amount of oxygen extracted by the tissues for respiration.)
9. *Oxygen Consumption:* the amount of oxygen utilized by the tissues ($\dot{V}_{O_2}$), which is the product of cardiac output and a-v_{O_2} difference.

GAS TRANSPORT. The transport of oxygen and carbon dioxide is of primary importance in exercise, thus necessitating examination of the mechanisms involved. Oxygen is carried in two forms in the blood. Some is *dissolved* in order to establish a pressure gradient from blood to the tissues, such that oxygen diffuses into the tissues. The majority of oxygen (approximately 65 times that dissolved), however, is carried *bound to hemoglobin.* A small amount of carbon dioxide is also carried dissolved in the blood, and about 25% is transported bound to hemoglobin. Approximately 60 to 80%, however, is carried in the form of the bicarbonate ion, HCO_3^-, which is soluble in blood. HCO_3^- is formed when carbon dioxide and water are combined, while the reaction is reversed at the lungs to liberate carbon dioxide to the environment.[74]

THE CARDIORESPIRATORY RESPONSE TO ACUTE EXERCISE

Although the respiratory and cardiovascular systems were separated to discuss basic structure and function, the two systems are actually physiologically integrated. Exercise presents the challenge of an increased requirement for oxygen, as well as an increased need for carbon di-

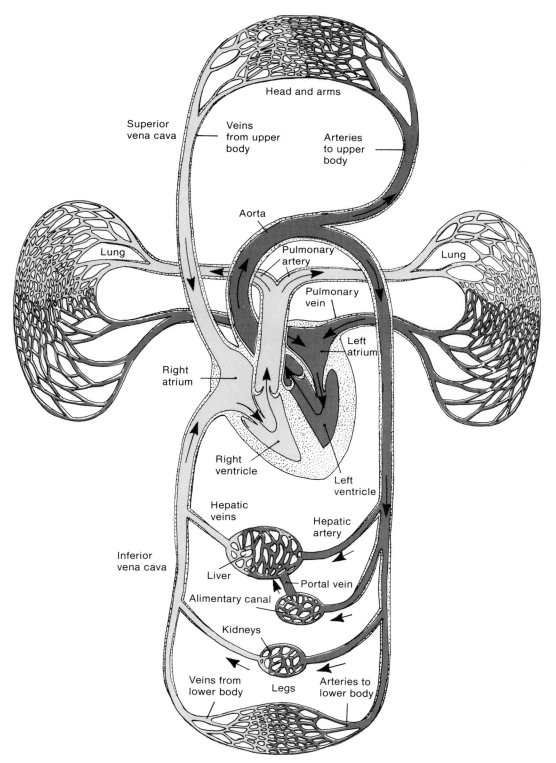

FIG. 3–5. Schematic view showing the flow of blood (direction indicated by arrows) to and from the heart via the pulmonary and systemic vascular circuits. The dark shading indicates oxygenated blood, while the paler shading indicates deoxygenated blood. (From McArdle, W.D. et al.: Exercise Physiology: Energy, Nutrition and Human Performance. 2nd ed. Philadelphia: Lea & Febiger, 1986, p. 244.)

oxide disposal to maintain a relatively normal blood acidity. Thus, oxygen intake at the lungs, delivery to working tissues, and uptake by the tissues must increase. Carbon dioxide diffusion from working tissues to the blood, delivery to the lungs, and removal at the lungs must also increase. These needs are met by the enhanced response of the respiratory and cardiovascular systems, the degree of which is dependent on the intensity and duration of exercise, as well as one's training level (which will be examined at length later in this chapter). Figure 3–6 illustrates important parameters of both systems which increase from rest to meet the challenge of maximal exercise.

The respiratory system responds by increases in both external and internal respiration. $\dot{V}_E$ is elevated by increases in both the depth (V_T) and frequency of breathing (f_B). Increased ventilation leads to increased pressure gradients for both gases, thus facilitating external respiration. Internal respiration is enhanced as the metabolic activity of the tissue cells increases, resulting in increased pressure gradients. Thus a-v_{O_2} difference increases as more oxygen is dropped off (Fig. 3–6), and more carbon dioxide is picked up for transport to the lungs.

The primary alterations made by the cardiovascular system include an increase in blood flow and a redistribution of the blood flow from tissues not involved in the effort to tissues such as the skeletal muscle and heart, which are primarily involved in exercise (Fig. 3–7). Note that blood flow to the brain remains constant, and that muscle blood flow represents the major portion of cardiac output during exercise. The total blood flow, or cardiac output, increases via a neurally mediated rise in heart rate and an increased stroke volume, which is caused by a variety of factors including increased venous return and increased contractility of the heart muscle. This, combined with the vasoconstriction in minimally active tissues, causes an elevation in systolic blood pressure which, along with vasodilation in the working tissues, results in increased oxygen delivery to the tissues. Perfusion of the lung capillaries is also enhanced to match the increase in ventilation and maintain an effective ventilation-perfusion ratio.

CONTROL OF THE CARDIORESPIRATORY EXERCISE RESPONSE. Several of the parameters discussed are controlled by the nervous system both in rest and exercise. Ventilation, for example, increases in several phases. Initially, there is an anticipatory rise stimulated by the cerebral cortex. Then a rapid rise occurs as muscle and joint proprioceptors signal the brain that movement (work) is occurring. Finally, control is sustained using sensory information provided by chemoreceptors in the pulmonary arteries, which are sensitive to metabolic changes in the blood (e.g., carbon dioxide and oxygen).[103]

Heart rate is regulated by sympathetic and parasympathetic nerves acting on the sino-atrial node in the heart (a specialized area where contraction is initiated). As with $\dot{V}_E$, heart rate first rises in response to anticipation. Then a rapid rise upon initiation of exercise occurs in response to proprioceptor stimulation. A further gradual rise occurs, again in response to the chemical characteristics of the blood. The rise in heart rate is somewhat slower than the rise in stroke volume, but continues after stroke volume has reached a maximal level. After several minutes of submaximal exercise, heart rate, stroke volume, and $\dot{V}_E$ all reach a near steady rate or plateau.

Redistribution of blood flow occurs via vasodilation in the working tissues and vasoconstriction in uninvolved tissues. These changes in vessel diameter are regulated by a vasomotor center in the midbrain. The center sends out impulses to maintain tone, while inhibition of these impulses results in vasodilation.[13]

PHYSIOLOGIC LIMITATIONS TO PHYSICAL PERFORMANCE

Achieving excellence in any athletic endeavor necessitates an effectively integrated composite of anatomic, biomechanical, physiologic, and psychologic factors. However, the actual amount of limitation imposed by any one factor varies with the performance and the individual, and is not

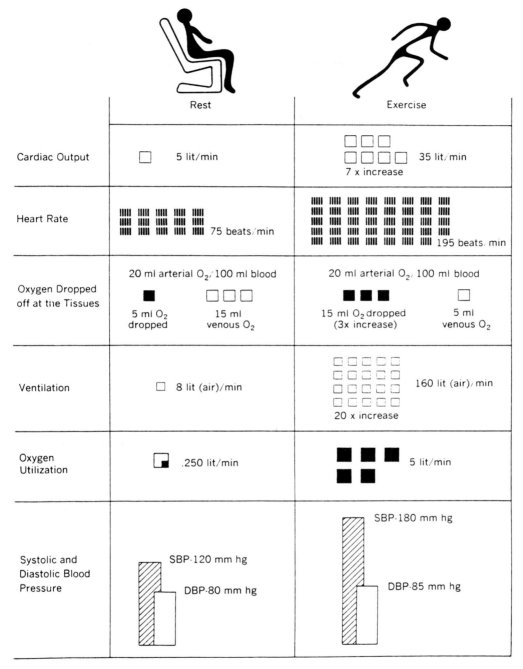

FIG. 3–6. The effects of maximal intensity exercise on various cardiorespiratory parameters. The increases represented for cardiac output, ventilation, and oxygen utilization would not be so great in the untrained person. (From Updyke, W.F., and P.B. Johnson: Principles of Modern Physical Education, Health, and Recreation. New York: Holt, Rinehart and Winston, 1970, p. 179.)

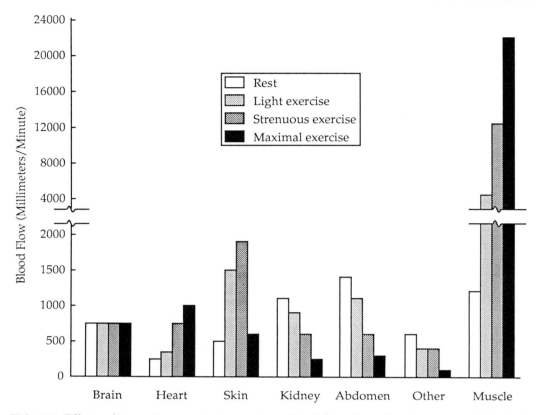

FIG. 3–7. Effects of increasing exercise intensity on blood flow through various parts of the body. Note that the scale for muscle blood flow has been expanded to show the very large increase during exercise. (Modified from Chapman, C.B., and J.H. Mitchell: The physiology of exercise. Sci. Amer. *212(5)*:88–96, 1965.)

possible, at present, to quantify. Hence, for simplification, this discussion is limited primarily to physiologic factors. Typically, athletic performances entail various combinations of muscular strength, power, endurance, and neuromuscular coordination. Again, differentiation between the relative effects of physiological factors on performance is not straightforward, though it is currently a primary research thrust in exercise and sport science.

Maximum muscular *strength* is defined as peak tension, or the amount of force that a muscle (or muscle group) can develop in a single maximal effort. Factors influencing muscle force production, including muscle length and angle of pull, were discussed in the previous chapter. However, muscular strength is primarily a function of

muscle cross-sectional area, being little different on this basis in males and females.[57] There is evidence, however, that strength training can increase maximum force production out of proportion to muscle hypertrophy, presumably through reduced inhibition and the resultant greater activation of motor units.[66] As shown in Figure 3–8, maximum muscular force is also a function of the rate of contraction, being greatest in rapid eccentric (lengthening) contraction, intermediate in isometric contraction, and lowest in fast concentric contraction. Since fast-twitch (type II) fibers produce greater force than do slow twitch (type I) fibers,[66] one might expect greater strength per unit area in the former. However, the relation between percentage cross-sectional area of fast-twitch fibers

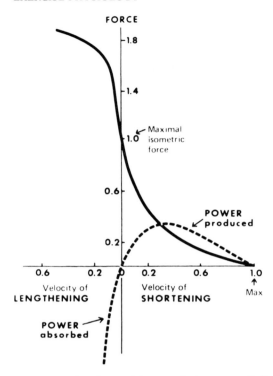

FIG. 3–8. The classical force-velocity curve (full line) obtained on an isolated muscle, showing that maximal force in a concentric activity is less than in an isometric contraction. Highest force can be attained in a rapid eccentric contraction. The dotted line gives the maximal power, i.e., the force times the velocity of contraction. (From Astrand, P.-O., and K. Rodahl: Textbook of Work Physiology. 3rd ed. New York: McGraw-Hill, 1986, p. 44.)

and strength is rather low,[68] meaning that other structural and functional factors are important in the expression of strength.

The advantage of greater strength in athletic performance, such as weight lifting is obvious, but strength also affects performances demanding primarily muscular power and endurance.[31] Power, which is the product of force times distance (i.e., work) per unit time is seen in Figure 3–8, to be maximum at about 30% of maximal isometric force. However, as shown in Figure 3–9, increased strength has the potential for not only increasing the maximum unloaded speed of movement, but more importantly, for effecting an increased speed for any given load. This explains the value of strength training in such field events as the discus and hammer throws, and the shot put. Improvements in the high and long jumps, and in sprinting, in which the whole body weight must be moved, are not as great.[21]

Muscular endurance is a factor of considerable importance in certain aspects of gymnastics (holding the iron cross position on the still rings) and wrestling. It is representative of maximum sustained effort of a relatively small portion of the body musculature and/or loads which occlude circulation during a large portion of each repetition (e.g., chin-ups, parallel bar dips, or push-ups). Maximum performance is not accompanied by breathlessness or respiratory discomfort, as is the case in intense running or swimming.

Single isometric muscular contraction to fatigue (muscular endurance) is well related to maximum voluntary contraction force (muscular strength). A person with great muscular strength will be able to use less motor units to sustain a given submaximal force than will a weaker person. Thus, more motor units can be resting at any one time, and it will take longer to fatigue all of the motor units. That circulation is also important in muscular endurance is evident in Figure 3–10, in which it is shown that isometric contraction holding time for the forearm flexor muscles is the same for both an occluded condition (with an inflated blood pressure cuff) and a non-occluded condition until approximately 50 seconds. At this point, which corresponds to approximately 60% of maximum contraction force, above which circulation is occluded in forearm muscle, the nonoccluded condition endurance time falls less rapidly. This is because sustained contraction of forearm muscle below 60% (without cuff occlusion) permits muscle blood flow with reestablished oxygen supply and removal of muscular contraction metabolic byproducts.

It should be recalled from previous discussion that muscular contraction necessitates continuous availability of ATP, either via anaerobic and/or aerobic metabolism. This is useful, in that aside from initial explosive contractions within 1 second limited primarily by neuromuscular

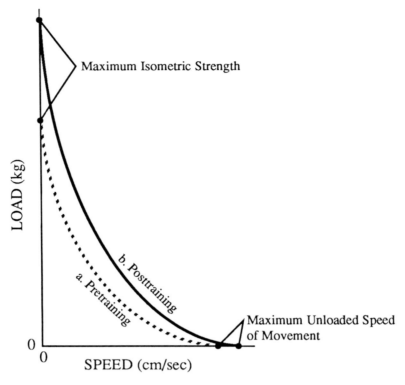

FIG. 3–9. Approximate effects of strength training on muscle force-velocity curves. (Modified from Lamb, D.R.: Physiology of Exercise: Responses and Adaptations. New York: Macmillan, 1984, p. 289.)

contractile elements, maximum performances in all athletic events in which excellence of performance is dependent on time can be characterized according to primary sources of energy supply. Table 3–2 summarizes this concept.

As suggested by the two transitional categories, one should consider primary energy sources as extending along a continuum with some overlap. That is, there is some oxidative metabolism in a 100 m sprint, though the primary energy source consists of ATP and CP. This notion, as well as the sequence of activation of energy sources in active muscle, is clearly evidenced in Figure 3–11. Both the immediate energy source (ATP and CP) and nonoxidative energy source (glycolysis) are anaerobic, while the oxidative energy supply system is aerobic. Figure 3–12 illustrates the relative percent contributions of aerobic and anaerobic energy for maximum physical performance of various durations.

This concept is of particular importance, in that all timed maximum performances, whether for bicycling, swimming, running, speed skating, or cross-country skiing, share a common dependence on this time-energy source relationship, though each has a unique muscular fitness component.

Identification of the time-energy source relationship gives a useful perspective of what limits maximum time-dependent performance, but does not address how this happens. That is, how do neuromuscular contractile elements, and the availability of various energy sources limit maximum time-dependent performance? Initial speed of movement performance is dependent on both the basic muscle velocity to load relationship and individual variation in the athlete's neuromuscular capability. Particularly important seem to be the maximum sliding velocity (contractile speed) of the myofibril filaments[22] and the

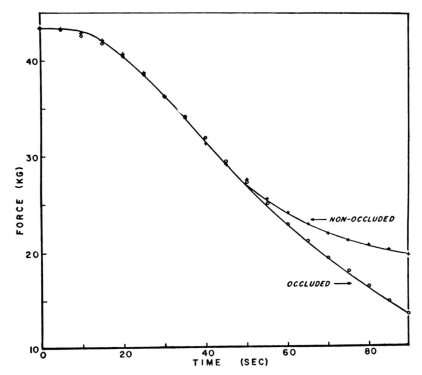

FIG. 3–10. Isometric fatigue curves for forearm muscles in subjects holding maximum voluntary contraction. (From Royce, J.: Isometric fatigue curves in human muscle with normal and occluded circulation. Res. Quart. *29*:204–12, 1958.)

high myosin ATP activity and nerve threshold for recruitment, as well as rapid nerve conduction velocity, all of which are characteristic of fast twitch, type II, muscle fibers.[66]

Energy source limitations for maximum time-dependent performances of 10 seconds or longer are more readily identified. Table 3–3 indicates the maximum energy supply for ATP, CP, glycogen and fat. Though the low content of ATP and CP in skeletal muscle, relative to the rate of their utilization, suggests that their depletion would account for fatigue and determination in maximal sprinting speed, it appears more likely from the data presented in Table 3–4 that it is due to the maximum glycolytic capacity of the muscle via accumulation of hydrogen ions caused by high lactate production. The high hydrogen ion accumulation may interfere with calcium ion effect on troponin, which regulates

Table 3–2. Primary Energy Sources at Selected Maximum Performance Time Intervals

Duration of Performance	Primary Energy Source
<1 sec	Neuromuscular contractile elements
1–10 sec	Immediate energy stores (ATP, CP)
10–30 sec	Transitional period
30 sec–2 min	Nonoxidative energy sources (glycogen and glucose)
2–10 min	Transitional period
10 min–2 + hrs	Oxidative energy sources (glycogen and fat)

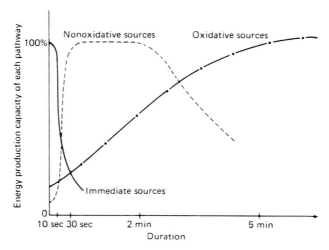

FIG. 3–11. Sequence of the activation of energy sources within an active muscle. (From Edington, D.W., and V.R. Edgerton: The Biology of Physical Activity. Boston: Houghton Mifflin, 1976, p. 8.)

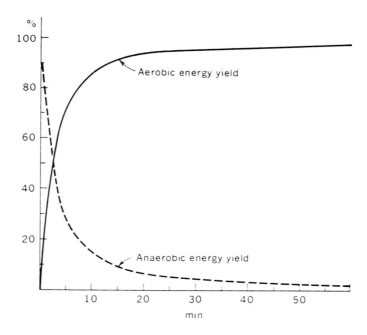

FIG. 3–12. Relative contribution in percent of total energy yield from aerobic and anaerobic processes, respectively, during maximal efforts of up to 60 min duration for an individual with high maximal power for both processes. Note that in a 2 to 3 min maximal effort both processes are equally important for success. (From Astrand, P.-O., and K. Rodahl: Textbook of Work Physiology. New York: McGraw-Hill, 1970, p. 304.)

Table 3–3.   Maximum Energy Supply Stores*

	Energy/Mole kcal	Concentration mmol/kg Wet Muscle	Total Energy in Humans (Body Weight 75 kg, Muscle Weight 20 kg) kcal
ATP	10	5	1
Phosphocreatine	10.5	17	3.6
Glycogen	700	80	1100
Fat	2400	—	75,000

*Modified from Astrand, P.-O. and K. Rodahl: Textbook of Work Physiology. Physiological Bases of Exercise. 3rd ed. New York: McGraw-Hill, 1986, p. 536.

cross-bridge cycling and thus would reduce tension generation and power output of the muscle.

In longer timed events, aerobic metabolism becomes increasingly important, constituting about 85% of the energy supply at 10 minutes, compared to only 20% in an event lasting 30 seconds. Shifting more to oxidative metabolism of glycogen is advantageous in two ways: (1) more ATP is produced per unit glycogen than during glycolysis, and (2) more blood flow to the working muscle provides increased amounts of oxygen, and also buffers and removes protons in the form of lactic acid. However, the rate of oxidative phosphorylized ATP production is slower.[13] Hence, speed must invariably fall off the longer the distance, though there is plenty of substrate fuel to permit resynthesis of ATP, for at least 60 minutes. The primary limiting factor in performances of from about 5 to 60 minutes is the capacity of one's heart, lungs and circulation to supply oxygen to the working muscle. In healthy young adults, it seems clear that maximal ventilatory capacity does not limit the body's ability to consume oxygen.[5] This means that the primary limiting factor must be due to oxygen supply (which is principally a function of maximal cardiac output) and/or the muscles' ability to extract oxygen (which is primarily a function of high muscle blood flow and highly active mitochondria). The rate of maximal oxygen uptake (which is abbreviated $\dot{V}O_{2max}$, where $\dot{V}O_2$ represents the volume of oxygen consumed) is highest in middle-distance runners and cross-country skiers.

In prolonged maximal performance, e.g., the marathon which is more than 99% aerobic, the primary limiting factor is provision of the optimum glycogen and fat fuel mix. The energy cost for running a marathon is approximately 2,600 kcal for a 70-kg man, which is slightly more than double that available in muscle (Table 3–3). While body fat stores are in plentiful supply, fat has two basic disadvantages as an exercise fuel supply: (1) the triglycerides are broken down into fatty acids and transported in combination with the protein, albumin, in the blood, at a rate equivalent only to about 50% that of glycogen for ATP phosphory-

Table 3–4.   Metabolic Analysis of Fatigue in Sprinting*

	Concentration of Fuels (μmole/g Fresh Muscle)	
	Muscle at Rest	Muscle Immediately After Exhaustive Sprinting
Glycogen	88	58
Phosphocreatine	17.0	3.7
ATP	4.6	3.4
Lactate	1.1	30.5
pH	7.1	6.3

*From Newsholme, E. and T. Leech: The Runner. Roosevelt, N.J.: Fitness Books, 1985, p. 83.

lation; and (2) fat requires about 15% more oxygen for oxidation than does glycogen.[78] It appears evident, then, that an optimum mix of glycogen and fat utilization is essential to maximize performance so that blood glucose levels are not compromised due to muscle glycogen depletion, which would also result in significant slowing of running pace due to increased reliance on rate limited fatty acid oxidative energy supply (i.e., "hitting the wall"). Lactic acid and amino acids (breakdown products of protein) can also be used in aerobic metabolism, but probably only account for 10 to 15% of substrate energy supply in healthy young adults engaged in heavy prolonged exercise.[13]

It was previously mentioned that fast-twitch (type II) muscle fibers produce greater force than do slow-twitch (type I) fibers. They also differ significantly in the means by which they facilitate resynthesis of ATP to power muscular contraction. Type I fibers are red, due to their high myoglobin content, have numerous and large mitochondria, and a high concentration of enzymes required to sustain aerobic metabolism for ATP resynthesis. Type II fibers, of which there are at least two subdivisions,[74] are white, and have a high capacity for anaerobic resynthesis of ATP via glycolysis.

Skeletal muscles contain both fiber types, but the ratio of type I to type II fibers differs, on average, in particular muscles according to their primary function. For example, the soleus consists of about 87% type I fibers, while the other major calf muscle, the gastrocnemius, has about 45%.[75] For a particular muscle, however, there is no gender difference in the ratio of fiber types,[45,64] although males have substantially larger type II fibers.

Large individual differences amongst both sexes exist in the ratio of type I to type II fibers for a given muscle, and there have been a number of studies showing that certain elite athletes have a high proportion of either type I or type II fibers in the leg muscles, for example, if they are runners. Table 3–5 gives the average percentage fiber composition for the vastus lateralis muscle of the quadriceps group for average young adult males, elite sprinters, middle

Table 3–5. Fiber Composition of Muscle in Man, Horses, and Dogs*

	Percentage Fiber Composition of Muscle	
	Type I	Type II
Men		
Elite marathon runner	79	21
Middle distance runner	62	38
Sprinters	24	76
Average individual	53	47
Horses		
Quarterhorse	7	93
Thoroughbred	12	88
Heavy hunter	31	69
Dogs		
Greyhound	3	97
Mongrel	31	69

*From Newsholme, E. and T. Leech: The Runner. Roosevelt, N.J.: Fitness Books, 1985, p. 71.

distance runners, and marathon runners. Also shown are comparisons of specially bred horses and dogs with their "average" counterparts.

It seems certain that elite sprinters and distance runners are genetically advantaged for success in their events by a predominance of type II or type I fibers, respectively.[25] However, athletes who are required to exercise at near maximum aerobic and anaerobic levels, such as in middle-distance running and swimming, or in sports such as basketball or soccer, require activation of both fiber types at a more equal level of energy production.[74] Further, the ratio of muscle fiber types is only one of a number of important elite performance physiologic requisites, and does not in itself, predict performance very well.[35,64] One of the reasons for this is that, though the muscle fiber composition does not change with training, certain intense training programs can alter the biochemical characteristics, particularly of the type II fiber, as well as their size.[43,58,70]

Success in many athletic performances is not primarily limited by physiologic factors discussed above, but rather by neuromuscular coordination (i.e., general motor ability and motor skill). That is, even average amounts of muscular strength and endurance are not required for championship level performance in such sports as bowling, archery, and golf. Here highly refined neuromuscular mechanisms affect the eye-hand coordination demanded for excellence. Success in many other sports, however, involves a unique mix of muscular strength, power and/or endurance, together with a significant neuromuscular skill component. Sports such as basketball, gymnastics, diving, soccer, and wrestling are examples of this blend of neuromuscular coordination with other physiologic limitations necessary to the achievement of excellence in performance.

If heavy, sustained performance is required, fatigue will become a primary consideration, regardless of the activity. This is due, in part, to failure of muscle to sustain its original ability to produce force. Other factors include psychologic aspects such as motivation, whether due to staleness or perhaps even boredom. So viewed, fatigue can be defined as the inability and/or unwillingness to continue work at the same intensity. Of interest here, however, is examination of the physiologic factors which might best explain this phenomenon. These could include any (or all) of the following: (1) the CNS; (2) the motor neuron(s); (3) the neuromuscular junction(s); and (4) the muscle(s). Even when so limited, it appears that the physiologic causes of fatigue in various athletic performances are multiple and complex.[85] Current evidence suggests that the CNS may account, in part, for neuromuscular fatigue, though mechanisms are uncertain.[66] It seems clear that the motor nerve is not the site of muscular fatigue, though there is some evidence that the neuromuscular junction may be.[99]

There is a growing body of knowledge that the principal site of fatigue is the muscle. However, because of the wide range of primary energy sources in events lasting only seconds to those of several hours duration, it is not possible to isolate a single cause. In fact, effective work output depends on maintenance of the functional integrity of several systems, as well as their interaction. Thus, muscular fatigue may occur due to depletion of essential metabolites such as ATP, CP, muscle glycogen, and blood glucose, and/or the interference with the rate of ATP resynthesis effected by accumulation of hydrogen ions, the resultant decreased muscle pH, increased lactic acid, and increased calcium ions in the muscle mitochondria. Heart muscle fatigue, even in prolonged work, is not a likely limit to exercise capacity in healthy individuals.[13] Prolonged activity of several hours, or even of shorter duration in ambient heat stress, can cause decreased performance (i.e., earlier onset of fatigue) due to increased peripheral blood flow demand, fluid and electrolyte redistribution, dehydration, and probable metabolic pattern alteration.[13]

EFFECTS OF SELECTED ENVIRONMENTAL FACTORS ON PHYSICAL PERFORMANCE

Numerous environmental factors, such as temperature, airflow, humidity, altitude (hypobaria), hyperbaria (as experienced in sport diving), deviations from earth's gravity, and air pollution, exert significant effects on man's physical performance capacity. Further, almost everyone encounters environmental stress at some time, and many on a regular basis. Fortunately, man has evolved with considerable physiologic ability to respond to acute exposure to environmental stress, as well as to improve tolerance via adaptations to repeated exposure. For example, exposure to cold induces reflex peripheral vasoconstriction and shivering in an attempt to prevent central body temperature from falling. Adverse effects, however, can follow which limit one's performance, including numbness in the hands affecting coordination and, with lowered body temperature, reduced muscle metabolism and maximal cardiac function. If the cold stress is not too great nor too little (i.e., above threshold), with repeated exposure, physiologic changes (adaptations) occur which enable one to cope with the same cold stress as if it were of less magnitude. In this section, the effects of commonly encountered environmental conditions, viz., heat, cold, altitude, and air pollution, on man's physical performance capacity, health and safety, are examined.

EXERCISE IN THE HEAT

Man is a homeotherm, who has developed a sophisticated temperature regulating system which enables him to maintain the body's core temperature relatively constant in spite of exposure to substantial variations in environmental temperature. During exercise, approximately 75% of total metabolic energy production appears as heat which, in order to maintain core temperature, must be lost from the body. This is much more difficult to achieve if the ambient environment is hot and humid than in moderate conditions. To understand why this is so, it is necessary to examine how man exchanges heat with the environment, the physiologic mechanisms available to facilitate this, as well as limitations to these responses.

Man continually produces metabolic heat, which rises from about 70 kcal/hr at rest to more than 1,100 kcal/hr for over 2 hours for a champion marathon runner. Dissipation of heat in cool and moderate temperatures is achieved at rest primarily by convection and radiation. Radiation is the exchange of heat via electromagnetic waves, while convection involves heat exchange of an object with moving currents of fluid (i.e., air or water). The rate of heat exchange via convection and radiation depends to a large extent on the temperature gradient between the skin and the ambient environment. In cool conditions, heat is lost to the environment, but in hot conditions, where the ambient temperature exceeds skin temperature, heat is gained via convection and radiation. It then becomes necessary to activate the body's evaporative heat loss mechanism. This is done by sweating, with heat loss occurring as the fluid is changed to the gaseous state during evaporation.

The interrelationship between exercise workload and heat exchange at a constant 21°C (Celsius) ambient temperature is shown in the left panel of Figure 3–13. Heat loss by convection and radiation is not affected by increasing workload with ambient temperature constant. Evaporative heat loss from the lungs increases with enhanced ventilatory demand of increasing workload, but is only 15% of sweat evap-

orative heat loss from the skin in heavy work. The latter can be seen to assume the greatest proportion of the total heat loss at about 900 kpm/min. In the right panel of Figure 3–13, workload remains constant (900 kpm/min), as does metabolic heat production, in a series of exposures at different room temperatures (5 to 37°C). With increasing room temperature, evaporative heat loss increases as a direct function of the resultant progressive decrease in skin surface to room temperature gradient. At 33°C, room temperature exceeds skin temperature and convection and radiation become avenues of heat gain at higher temperatures, which necessitates further increases in sweating and evaporative heat loss. Thus, sweat evaporation represents man's primary defense against hyperthermia (when core temperature rises above 41°C due to continued imbalance of heat gain over heat loss).

Central body (core) temperature is controlled by balancing heat gain and heat loss. This is done by integration of peripheral and central blood temperature inputs to the hypothalamus, which functions much as a thermostat. If heat loss is too great, mechanisms of heat conservation will be activated; if heat gain exceeds heat loss, the hypothalamus initiates peripheral vasodilation and sweating. The two principal physiologic responses to work in the heat, viz., increased circulatory demand to transport heat to the periphery and sweating, are strikingly evidenced in the comparison shown in Table 3–6. The increased circulatory demand for doing the same moderate bicycle ergometer exercise in the hot steel mill is evidenced by a heart rate of 166 beats/min, compared to 104 in the cool condition. A near 5 times increase in sweating is evidenced by the difference in body weight loss for the two conditions.

Had the exercise workload in the previous comparison been doubled, the oxygen uptake would become 3.0 l/min., with the heart rate in the cool condition increased to about 170 beats/min. The core temperature would rise steadily to about 39°C within 30 minutes of exercise, reflecting greater heat production in the muscles which is thought to facilitate faster enzymatic action for increased energy produc-

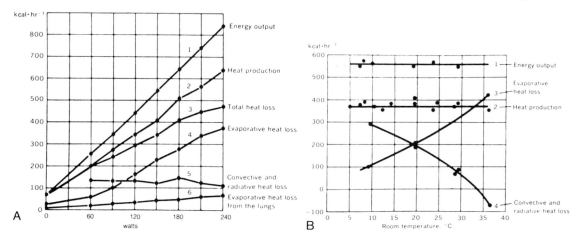

FIG. 3–13. A. Heat exchange at rest and during increasing work intensities (expressed in watts along the abscissa) in a nude subject at a room temperature of 21 degrees C. B. Heat exchange during work (150 watts) at different room temperatures in a nude subject. (Both from Nielsen, M.: Die regulation der korpertemperatur bei muskelarbeit. Skand. Arch. Physiol. 79:193–230, 1938, as modified by Astrand, P.-O., and K. Rodahl: Textbook of Work Physiology. 3rd ed. New York: McGraw-Hill, 1986, pp. 595 and 598.)

tion inherent in heavy work.[5] This increased metabolic heat production would necessitate increased sweating and a body weight loss of perhaps 1 kg. If this greater work level were now attempted in the hot steel mill condition, the combined circulatory demand for metabolism and heat dissipation would likely result in a near maximal heart rate, with evaporative heat loss demand increasing beyond the sweating capacity of the subject. If this occurred, the subject would not be able to complete the full 45 minutes of exercise in these conditions.

The amount of ambient heat stress imposed on the body is primarily a function of the air temperature. However, significant heat gain via radiation can occur, even in moderate air temperatures, in unob-

structed direct sun exposure. In hot-dry conditions, sweat evaporates readily provided there is adequate airflow (generally one's body movement through space provides this, even in the absence of wind). However, in hot-humid conditions, the gradient for sweat evaporation from the skin to the already highly saturated air molecules is reduced and sweat drips from the body without cooling it. Clothing in the heat during exercise is an important consideration, in that it represents a barrier to heat exchange. Light clothing assemblies of material that wicks sweat to the surface for evaporation is preferred. Sweat or vapor barrier suits create an intensely hot microenvironment, in that heat loss via sweat evaporation is drastically reduced.[17]

Prolonged work in the heat imposes a

Table 3–6.   Effect of Environmental Temperature on Human Response to Standard Work on a Bicycle Ergometer for 45 Min*

Environmental Temp.	Heart Rate beats/min	Rectal Temp degrees Celsius	Oxygen Uptake liters/min	Weight Loss kg
Cool	104	37.7	1.5	0.25
Hot steel mill, air temp 40 to 50 degrees Celsius + radiation	166	38.5	1.5	1.15

*Modified from Astrand, P.-O. and K. Rodahl: Textbook of Work Physiology. Physiological Bases of Exercise. 3rd ed. New York: McGraw-Hill, 1986, p. 626.

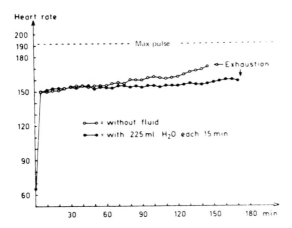

FIG. 3–14. Mean heart rates in subjects running on the treadmill at 70 percent of maximum oxygen uptake until exhaustion, with and without fluid. (From Staff, P.H., and S. Nilsson: Vaeske- og sukkertilforsel under langvarig intens fysisk activitet. Tidsskrift Den Norske Laegeforening. *16:*1235–1239, 1971, as modified by Astrand, P.-O., and K. Rodahl: Textbook of Work Physiology. 3rd ed. New York: McGraw-Hill, 1986, p. 558.)

gradually increasing strain on the body's resources. Sweat production, necessary for effective evaporation and body cooling, results in progressive dehydration which will reduce plasma volume, cardiac output and transport of heat to the periphery, thus resulting in a secondary rise in core temperature. As shown in Figure 3–14, progressive dehydration during prolonged running without fluid replenishment results in greater circulatory strain after the first hour and exhaustion nearly 30 minutes earlier than when 8 oz. of water is taken every 15 minutes. Heavy sweating also results in significant loss in electrolytes (primarily sodium, chloride, and potassium), but not to the same degree as water loss. Thus, in most instances, electrolyte replacement can occur following exercise without deleterious effects on performance. However, rehydration is achieved more quickly if the fluid solution contains sodium chloride than water alone.[79] As a general rule, salt tablets are not necessary, as a normal diet lightly supplemented with table salt, will provide sufficient replacement in a timely fashion.

When the total thermal stress exceeds the body's thermoregulatory capacity, disabilities of varying magnitude occur. These can be classified into three major categories in order of increasing severity: (1) heat cramps; (2) heat exhaustion; and (3) heat stroke. It is important to realize that they may overlap or follow each other in sequence. The first two are not dangerous if one recognizes their symptoms and takes appropriate precautions. A highly motivated person, however, may overextend himself when heat exhaustion due to circulatory inadequacy occurs, thus resulting in core temperature rising to hyperthermic levels (in excess of 40.5°C). Further persistence will result in breakdown of the body's temperature regulation center, a distinct drop, or cessation of sweating, and a further rise in core temperature. If core temperature remains at such a high level for sufficient time, it will cause irreversible damage to the central nervous system and possibly even death.[17,74]

Man has a potent capability to make significant improvements in heat tolerance via the process of heat acclimatization. This process involves 4 to 8 daily exposures to heat, usually of 1 to 2 hours' duration, while engaged in moderate exercise. As shown in Figure 3–15, sweat rate for a standard work-in-the-heat exposure increases rapidly during the first 5 days. This provides for better evaporative cooling at the skin surface, which results in decreased skin temperature (not shown). This means that blood returning to the core is cooler, thus helping to reduce core temperature and reflexly, heart rate. Another important change is the expansion of plasma volume which, together with better control of peripheral blood flow, results in an increased central blood volume. Both help to further reduce heart rate due to increased stroke volume. Nonetheless, individuals have markedly different capabilities to tolerate heat stress. Part of this is due to inherent variations in number of sweat glands, as well as in body fat and fitness level. Recent evidence suggests that women are not less tolerant of heat stress when exercise workloads are adjusted to gender differences in body size and equal heat acclimatization effects are assured.[49]

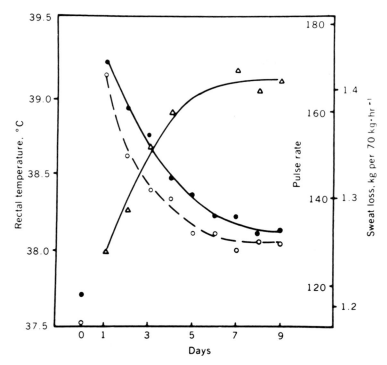

FIG. 3–15. Mean rectal temperature (●), heart rates (o), and sweat losses (Δ) in a group of men during a 9-day acclimatization to heat. On day 0 they worked for 100 min. at a rate of energy expenditure of 300 kcal/hr in a cool climate. On the following days they worked in a hot climate (48.9 degrees C dry-bulb and 26.7 degrees C wet-bulb temperature). (From Lind, A.R., and D.E. Bass: Optimal exposure time for development of acclimatization to heat. Federat. Proc. 22:704–708, 1963, as modified by Astrand, P.-O., and K. Rodahl: Textbook of Work Physiology. 3rd ed. New York: McGraw-Hill, 1986, p. 606.)

A prevalent notion still exists that elite, highly-trained and heat-acclimatized athletes are immune to hyperthermia and heat stroke. Actually there are numerous case studies of such individuals whose cerebral will to exceed an appropriately rational pace for the existent ambient conditions has resulted in classic heat stroke, sometimes resulting in death despite readily available first aid and subsequent medical care.[94]

The American College of Sports Medicine has advanced a position statement which can aid in the prevention of heat injuries to all who engage in distance running competition during ambient heat stress conditions.[4] It includes guidelines relative to ambient temperature and humidity conditions, time of day to hold athletic events, advice on fluid replenishment, and the provision of well-trained personnel at aid stations, as well as medical supervision. Similar procedures have resulted in substantial reduction of heat stroke problems in football players initiating practice during the late summer.[77]

EXERCISE IN THE COLD

The same body core temperature regulating system operates during cold stress, which is defined as a condition in which the rate of heat loss exceeds heat production for a given period of time. Ambient cold stress is not usually a significant problem for one engaged in prolonged heavy exercise because of high metabolic heat production and since appropriate clothing can effectively prevent high rates of heat loss. However, occasional cold survival problems attendant to hiking, boating, and camping mishaps, in which one is immersed in cool water or has clothing inadequate to prevent excessive heat loss due to extreme deterioration in the weather, do occur.

When one experiences ambient cold stress, the hypothalamus initially activates a decrease in peripheral blood flow (vasoconstriction) which increases the body's insulation and aids in keeping the deep body tissues warm enough to continue the function of vital life processes. This response is particularly effective in individuals with a substantial subcutaneous fat layer. In more severe cold stress, shivering (involuntary muscle contraction) is activated to increase metabolic heat production. Thus, the body responds both to decrease the rate of heat loss and to increase the rate of heat production.

The degree of ambient cold stress in air depends on the air temperature and the amount of solar radiation, but is greatly increased by wind (i.e., the "wind chill" effect). Further, clothing must remain dry in order to retain its full protective insulative properties. When rain or snow (which melts when it hits exposed body parts) occur, they evaporate and increase the rate of heat loss. Cold exposure in water results in a near 4 times greater rate of heat loss than in air at the same temperature. Thus, even moderate water temperatures (65 to 80°F) can result in excessive heat loss in lightly clad individuals. The rate of heat loss in cold water may exceed that of even maximal metabolic heat production during swimming.

The proper choice of clothing is usually man's best defense against excessive heat loss and the development of hypothermia (when body core temperature falls below 35°C). Generally, it is best to use several relatively thin layers of clothing so that the rate of heat loss through several warm air pockets between layers is reduced. This also permits ready adjustment of the clothing assembly insulation while exercising in cold air. Indeed, heavily exercising man can become a tropical man sweating heavily in a microclimate of clothing insulation too great for the metabolic heat production.

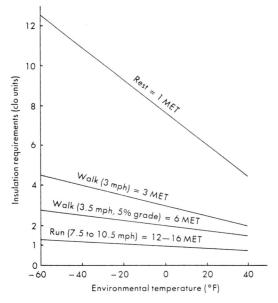

FIG. 3–16. Illustration of the insulation requirements for clothing (clo units) at rest and at various exercise intensities when a person is exposed to a variety of environmental temperatures. One MET is defined as the energy requirement for resting metabolism. (From Claremont, A.D.: Taking winter in stride requires proper attire. Physician Sportsmed. 4(12):65–68, 1976.)

The appropriate clothing insulation to maintain body core temperature for any ambient air temperature is shown in Figure 3–16 to be greatly influenced by increasing levels of metabolic heat production during exercise. These relationships apply when effects of wind chill and rain are minimized by the use of wind-breaker and water repellent garments, respectively.

When clothing protection is inadequate to balance heat loss and heat production during cold exposure, the fit person has an advantage in delaying or preventing the development of hypothermia. This is because the environmental conditions affect the rate of heat loss which will be nearly the same for the fit and unfit individuals. However, the fit person will be able to work at a higher metabolic heat production and thus, more adequately maintain body core temperature than his unfit counterpart.

It appears that man's ability to adapt to repeated cold exposure is of less magnitude and functional importance than that effected in heat acclimatization. This appears due, in part, to the fact that individuals who reside in cold climates minimize its effect by employing clothing assemblies which, in essence, form a moderate microclimate. This is also evidenced in the loss of cold acclimatization developed by the previously lightly clad Korean diving women foraging for seafood several hours per day in 10°C water, who now wear neoprene wet suits.[80]

Physical performance during prolonged exposure to cold stress can become significantly compromised. If the hands are exposed, they can become numb and the sensory receptors essentially anesthetized so that manipulative skills such as throwing and catching become much more difficult. Reduced core temperature results in lowered muscle temperature and a slowing of muscle enzymatic function, as well as reduced maximal heart rate and cardiac output. Both factors contribute to a substantially reduced maximal aerobic capacity and work performance.[8]

The two primary cold injuries upon prolonged exposure are frostbite and hypothermia.[49] Frostbite usually occurs in exposed body parts, such as the earlobes, fingers and toes, where blood circulation has been substantially reduced. Effective initial treatment entails immersing the affected body part in water between 99 to 106°F until thawed. Frostbite can usually be prevented by wearing gloves and boots with good insulation, a cap that covers the ears and a mask or cloth covering over the nose. As hypothermia progresses with the body core temperature falling below 35°C, one becomes progressively weaker and ill-coordinated. Shivering actually stops around 33°C as effective temperature regulation fails. With further exposure, the central nervous system becomes depressed, and fatigue, sleepiness, collapse, and coma follow. Severe hypothermia is a medical emergency condition which demands rewarming, preferably in a stirred water bath between 105° to 108°F, as soon as possible. Hypothermia is best prevented by taking appropriate precautions regarding possible adverse weather conditions, including clothing and shelter.

ATHLETIC PERFORMANCE AT ALTITUDE

The barometric pressure and air density are reduced by about 25% from sea level at an elevation of 7,000 ft. Thus, athletic performances in which air presents a resistance to be overcome, is facilitated at altitude. Faster sprint times and longer jumps, as well as improved skating and sprint cycling performances occur because of reduced air density (i.e., thinner air). However, the most significant impact on athletic performance at altitude is the reduced aerobic capacity induced by the proportional decrease in the partial pressure of oxygen at reduced barometric pressure. This results from less "driving force" of oxygen into the blood in the lungs and thus, less oxygen transported to the working muscles during maximum exercise. The effect is substantial, resulting in a near 5% greater time to run 10,000 meters at 7,000 ft. compared to sea level performance.[28]

If the distance runner continues to train at altitude, within several weeks an increased hemoglobin concentration and ventilatory capacity which results in enhanced oxygen transport, increased aerobic capacity, and improved performance, will occur. However, the acclimatization increase in aerobic capacity generally represents less than 20% recovery of the decrement upon initial exposure. Somewhat surprisingly, these changes do not translate into an automatically enhanced performance on return to sea level.[2]

EXERCISE IN ENVIRONMENTAL AIR POLLUTION

Air pollution is now a problem of considerable concern in many metropolitan areas. It arises primarily from industrial and motor vehicular emissions into the atmosphere. Directly emitted air pollutants are termed primary, while those which arise from chemical reactions of primary pollutants induced by sunlight are classified as secondary pollutants. While photochemical smog includes numerous air pollutants, only carbon monoxide and ozone currently exceed federal air quality standards for public health protection on a routine basis in numerous urban areas in the United States.[49] Both have been found to adversely affect physical performance, although by different mechanisms.

Carbon monoxide is a colorless, odorless gas directly emitted into the atmosphere via incomplete combustion processes. Upon inhalation, it diffuses across the lung alveolar membranes and readily binds with circulating blood hemoglobin. This reduces the amount of hemoglobin available for oxygen transport, as it has an affinity for carbon monoxide about 250 times greater than for oxygen. The result is the formation of blood carboxyhemoglobin at a level which is dependent on the ambient concentration of carbon monoxide, duration of exposure, and the individual's breathing rate. Thus, if one exercises at a workload necessitating 10 times greater ventilation than at rest at the same concentration and exposure time, the carboxyhemoglobin level will be accordingly higher. This could have important consequences in reducing one's blood oxygen transport capacity, though with several hours breathing of non-polluted air the effect will be reversed.

Smokers have, in addition to many other adverse health effects inherent in this form of personal air pollution, chronically elevated carboxyhemoglobin levels. For example, a person who smokes 1 pack of cigarettes per day would have a carboxyhemoglobin level at mid-day of approximately 6½%. If he should ride a bicycle at moderate effort through heavily traveled downtown streets for 1 hour, his carboxyhemoglobin level might well rise to 10%, which would result in a near 10% reduction in maximal aerobic capacity.[87]

Ozone is a secondary pollutant of principal importance in the photochemical air pollution mix prevalent in numerous metropolitan areas during the summer months. When inhaled by humans in sufficient dose, it induces irritant effects on the respiratory tract which impair pulmonary function, result in subjective symptoms of respiratory discomfort, including cough and shortness of breath, and can limit exercise performance.[1]

As is true with any air pollutant, exercise enhances the total dose over that at rest for any concentration exposure time product via metabolically induced increase in ventilation. The results of recent studies indicate that significant impairment of exercise performance, accompanied by pulmonary function changes and symptoms of respiratory discomfort, can occur upon engaging in heavy aerobic exercise for 1 hour at 0.18 ppm ozone, a level reached for 1 hour, or more, on about 180 days per year in the Los Angeles basin.[1] This suggests that highly trained endurance athletes are likely to be more susceptible to the effects of ozone than other population groups. Indeed, this has been observed, in that 5 of 10 athletes were unable to complete the prescribed 1 hour exposures to 0.18 ppm ozone.[92] With the addition of heat, typical of photochemical smog episodes, decrements in performance have been observed at even lower ozone concentrations.[38]

Mechanisms accounting for reduced maximum exercise performance upon significant ozone exposure have not been precisely identified. Though significant pulmonary function impairment (primarily reduced inspiratory capacity) has been routinely observed, as well as enhanced subjective symptoms of respiratory discomfort, no consistent objective evidence of effect on oxygen diffusion, transport and delivery has been observed. Hence, it appears that factors associated with ventilatory limitation impair both $\dot{V}O_{2max}$ and prolonged heavy exercise ($>65\%$ $\dot{V}O_{2max}$) performance. It is not certain whether this ventilatory limitation is due to an inability or unwillingness to inspire fully as a result of subjective respiratory discomfort.

Given that ozone can adversely affect the athlete's performance, what can one do to minimize this effect? One strategy is to avoid peak periods of photochemical smog episodes which typically occur for several hours in the middle of the day. This is essentially the strategy adopted by the California South Coast Air Quality District, which advises that school physical education and athletic practice and competition be terminated when a first-stage alert (ozone concentration in excess of 0.20 ppm) occurs. Thus one is advised to exercise early in the morning or in the evening to avoid ozone concentrations in excess of 0.20 ppm. Though there is some evidence that several days of repeated exposure at greater ozone concentrations produce an adaptive, reduced response effect including improved exercise performance,[37] this may not be without long-term adverse health effects.[12]

ERGOGENIC AIDS AND PHYSICAL PERFORMANCE

Ergogenic aids are substances and phenomena utilized to enhance performance above levels anticipated under normal conditions.[76] They are used in an attempt to enhance physiologic capacities and reduce psychologic inhibitions. The search by athletes for substances and methods which might enhance performance and thus yield a competitive edge is not new, but their use appears now to be more widespread than ever.

The International Olympic Committee (IOC) uses the term doping to identify ergogenic practices that are illegal. The principal aspects of their definition of doping are as follows:[107]

1. Doping involves taking a foreign substance into the body, or
2. "Physiological substances taken in abnormal quantities," or "taken by an abnormal route of entry."
3. Taking a foreign substance for the purpose of gaining a performance advantage in an "artificial manner."
4. Also, any medical intervention that "boosts the athlete's performance" is thought to be doping.

The IOC, has banned numerous alleged performance enhancing substances under several classifications, including (1) psychomotor stimulants, (2) sympathomimetic amines, (3) miscellaneous CNS stimulants, (4) narcotic analgesics, and (5) anabolic steroids. A urine sampling procedure of medal winners, or randomly selected athletes, has been developed to determine if banned substances are present.

Unfortunately, though, many of these substances are found in numerous over-the-counter and prescribed medications.

In addition to the moral question alluded to above, there is the fundamental issue of whether any ergogenic aids induce effects which enhance performance beyond that attributed to the placebo effect, i.e., the performer thinks the substance will improve performance (though it is inert), so it does. A further problem of importance is whether substances which may actually produce physiologic changes inducing enhanced performance also have harmful side effects. Both of these issues will be examined in the ensuing discussion of the most routinely used ergogenic aids under four classifications: (1) nutritional supplements, (2) CNS stimulants, (3) cardiovascular enhancers, and (4) muscle system effectors.

NUTRITIONAL SUPPLEMENTS

It should be realized that sound nutrition for the athlete is essentially the same as for the sedentary individual. That is, once essential requirements for protein, vitamins, and minerals have been met via a well-balanced diet, the competing athlete has few exceptional dietary needs other than elevated caloric intake.[82] Nonetheless, there are still many athletes who pursue the ill-advised notion that if some is good, more must be better.

One persistent notion is that those who initiate a high intensity strength training program need substantially greater amounts of protein beyond the normal daily recommended allowance of 0.8 g per kg of body weight. There is some evidence to substantiate this contention, though the still existent notion that one can automatically convert a high-protein pre-game steak meal into exceptional performance is not substantiated.[66] In one study[33] total protein breakdown was elevated by 30% in subjects engaged in 2 hours of heavy exercise. In the view of some,[14] there is inadequate information available on the dietary protein content necessary for athletes who wish to "bulk up." This is further compounded by the notion existent among many weight lifters, throwers in track and field, and football linemen that bulking up demands high dietary protein content in addition to anabolic steroid supplementation to maximize body mass gain and performance enhancement.[13] However, for individuals who initiate a personal fitness exercise program, no increase in the normal recommended daily protein intake is necessary.[74]

Vitamins are organic compounds that do not furnish energy or build tissue, but act as catalysts in the transformation of other organic compounds into energy. They are essential to adequate nutrition and, when deficient, result in a variety of clinical problems. It has been asserted that, since organic foodstuffs are used in large quantities to supply energy for strenuous physical activities, it might be difficult for an individual in training to obtain sufficient vitamins in his diet. Vitamin deficiency has not been demonstrated in athletes. Nonetheless, many athletes and coaches suspect that a vitamin shortage occurs to the extent that it might become a limiting factor in one's performance. However, an increase in activity increases the need for vitamins only in near direct proportion to the increase in the expenditure of energy. There is no consistent evidence that vitamin supplementation above that obtained in one's normal well-balanced diet aids work performance. Nonetheless, many athletes take vitamin supplements regularly, with some imbibing 10 to 1,000 times the recommended daily requirement.[74] Excess intake of fat soluble vitamins (A, D, E and K) can be toxic as they are stored in body tissues, primarily in the liver. Excess intake of water soluble vitamins (B complex and C) is not generally a problem as the excess is removed by the kidney and excreted. However, megadoses of vitamin C have been observed to cause several toxic responses.[51] Hence, megadose vitamin supplementation in healthy people is ill advised.

Minerals are inorganic elements which are vital to life via their roles in bone formation, heart, muscle and nerve function, and in regulating cellular metabolism in combination with certain enzymes and hormones. Adequate intake of minerals is generally assured when one imbibes a balanced diet. There is no evidence of performance enhancement via mineral supplementation of already well-nourished individuals. However, some athletes may have slight deficiencies in one or more minerals due to their intense training programs if undertaken with dietary restriction.

The development of osteoporosis, particularly evident in postmenopausal women, actually is initiated in many adults because of years of inadequate calcium intake.[71] Although regular exercise has been found to help slow the rate of aging (and loss of calcium) from the skeleton,[11,65] intense exercise in young adult female distance runners may induce secondary amenorrhea, and makes these women vulnerable to calcium loss and decreased bone mass.[18] It is clear that increased attention to insuring more adequate calcium intake is needed, especially in females,[50] even to the point of supplementation of calcium in the diet.

Iron is another mineral deficiency of significant proportion in American women.[48] This is especially true of regularly menstruating women who lose increased amounts of iron in menstrual discharge. Many of these women develop iron deficiency anemia which adversely affects endurance capacity. For female athletes engaged in heavy endurance training, iron supplementation of 15 to 20 mg per day should suffice. Significantly more than this is ill advised, as excess iron cannot be stored but can accumulate in the liver where it can cause toxic side effects.[48,66]

As mentioned in an earlier section, ingestion of water, both 30 minutes before and at 15- to 20-minute intervals during prolonged work in the heat, significantly increased performance time over that when no fluids are imbibed. Because heavy, prolonged exercise ($\geq 70\%$ of $\dot{V}O_{2max}$) can deplete muscle glycogen within 60 to 75 minutes[9] and encroach on liver glycogen reserves necessary to sustain blood glucose levels, comparisons between glucose solutions and water only drinking have been conducted. Lamb and Brodowicz[67] reviewed these studies and found that beverages containing glucose, sucrose, or glucose polymers yielded similar beneficial effects in the maintenance of temperature regulation as water, but that blood glucose levels were better maintained and associated with improved performance time relative to water. However, glucose solutions should not be taken within 1 to 2 hours of prolonged endurance performance, as they induce high insulin levels which lower fatty acid mobilization, and also eventually result in somewhat lower blood glucose levels during exercise.[26]

There still exists belief amongst some coaches and athletes that a high protein pregame meal is best. However, numerous studies of pre-event meal regimens have failed, with one notable exception (carbohydrate loading enhancement of prolonged endurance performance), to demonstrate any significant effect on athletic performance.[108]

Prolonged endurance performance (60 minutes, or longer) presents a special pre-event nutritional concern, in that this type of performance induces muscle glycogen depletion in subjects who have been on a normal mixed diet.[52] Further, the effects of carbohydrate loading (a diet especially high in carbohydrates) on muscle glycogen levels appears to be interrelated with work induced depletion and other dietary manipulations (Fig. 3–17). It can be seen that the 7-day multiple intervention method resulted in a muscle glycogen content more than double that achieved on the control mixed diet. The effect of dietary manipulated muscle glycogen level on exercise performance time at a workload of 75% of VO_{2max} is substantial and consistent, as can be seen in Figure 3–18.

These observations have led to an almost universal use of carbohydrate loading by both competitive long-distance runners and "recreational" road runners. Experience has shown over the past 15 to 20 years that the procedure does not produce universally successful results. Though it appears that an increased sensitivity of the enzyme glycogen synthase, which converts glucose to muscle glycogen, may occur with glycogen depletion,[63] repeated supercompensation attempts may not be so successful. Further, potentially negative effects on performance can occur if (1) adequate vitamins and minerals are not included in the altered diet, (2) the low carbohydrate period results in significant lethargy and possible use of lean tissue to maintain blood glucose levels, (3) the dietary manipulations are not tolerated gastrointestinally, and (4) there is gain in body weight, which occurs with the storage of about 3 g of water per g of muscle glycogen added. Many of these negative effects can be avoided by employing a less stringent pre-event protocol, which includes 6 days of reduced training (tapering) prior to competition, accompanied by 50% carbohydrate diet for the first 3 days and 70% carbohydrate for the last 3 days. This protocol has been found to yield similar muscle glycogen levels as those shown in Figure 3–17.[93]

CENTRAL NERVOUS SYSTEM STIMULANTS

Amphetamines are drugs that stimulate CNS function and elicit physiologic responses characteristic of enhanced sympathetic nervous system effects. CNS changes include increased arousal, wakefulness, confidence, and masking fatigue. Sympathomimetic effects include increased cardiac output, blood pressure, and glycolysis in muscle and liver, vasodilation in skeletal muscle, and vasoconstriction of peripheral blood vessels. The results from experimental studies of amphetamines utilizing human volunteers do not provide convincing evidence of an enhancing effect on performance.[42] There is, however, suggestive evidence that amphetamines facilitate longer submaximal work performance, perhaps due to a lower sense of fatigue.[69] A more recent, well-controlled study (double-blind method)[20] utilized 15 mg of amphetamine sulfate ingested 2 hours before an endurance performance task. Though no change in VO_{2max} was observed, peak lactic aid levels and performance time were increased, again suggesting a masked fatigue effect. There is also suggestive evidence that amphetamine ingestion is associated with improved performance in large muscle, power performance, but impairs more complex skill performance requiring continued concentration and judgment.[14]

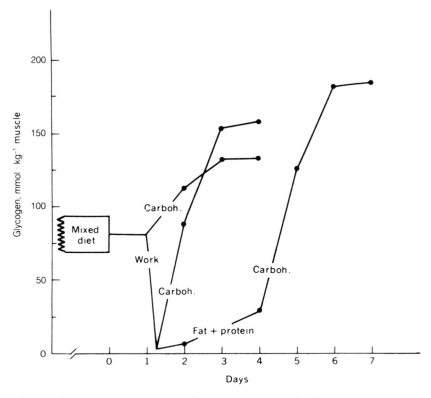

FIG. 3–17. Diet and exercise combinations for increasing muscle glycogen content. (From Saltin, B., and L. Hermansen: Glycogen stores and prolonged severe exercise. In Nutrition and Physical Activity. Edited by G. Blix. Stockholm: Almqvist & Wiksell, 1967, pp. 32–43, as modified by Astrand, P.-O., and K. Rodahl. Textbook of Work Physiology. 3rd ed. New York: McGraw-Hill, 1986, p. 553.)

While there is suggestive research evidence of improved performance with amphetamines, there are important reasons to avoid their use. In major athletic competition, e.g., the IOC, their use is banned due both to potential for unfair competitive advantage and serious side effects. The latter include: (1) physiologic or psychologic drug dependency with continued use; (2) resultant need for larger doses upon continued use, which may potentiate cardiac arrhythmias and psychic distress; (3) undesirable immediate effects, including headaches, dizziness, and confusion, which impair mental concentration and effective judgment; and (4) compromises normal body awareness of extreme fatigue. The latter is of particular importance, in that there are well-documented accounts of endurance cyclists who have died while competing in events under conditions of ambient heat stress, where the effects of masked fatigue awareness and reduced heat dissipation capability form a deadly combination.[42]

CARDIORESPIRATORY ENHANCERS

Oxygen breathing at higher concentrations than that at earth's atmosphere (hyperoxia) has frequently been used since its employment before competition and during recovery by the Japanese swimmers, who experienced unexpected success at the 1932 Olympics. While improved short-term combined anaerobic/aerobic performance has been observed upon immediately prior inhalation of hyperoxic gas, practical considerations prevent its effective utility

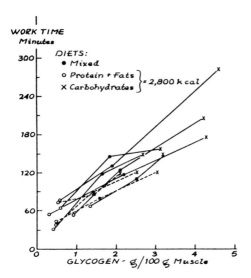

FIG. 3–18. Relation between initial glycogen content in the quadriceps muscle in nine subjects who had been on different diets, and maximal work time when working at a given load demanding 75 per cent of maximal aerobic power. (From Bergstrom, J. et al.: Diet, muscle glycogen, and physical performance. Acta Physiol. Scand. 71:140–150, 1967.)

in athletic competition, in that the physiologic advantage would be largely compromised by again breathing ambient air before the race actually starts.

There is consistent evidence that continuous breathing of hyperoxic gas during submaximal and maximal aerobic exercise enhances performance.[74] This effect appears to be due to a slightly increased arterial oxygen content, reduced lactic acid production, as well as to reduced oxygen cost of breathing. Again, however, practical considerations inhibit the effective utility of pressurized oxygen in competitive athletics, though it has great value for high altitude mountaineers, fire fighters, and for those with lung disease who would remain bedridden without their portable oxygen cannisters.[66]

Where practical considerations do not prohibit the inhalation of hyperoxic gas during recovery from intense work (and prior to reinitiation of similar effort), is where its continued use prevails. No physiologic or enhanced performance efficacy

to this procedure has been observed in well-designed laboratory studies.[10,105]

Blood doping is an ergogenic procedure of comparatively recent origin used to increase oxygen transport capacity and enhance endurance performance. As indicated in Figure 3–19, 900 ml (about 1 quart) of blood is withdrawn, the plasma is separated and immediately reinfused, and the red blood cells (RBC) stored in a freezer for 5 to 6 weeks. Meanwhile, the athlete's RBC volume and hemoglobin (Hb) concentration have returned to normal levels. The stored blood cells are then reinfused from one to several days prior to a championship event, although the elevated RBC volume and Hb concentration appear to persist for at least 2 weeks.[88] The procedure provides an immediate increase in total blood volume, as well as RBC volume and Hb concentration. It is theorized that oxygen transport will be increased in maximum work due to the blood's enhanced oxygen carrying capacity. On the other hand, the immediate increase in RBC upon reinfusion results in an increased cellular concentration, which could increase blood viscosity and decrease maximal cardiac output and muscle blood flow velocity.[88] Further, some athletes' maximum aerobic capacity may be limited by their muscles' ability to extract oxygen from an already adequate central oxygen transport mechanism.

Results from early RBC reinfusion investigations were equivocal due to either inadequate amounts of blood withdrawal and/or deterioration in RBC over several weeks of refrigeration.[39] In every study since 1980 in which 900 ml, or more, blood has been withdrawn and placed in freezer storage for 5 or more weeks, significant increases in Hb concentration, VO_{2max} and endurance performance have been observed.[74] The increased total blood volume appears to preserve, or slightly increase maximal cardiac output, while the elevated Hb concentration ensures an increased arterial oxygen content. This means that more oxygen per unit time arrives at the working muscle, of which only a portion (less than 50% in one study of highly trained endurance athletes[98]), is actually used.

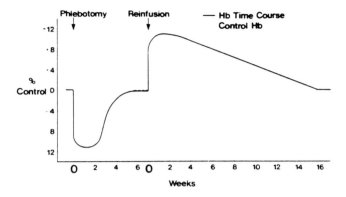

FIG. 3–19. Time course of hematology changes following the removal and reinfusion of ~900 ml of autologous freeze-preserved blood. (From Gledhill, N.: Blood doping and related issues: a brief review. Med. Sci. Sports Exer. *14*:183–189, 1982.)

The reinfusion procedure, utilizing one's own blood, when done under appropriate medical supervision is of low risk. The procedure is clearly at variance with the intent of the antidoping regulations of the IOC, but there is no means available to enforce a ban on its use.[14] This is because there is no test to detect blood doping, as the changes in Hb concentration are similar to those seen in short term altitude acclimatization (where there is, however, no increase in total blood volume).

MUSCLE FUNCTION ENHANCERS

Exhaustive short-term exercise, in which glycolysis is the primary energy source, results in significant accumulation of lactic acid, a resultant fall in intracellular pH and ultimately, inhibition of energy resynthesis and contractile capability of the muscles.[23,81] These events are deterred in part by the body's bicarbonate buffering system, which has led to speculation that inducement of alkalosis prior to exercise might delay the onset of fatigue via an enhanced buffering effect and promotion of lactic acid efflux from muscle, thus delaying a decrease in intracellular pH.[14]

Results from recent studies, in which the ingestion of bicarbonate 1 to 3 hours prior to maximum exercise of from 1 to 10 minutes, have nearly always shown improved performance over that achieved in control conditions.[67] In one study, utilizing the double-blind method, ingestion of sodium bicarbonate resulted in a significant pre-race elevation in blood pH and bicarbonate levels, which remained significantly higher than control and placebo condition values following an 800-meter race.[106] In the alkalotic condition, subjects ran significantly faster (2.9 seconds) and had significantly higher post-race blood lactate and extracellular hydrogen ions, which suggests a higher anaerobic energy contribution than for the control conditions.

Lamb and Brodowicz[67] report some negative observations of bicarbonate loading, including: (1) development of nausea and/or diarrhea about 3 hours postingestion in about 50% of the subjects; and (2) the danger of ill-advised excessive dosing by individual athletes which could lead to severe alkalosis and even death. Bicarbonate loading also appears to be at variance with the antidoping regulations of the IOC. If so, significant loads could easily be detected by pre-race blood sampling for pH and bicarbonate levels.[40]

Caffeine is a compound found in a variety of foods, such as coffee, tea, cocoa and cola nuts, as well as in numerous nonprescription medicines. It is a CNS stimulant, but also increases heart rate and contractility, causes peripheral vasodilation, and influences fatty acid mobilization.[13] Several investigators have found that caffeine equivalent to between 2½ to 3 cups of coffee taken about 60 minutes prior to prolonged exercise enhances performance.[86] Whether this is due to (1) increased free fatty acid supply to the muscles, thereby sparing muscle glycogen, (2) stimulation of the central nervous system, (3) suppressing intramuscular glycolysis, (4) direct action on the muscle, possibly by enhancement of calcium release from the sarcoplasmic reticulum, or (5) by some other mechanism, is unclear.[86]

Caffeine induces rather a wide magnitude of effects in humans and, because of its cardiac stimulatory properties, it can cause increased risk of arrhythmias, making its use ill-advised in older, less well-conditioned individuals.[13] Caffeine is on the list of drugs banned by the IOC, but the plasma levels required to disqualify one from competition are so high that oral ingestion of caffeine is unlikely to result in doping detection.[86]

Anabolic steroids are synthetic derivatives of the male hormone testosterone, which has both anabolic (growth enhancing) and androgenic (promotion of secondary sexual characteristics) properties. Drug manufacturers have reduced but not fully eliminated the androgenic effects of these products. Early clinical studies revealed that anabolic steroids induced protein retention and tissue growth in late maturing prepubertal males and in older males who had no testes or malfunctioning testes.[14]

Because of their presumed muscle building qualities in already mature individuals, numerous athletes have used these drugs with the intent of increasing strength, power, and speed. In a survey study reported in 1983,[100] 99% of male competitive powerlifters admitted to having taken steroids at some point in their career. An 80% incidence of top-level male shot putters, discus, hammer and javelin throwers was reported, followed by 70% of the football players surveyed. Twenty-five percent of female powerlifters reported taking steroids.

Well-controlled (double-blind method with placebo control) laboratory studies, utilizing therapeutic doses (5 to 20 mg per day), have yielded equivocal results, with about as many showing significant gains in strength as those reporting no changes.[109] Almost all report gains in weight, but it is not clear how much is muscle tissue. Testimonials from top-level strength and power athletes indicate that typical anabolic steroid dosage may be 10 to 20 times therapeutic dosage,[109] and taken in oral and injectable form.[16] Limited data obtained on these highly trained athletes suggest that weight and strength gains, like those in some patients,[90] are greater at these high dose levels.

In addition to the banning of anabolic steroids by the IOC, track and field federations, and the National Collegiate Athletic Association, use of these drugs is ill-advised because of numerous side effects. Clinical reports from extended use in patients indicate unusually high incidence of liver dysfunction, as well as the development of several potentially fatal liver and blood diseases.[60] Other side effects observed in males include significant mood changes and the development of aggressiveness, temporarily reduced sperm production, and increased risk for coronary heart disease.[83] Females who use steroids frequently develop menstrual irregularity and experience masculinization effects (i.e., deepening of the voice and hair growth on the face and chest), some of which may not be entirely reversible.[14]

PHYSIOLOGIC PRINCIPLES OF TRAINING

Inherent in repeated performance of a sufficiently stressful workload is what is referred to as the training effect. It occurs every day in both elite athletes' efforts at obtaining the maximum competitive edge, as well as in an increasing number of individuals who elect a more active lifestyle after numerous years of sedentary existence. Though the effort involved and, indeed, some of the subtleties inherent in the primary purpose of those who engage in repeated exercise sessions differ, the basic physiologic processes and thus, the principles of training are in many respects essentially similar.

Figure 3-20 presents a schematic interrelationship of several important training principles. Fundamental aspects include the training overload (and the lack of it) on the x axis and the body's response on the y axis. Overload refers to an increase in activity level above that which one is routinely accustomed to. In essence, it means that the body's muscles are required to do more work. This can be accomplished via lifting more weight, lifting the same weight

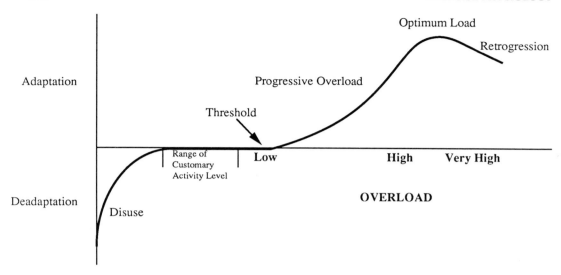

FIG. 3–20. Illustration of the effects of decreased (disuse) and increased (overload) levels of physical activity (compared to one's customary activity level) on deadaptation and adaptation, respectively, and their relation to several important training principles. See text for further explanation.

faster, or lifting it for a longer period of time during a single work session.

As mentioned earlier, however, it is necessary to repeat this process for some period of time before noticeable training effects will occur. Further, it is essential to achieve a sufficient stimulus, termed the training threshold, which is of particular importance to those who initiate training without the intent to compete in athletics. The most frequently used barometer to assess this point of initial training stimulus in previously sedentary individuals is the heart rate response to a given workload. In a now classic experiment, Karvonen[62] found that when sedentary young adult subjects trained for 30 minutes per day, 5 days per week, and their heart rate was not above 70% of maximal heart rate during exercise, they experienced no submaximal workload heart rate reduction during the 4-week training period. If their exercise heart rate fell below this level (about 140 beats/min), then the running speed was increased and a training effect ensued. This observation has been confirmed on numerous occasions with healthy but sedentary young and middle-aged adults. It has also been found that a minimum duration of 20 minutes per day and a fre-

quency of at least 3 times per week are necessary to initiate aerobic training effects. Some studies suggest that training effects can occur in elderly, less fit adults and cardiac rehabilitation patients at a somewhat lower percent of maximal heart rate when minimum duration and frequency are adhered to.[46,84,95]

Adaptation, both in body structure and function, occurs during a training program following establishment of a training threshold. It increases in magnitude with progressive overload, as an interrelated effect of intensity and duration. Figure 3–21 depicts blood lactate response to a standard treadmill exercise test, in which the first 20 days of running at 7 miles per hour for 30 minutes per day showed an initially rapid decline with leveling off by day 15. At day 20, the intensity of running was increased to 8½ mph, and another less precipitous decrease in blood lactate followed for a week before again plateauing. While an athlete seeks to increase progressively the training volume and intensity over a season, it appears that maximum performance improvement at the end of the season may occur when one alternates periods of several days intense with less intense training[13] (Fig. 3–22).

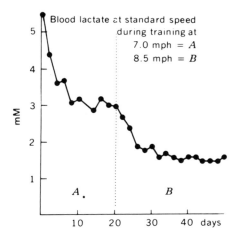

FIG. 3–21. Progressive decrease of blood lactate for a standard amount of exercise: running on a treadmill at 7 mph for 10 min. (From Edwards, H.T., L. Brouha, and R.E. Johnson: Effets de l'entrainement sur le taux de l'acide latique sanguin au cours du travail musculaire. Le Travail Humain. 8:1–9, 1939, as modified by Astrand, P.-O., and K. Rodahl: Textbook of Work Physiology. 3rd ed. New York: McGraw-Hill, 1986, p. 437.)

As depicted in Figure 3–20, an optimum training load is reached when further improvement, usually assessed by performance, is not achieved with additional overload. This point has not been accurately identified for either strength, anaerobic or aerobic exercise training. However, in each case too much training at any point in time can lead to retrogression in the athlete's performance. This appears to be a complex phenomenon in which a further increase in training load would be productive if other interrelated factors were at an optimal level. For example, the body's energy reconstitution processes may be unable to keep pace with the training stimulus due to other factors such as inadequate sleep and nutrition.

Most of us have observed the "natural athlete" who seems to excel in a wide spectrum of athletic activity. This is due, in part, to the fact that many athletic performances usually demand varying degrees of common physical requisites, such as hand/eye coordination, muscular strength, power, endurance, and agility. In addition, the "natural" athlete usually has a rich (diverse) physical activity participation background. However, when tested on unique motor tasks, they evidence no consistent superiority above non-athletes.[96] This observation led to the development of a now fundamental principle of training—specificity, in which adaptations occur when the training activity utilizes the same muscles as those employed in performance. Thus, it is obvious that a jogging program will elicit quite different physiologic adaptations than a weight training program. Not usually appreciated, however, is that participation in a particular type of activity—for example, cardiorespiratory endurance—also yields specific effects. This is illustrated in an experiment in which swimmers demonstrated an 11% gain over the season of training in a swimming ergometry test, but no change in a treadmill

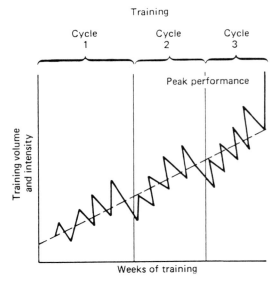

FIG. 3–22. Over the course of a training season, training volume and intensity should increase in a cyclic, discontinuous manner. Days and weeks of heightened training should be followed by recovery days and weeks of lesser intensity. Similarly, each training cycle begins at an intensity less than that at the end of the previous cycle. In this system the stimulus of progressive training is accompanied by periods of recovery and adaptation. (From Brooks, G.A. and T.D. Fahey: Exercise Physiology. New York: Macmillan, 1985, p. 430.)

run test to exhaustion.[73] Thus, it appears that peripheral muscular adaptations are important in maximizing the training effect of rhythmic cardiorespiratory exercise training. Specificity also entails utilizing the same neural patterns and energy delivery systems to maximize training adaptations for competitive performance. This means that training activities should be performed at near the same intensity (speed) of competition. Appropriate rest intervals in high intensity exercise also permit more total stress on the primary energy supply systems than would be possible in continuous training.[66]

Even when other important principles discussed above are adhered to, it is necessary to understand that a group of seemingly similar individuals will respond to a training program in many different orders of magnitude. That is, some will experience striking physiologic adaptations and improved performance, whereas others will not. This difference in response is thought to be due, in part, to hereditarian factors, such as differences in muscle fiber types and enzyme systems.[84] Also of importance is the individual's immediately prior activity level, which is strikingly exemplified in Figure 3–23. Five normally active young adult males demonstrated different maximal oxygen uptake responses to 8 weeks of hard aerobic endurance training. In general, those who had lower initial values (far left panel) experienced greater increases, the mean for the group being about 4.0 liters per minute, post-training. When this value is compared to the mean pre-experiment value (3.35 liters per minute), the improvement was 19% (0.65/3.35). However, when compared to the mean value of 2.5 liters per minute following 21 days bed rest, the group increase was 60% (1.5/2.5).

In some activities, individual differences in initial skill level can play a substantial role in providing an appropriate training stimulus. That is, poorly-skilled swimmers can improve performance faster and need greater increases in training speed, since they will be improving via better neuromuscular coordination as well as by training induced physiologic adaptations. This phenomenon is less evident in other rhythmic endurance activities such as walking, running, and bicycling.

Everyone is aware of the effects of prolonged inactivity as evidenced by the appearance of a broken limb following casting. In addition to clearly apparent atrophy, there is a loss in muscular strength, endurance, and flexibility. The effect of disuse, or decrease in the accustomed level of activity, indicates that training benefits cannot be stored. This principle of reversibility, or transiency of training effect, is evidenced within only 6 days of nontraining in some physiologic parameters.[27] In this same study, $\dot{V}O_{2max}$ following prolonged endurance training (1 year or more) was measured at 12, 21, 56, and 84 days after training cessation. The most rapid drop (7%) was observed at 12 days, but with a continued decline to 16% at 84 days following training cessation. Further, what is lost is harder to gain back, in that 2 weeks of retraining following 2 weeks of training cessation did not fully restore losses in aerobic work performance or maximal oxygen uptake.[55]

PHYSIOLOGIC EFFECTS OF TRAINING

As suggested in the previous section on training principles, adherence to properly prescribed training programs will induce both structural and functional changes. In athletes training for competition, it is necessary to make the program highly specific to maximize the rate of changes and improvement in performance. In this section, major physiologic adaptations induced by specialized training will be described. It should be appreciated, however, that a previously sedentary individual could experience some degree of each of these training adaptations by undertaking a carefully designed general training program.

STRENGTH ADAPTATIONS

Repeated sessions of heavy resistance work induce neuromuscular adaptations which increase strength. Though it is well known that the primary structural change

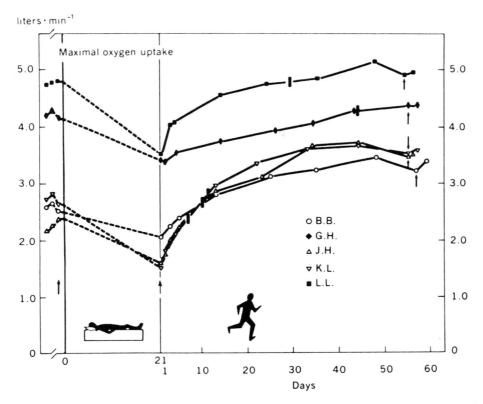

FIG. 3–23. Changes in maximal oxygen uptake, measured during running on a motor-driven treadmill, before and after bed rest and at various intervals during training; individual data on five subjects. Heavy bars mark the time during the training period at which the maximal oxygen uptake had returned to the control value before bed rest. (From Saltin, B. et al.: Response to exercise after bed rest and after training. Circulation. *38* (Suppl. 7):1–78, 1968.)

induced by strength training is hypertrophy, i.e., increase in size of already existing muscle cells, it appears that strength actually improves more during the first several weeks via neural factors (Fig. 3–24). The reversal of primary contributions to strength gains from the neural component first and then by muscular hypertrophy during 8 weeks of training was determined using an integrated electromyogram (EMG) procedure. During the first 2 weeks, increases in maximum force development were associated with directly proportional increases in EMG activity. This meant that more motor units were being recruited, and/or that motor units were being recruited more frequently. During the last 2 weeks, increases in maximum force (strength) were achieved without additional change in EMG neural activity, but with evidence of muscle hypertrophy.

Muscle hypertrophy is associated with an increased synthesis of cellular material, especially the proteins which comprise the contractile elements. Specifically, this involves the enlargement of myofibrils via the production of actin and myosin filaments.[41] The diameter of the muscle increases because of greater amounts of actin, myosin, and other intracellular proteins in the myofibrils. Muscles also increase in size due to proliferation of connective tissue surrounding the muscle fibers. The strength of tendons is also enhanced with heavy resistance training.[102]

There have been several reports which suggested that heavy resistance training induced muscle cell hyperplasia (increased

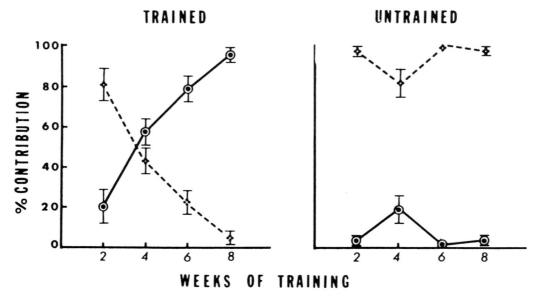

FIG. 3–24. The time course of strength gain, showing the percent contributions of neural factors (◇) and hypertrophy (◉) in the trained and untrained arms of young adult males. (From Moritani, T., and H.A. deVries: Neural factors versus hypertrophy in the time course of muscle strength gain. Am. J. Phys. Med. 50:115–130, 1979.)

number of cells) via longitudinal splitting of the muscle fibers. It now appears that this conclusion is in error due to inappropriate methodologic assumptions.[44]

Heavy resistance training does not appear to alter the ratio of fast twitch to slow twitch fibers. However, it does appear to selectively enhance the area of the fast-twitch fibers with no significant change in the size of slow twitch fibers.[101] Mitochondrial number and size are unaffected so that the muscle's oxidative capacity per unit of muscle is reduced.[74]

ANAEROBIC TRAINING MUSCLE
ADAPTATIONS

Improvements in strength via training mean that the same force can be developed while contracting fewer motor units at the same time. Thus, strength adaptations almost invariably improve power in anaerobic performance.[66] There are, however, energy supply and utilization factors which become increasingly important in performances where speed of movement

against a given force over time become paramount.

Studies of muscle structural and functional adaptations consequent to anaerobic training programs are of recent origin.[14] Thus, there is a less complete picture of adaptations that facilitate improved anaerobic performance than for predominantly aerobic performances. Strength training has been shown to increase muscle concentrations of ATP, PC, and glycogen,[72] which has the potential for facilitating anaerobic performance. However, improvement would necessitate increases in key glycolytic enzymes, as has been observed in strength training[24] and in sprint training.[36] Trained individuals show greater muscle glycogen depletion and elevated muscle and blood lactate levels following maximal anaerobic performance on a bicycle ergometer than do untrained subjects.[61] It is not clear whether anaerobic training improves performance primarily via increased anaerobic substrates, enhanced glycolytic enzyme activity, or greater capacity for lactic acid tolerance. At present, it seems that all may have an important role.[74]

AEROBIC TRAINING MUSCLE ADAPTATIONS

Profound changes in skeletal muscle structure and function occur with endurance exercise (low resistance, high repetition) training. There is little, if any increase in muscle size, and no change of basic muscle fiber types, but the muscles' oxidative capacity for generating ATP (via phosphorylation) is significantly enhanced via substantial increase in mitochondria size and number. A near doubling of key energy liberating enzymes of the Krebs cycle, the electron transport chain, and fatty acid oxidation have been observed in endurance trained animals.[14] This results in a slower utilization of muscle glycogen and blood glucose, a greater reliance on fat oxidation, and lower lactate levels during prolonged submaximal exercise of a given intensity.[53] Endurance training of animals significantly increases muscle myoglobin which, if also true in humans, would facilitate increased oxygen diffusion to the mitochondria.[14] It appears that endurance training induced increases in mitochondrial oxidative capacity of rats are better related to improved endurance performance than is maximal oxygen uptake, though the latter is well related, ($r = 0.82$) to the maximum workload intensity.[29]

AEROBIC TRAINING CARDIORESPIRATORY ADAPTATIONS

Repeated stress upon a large portion of the skeletal muscle mass (usually including the legs), at low resistance with high repetition, induces significant central cardiorespiratory adaptations. In terms of the need to increase oxygen pick-up, transport and delivery, it is physiologic to proceed accordingly.

Even with frequent repetition of deep labored breathing inherent in aerobic endurance exercise, there is little evidence of significant structural change in the lung that facilitates enhanced oxygen pick-up and carbon dioxide exhalation following training.[31] However, there appears to be some hypertrophy of the respiratory musculature as well as increased respiratory enzymes, mitochondrial size, and thus oxidative capacity, which facilitates increased maximal ventilation ($\dot{V}_{Emax}$). There is also an increased efficiency of breathing (i.e., less ventilation is required per unit of oxygen loaded into the blood). As efficiency increases, the ventilation perfusion ratio nears unity (i.e., more closely matched to lung blood flow and thus, increased diffusion capacity). This change in the ratio is due to enhanced alveolar ventilation and a concomitant increase in lung capillary perfusion resulting from an increase in cardiac output. As breathing efficiency rises with training, there is also less metabolic acidosis to drive ventilation at any given submaximal workload and thus decreased ventilation.[5,74]

Part of this enhanced O_2 diffusion in the lung alveoli, as well as increased O_2 transport capacity, is due to an increased red blood cell volume and thus, in hemoglobin content of the blood. Plasma volume increases even more, apparently to facilitate transport of increased metabolic heat production to the periphery.[32]

Endurance exercise training also results in a decreased heart rate at rest and at a given submaximal workload, due primarily to a shift in ANS stimulation. On the other hand, stroke volume is increased both in submaximal and maximal work. There are several factors possibly responsible for this increase including: (1) increased plasma volume, with consequent increased venous return; (2) decreased heart rate allowing greater time between beats for ventricular filling; and (3) increased contractility or force of contraction, resulting in greater emptying of the ventricles with each contraction.[31,46]

In submaximal work, cardiac output is lowered by endurance training, apparently because the working muscles become more efficient in extracting oxygen. However, during maximal work, endurance training enhances cardiac output as a function of an increased stroke volume, as maximum heart rate changes little and, if so, decreases slightly. Systolic blood pressure changes with aerobic training usually parallel heart rate responses, while diastolic blood pressure does not change, either in submaximal or maximal exercise.

The peripheral changes consequent to

endurance training in skeletal musculature noted earlier, including increased capillarization, myoglobin, and mitochondria size and number, all contribute to more efficient oxygen diffusion to the muscle cells. Though, for a given submaximal workload, the same *amount* of oxygen is needed, more is extracted per unit of blood, thus reducing heart rate and cardiac output. This improved oxygen extraction at the muscle is also important in increasing maximal work performance, as a greater maximal a-v$_{O_2}$ difference contributes to an increased $\dot{V}O_{2max}$.[46,89]

Table 3–7 presents a qualitative summary of the major cardiorespiratory adaptations consequent to endurance training. In integrative terms, two factors should be evident: (1) submaximal work is done at the same metabolic demand (i.e., $\dot{V}O_2$ is the same), but there is less stress on the system as it is now more efficient; and (2) maximal performance is enhanced, both due to increased cardiac output and a-v$_{O_2}$ difference.

OTHER TRAINING ADAPTATIONS

There are numerous other structural and functional changes effected via persistent adherence to exercise training. In this section, the effects of endocrine function on exercise response and training adaptations, as well as training changes in body composition and joint flexibility will be examined briefly.

The endocrine system functions in a highly integrated manner with the nervous system to coordinate various physiologic responses essential to effective exercise performance. The nervous system provides immediate stimuli, while the endocrine system usually acts to fine-tune these immediate effects. The endocrine system, via secretion of numerous hormones, exerts profound effects on the rates of cellular activity, either by affecting intracellular protein synthesis, enzyme activity, or by directly altering cell membrane permeability.[66] The effects of hormonal response to exercise have only recently been investigated, and the effects of exercise training on endocrine function relative to human performance and health are poorly understood.[66]

It appears that there are few consistent important changes induced by training in resting hormone concentrations. For example, resting total thyroxine (a potent stimulus on basal metabolic rate) levels are slightly decreased, while free thyroxine levels are elevated.[66] Further, hormone response levels during the same submaximal workload following training appear to be influenced by the associated reduction of sympathoadrenal hormones (epinephrine and norepinephrine), though resting levels of these hormones are not reduced.[66]

Exercise training can have varied effects on body composition, depending on its intensity and particularly its duration. Heavy resistance training results in substantial increases in lean body mass, though body fat may not change.[31] Aerobic endurance training induces a much greater caloric cost and appears to produce for some time a systematic imbalance between caloric in-

Table 3–7. Summary of Cardiorespiratory Adaptations to Endurance Training

Parameter	Submaximal Exercise	Maximal Exercise
1. $\dot{V}_E$	−	+
2. Blood lactate	−	+
3. Heart rate	−	0
4. Stroke volume	+	+
5. Cardiac output	−	+
6. a–v$_{O_2}$ difference	+	+
7. $\dot{V}O_2$	0	+
8. Systolic blood pressure	−	0
9. Diastolic blood pressure	0	0

− Indicates decrease; + indicates increase; and 0 indicates no change.

take and cost, thus resulting in a loss of body fat without significant increase in muscle mass.[3] This relationship will be examined at length in a later chapter. While the length of bone cell growth appears almost totally determined by genetic factors, there is substantial evidence indicating that bone diameter and density can be increased by exercise training in the presence of adequate diet.[97]

Flexibility refers to the range of movement in a joint, or in the case of the spinal column, a series of joints. It is, perhaps surprisingly, a rather highly specific quality—that is, one who is extremely flexible in one joint may be average or less in flexibility of other joints.[31] Excellent flexibility is of primary importance in certain joints for success in particular sports, e.g., the trunk in gymnastics, diving, and for a hurdler on the track.

Increased flexibility, achieved via appropriate stretching regimens, is of value to those recovering from injury, such as prolonged immobilization of a limb requiring casting, as well as in relieving unusual exercise induced muscle soreness. Further, enhanced flexibility is thought to have an important role in injury prevention during athletic performance because it permits the musculotendon unit to move through its range of motion with less strain.[14] Nonetheless, physiologic mechanisms attendant to improved flexibility are not well understood.

Flexibility at a joint is limited in part by its bony structure which is not modifiable. In many joints, such as the hip or ankle, range of motion is limited primarily by connective tissue, including the fascial sheath of the muscle but not its contractile elements.[31] A primary factor that complicates the stretching of connective tissue to improve joint flexibility is that it has both elastic (rubber band-like) and viscous (putty-like) properties. To improve range of motion, it is necessary to increase the viscous, or plastic elongation.[66]

Results from animal experiments show that the proportion of elongation that remains after stretching is greater for low-force, long duration stretch.[104] These authors also found that for the same amount of tissue elongation, the high-force stretch method induced more structural tissue weakening than the slow, low-force method. de Vries[30] compared static (low force, long duration) stretch with dynamic (high force, short duration) ballistic stretch effects on flexibility of young adults, and found no significant difference between flexibility improvements induced by the two methods. In view of the myotatic reflex of the stretched muscle being stronger in ballistic stretching, as well as the suggested increase in tissue weakening and possible muscle soreness, static stretching held for 30 to 60 seconds was advocated as the preferred method for enhancing flexibility.

More recent experiments show that elevated temperature (101° to 103°F) enhances the degree of plastic elongation effected by low-force, prolonged stretching.[91] This suggests that stretching preceding athletic performance would be best done after 5 to 10 minutes of slow jogging to elevate muscle temperature. If injured, muscle temperature prior to stretching can be artificially elevated by hot packs, diathermy, or ultrasound.

Use of biofeedback techniques to aid the injured patient in achieving maximum relaxation prior to prolonged stretching has been found to minimize voluntary muscular resistance.[91] Use of proprioceptive neuromuscular facilitation (PNF) to stimulate muscle relaxation via golgi tendon organs of the muscle by maximum contraction prior to stretch has not been found to produce greater hip flexibility than that induced by more conventional methods.[47]

SUMMARY

1. Exercise physiology has well-evidenced roots in physiology during the first half of the 20th century, in which leading physiologists demonstrated the extent of primary organ systems' response to the

stress of exercise and accompanying environmental conditions.

2. Energy supply for muscular work entails an intricate metabolic response system, which provides impressive versatility in meeting the demands for intense, short duration (anaerobic) exercise and prolonged (aerobic) exercise.

3. While ATP, glycogen and fat are utilized as metabolic fuels in different proportions during anaerobic and aerobic work, oxygen is required in an amount needed to meet the overall energy demands according to the combined intensity and duration of activity.

4. The energy requirement for exercise can be closely estimated by the amount of oxygen consumed and less exactly by heart rate, which is affected by environmental conditions and one's emotional state.

5. The cardiorespiratory system provides essential support for sustaining exercise beyond several minutes duration (i.e., aerobic). This is accomplished by increases in cardiac output, pulmonary ventilation, and oxygen extraction from the blood in the muscle tissue.

6. Maximum muscular strength is defined as the amount of force developed in a single maximal effort. With greater strength, fewer motor units are required to effect the same amount of power (explosive performance) and endurance (aerobic performance).

7. In athletic performance where quality of performance is assessed on the basis of time, the relationship of anaerobic and aerobic energy supply is critical. These energy supply processes are intimately tied to the muscle structure and function, which appear to be affected largely by genetic factors.

8. Physiologic explanations for fatigue during sustained performance are incomplete though, in healthy persons, it seems certain that heart function and motor nerves are not important factors. While there is some evidence that the neuromuscular junction is of importance, the principal site of fatigue appears to be within the muscle.

9. Numerous environmental factors exert important limitations in man's capacity for work, some of which can also significantly affect one's safety and well-being.

10. Environmental heat presents a dual stress on the body's circulatory capacity to deliver adequate blood supply to the working muscles and to the periphery for heat dissipation. Sweating, and its effective evaporation, is man's primary defense against hyperthermia.

11. Cold stress signifies that heat loss from the body exceeds metabolic heat production. This can usually be obviated by intelligent choice of clothing, including protection against wind chill and moisture.

12. Altitude has both a facilitating effect on athletic performance because of reduced air density and a negative impact on aerobic endurance because of reduced oxygen pressure and pick-up in the lungs.

13. Air pollution is a problem of increasing environmental concern. Both carbon monoxide and ozone impair aerobic performance, though by different mechanisms.

14. Ergogenic aids are substances utilized to enhance performance. Sports governing bodies, such as the International Olympic Committee and the National Collegiate Athletic Association, have legislated against their use. Amphetamines and anabolic steroids are of particular concern because of deleterious side effects.

15. In most sports, athletes need only a well-balanced diet with increased caloric intake to meet the enhanced energy demands of training and competition. In prolonged endurance activities, utilization of a high carbohydrate diet (i.e., carbohydrate loading) for several days prior to competition has been found to increase muscle glycogen levels and improve performance.

16. Physiologic adaptations to persistent exercise stress occur most readily in accord with effective application of training principles, including (a) training threshold, (b) progressive overload, (c) retrogression due to overtraining, (d) specificity, and (e) individual differences in response to a given training stimulus. Training changes are transient, being lost rapidly following several days, or more, of inactivity.

17. Heavy resistance, low repetition exercise training induces muscle hypertro-

phy and neural changes that increase strength. Limited improvements in muscular power and endurance also occur with this training stimulus.

18. Low resistance, high repetition exercise training induces changes in muscle structure and function, as well as central cardiorespiratory function, which facilitate increased oxygen pick-up in the lungs, transport, and delivery to the muscles, thus effecting significant improvement in endurance performance.

19. An important byproduct of endurance training changes is that it enables one to do the same amount of work with less physiologic strain than before training. This is because it represents a lower percentage of the training induced enhancement of maximum capacity.

20. Flexibility at major joints of the body can be increased by utilization of static (low force, long duration) stretch of the musculotendinous complex.

REFERENCES

1. Adams, W.C.: Effects of ozone exposure at ambient air pollution episode levels on exercise performance. Sports Med. 4:395–424, 1987.
2. Adams, W.C., E.M. Bernauer, D.B. Dill, and J.B. Bomar, Jr.: Effects of equivalent sea-level and altitude training on $\dot{V}O_{2max}$ and running performance. J. Appl. Physiol. 39:262–266, 1975.
3. Adams, W.C., M.M. McHenry, and E.M. Bernauer: Long-term physiologic adaptations to exercise with special reference to performance and cardiorespiratory function in health and disease. Am. J. Cardiol. 33:765–775, 1974.
4. American College of Sports Medicine position stand on prevention of thermal injuries during distance running. Med. Sci. Sports Exer. 16(5):ix–xiv, 1984.
5. Astrand, P-O., and K. Rodahl: Textbook of Work Physiology. Physiological Bases of Exercise. 3rd ed. New York: McGraw-Hill, 1986.
6. Banister, E.W., P.M. Ribisl, G.H. Porter, and A.R. Cillo: The caloric cost of playing handball. Res. Quart. 35:236–240, 1964.
7. Benedict, F.G., and E.P. Cathcart: Muscular Work. Carnegie Inst. of Washington, Publ. No. 187, 1913.
8. Bergh, U., and B. Ekblom: Physical performance and peak aerobic power at different body temperatures. J. Appl. Physiol. 46:885–889, 1979.
9. Bergstrom, J., and E. Hultman: Nutrition for

10. Bjorgum, R.K., and B.J. Sharkey: Inhalation of oxygen as an aid to recovery after exertion. Res. Quart. 37:462–467, 1966.
11. Brewer, V., et al.: Role of exercise in prevention of involutional bone loss. Med. Sci. Sports Exer. 15:445–449, 1983.
12. Bromberg, P.A., and M.J. Hazucha: Is adaptation to ozone protective? Am. Rev. Respir. Dis. 125:489–490, 1982.
13. Brooks, G.A., and T.D. Fahey: Exercise Physiology: Human Bioenergetics and Its Applications. New York: Macmillan, 1985.
14. Brooks, G.A., and T.D. Fahey: Fundamentals of Human Performance. New York: Macmillan, 1987.
15. Brooks, G.A., K.J. Hittelman, J.A. Faulkner, and R.E. Beyer: Temperature, skeletal muscle mitochondrial functions, and oxygen debt. Am. J. Physiol. 220:1053–1059, 1971.
16. Burkett, L.N., and M.T. Falduto: Steroid use by athletes in a metropolitan area. Physician Sportsmed. 12(8):69–74, 1984.
17. Buskirk, E.R., and D.E. Bass: Climate and exercise. In Science and Medicine of Exercise and Sports. Edited by W.R. Johnson. New York: Harper & Brothers, 1960, pp. 311–338.
18. Cann, C.E., M.C. Martin, H.K. Genant, and R.B. Jaffe: Decreased spinal mineral content in amenorrheic women. JAMA. 251:626–629, 1984.
19. Cannon, W.B.: The Wisdom of the Body. 2nd ed. New York: Norton & Co., 1939.
20. Chandler, J.V., and S.N. Blair: The effect of amphetamines on selected physiological components related to athletic success. Med. Sci. Sports Exer. 12:65–69, 1980.
21. Clarke, D.H.: Adaptations in strength and muscular endurance resulting from exercise. In Exercise and Sport Science Reviews. Vol. 1. Edited by J.H. Wilmore. New York: Academic, 1973, pp. 74–102.
22. Close, R.I.: Dynamic properties of mammalian skeletal muscles. Physiol. Rev. 52:129–197, 1972.
23. Costill, D.L., et al.: Leg muscle pH following sprint running. Med. Sci. Sports Exer. 15:325–329, 1983.
24. Costill, D.L., et al.: Adaptations in skeletal muscle following strength training. J. Appl. Physiol. 46:96–99, 1979.
25. Costill, D.L., et al.: Skeletal muscle enzymes and fiber composition in male and female track athletes. J. Appl. Physiol. 40:149–154, 1976.
26. Costill, D.L., and J.M. Miller: Nutrition for endurance sport: carbohydrate and fluid balance. Internat. J. Sports Med. 1:2–14, 1980.
27. Coyle, E.F., et al.: Time course of loss of adaptations after stopping prolonged intense endurance training. J. Appl. Physiol. 57:1857–1864, 1984.

maximal sports performance. JAMA. 221:999–1006, 1972.

28. Daniels, J.: Equating sea-level and altitude distance running times. Track & Field Quart. Rev. *75(4)*:38–39, 1975.

29. Davies, K.J.A., L. Packer, and G.A. Brooks: Biochemical adaptations of mitochondria, muscle, and whole-animal respiration to endurance training. Arch. Biochem. Biophys. *209*:538–553, 1981.

30. de Vries, H.A.: Evaluation of static stretching procedures for improvement of flexibility. Res. Quart. *33*:222–229, 1962.

31. de Vries, H.A.: Physiology of Exercise For Physical Education and Athletics. 4th ed. Dubuque, Iowa: Wm. C. Brown, 1986.

32. Dill, D.B., K. Braithwaite, W.C. Adams, and E.M. Bernauer: Blood volume of middle-distance runners: effect of 2,300-m altitude and comparison with non-athletes. Med. Sci. Sports. *6*:1–7, 1974.

33. Durnin, J.V.G.A.: Protein requirements and physical activity. In Nutrition, Physical Fitness, and Health. Edited by J. Parizkova and V.A. Rogozkin. Baltimore: University Park Press, 1978, pp. 53–60.

34. Felig, P., and J. Wahren: Amino acid metabolism in exercising man. J. Clin. Invest. 50:2703–2714, 1971.

35. Foster, C., D.L. Costill, J.T. Daniels, and W.J. Fink: Skeletal muscle enzyme activity, fiber composition and $\dot{V}O_{2max}$ in relation to distance running performance. Eur. J. Appl. Physiol. *39*:73–80, 1978.

36. Fournier, M., et al.: Skeletal muscle adaptation in adolescent boys: sprint and endurance training and detraining. Med. Sci. Sports Exer. *14*:453–456, 1982.

37. Foxcroft, W.J., and W.C. Adams: Effects of ozone exposure on four consecutive days on work performance and $\dot{V}O_{2max}$. J. Appl. Physiol. *61*:960–966, 1986.

38. Gibbons, S.I., and W.C. Adams: Combined effects of ozone exposure and ambient heat on exercising females. J. Appl. Physiol. *57*:450–456, 1984.

39. Gledhill, N.: Blood doping and related issues: a brief review. Med. Sci. Sports Exer. *14*:183–189, 1982.

40. Gledhill, N.: Bicarbonate ingestion and anaerobic performance. Sports Med. *1*:177–180, 1984.

41. Goldberg, A.L., J.D. Etlinger, D.F. Goldspink, and C. Jablecki: Mechanism of work-induced hypertrophy of skeletal muscle. Med. Sci. Sports. *7*:248–261, 1975.

42. Golding, L.A.: Drugs and hormones. In Ergogenic Aids and Muscular Performance. Edited by W.P. Morgan. New York: Academic Press, 1972, pp. 367–397.

43. Gollnick, P.D., and B. Saltin: Significance of skeletal muscle oxidative enzyme enhancement with endurance training. Clin. Physiol. *2*:1–12, 1982.

44. Gollnick, P.D., B.F. Timson, R.L. Moore, and M. Riedy: Muscular enlargement and number of fibers in skeletal muscles of rats. J. Appl. Physiol. *50*:936–943, 1981.

45. Grimby, G., B. Danneskiold-Samsoe, K. Hvid, and B. Saltin: Morphology and enzymatic capacity in arm and leg muscles in 78–82 year-old men and women. Acta Physiol. Scand. *115*:124–134, 1982.

46. Grimby, G., and B. Saltin: Physiological effects of physical training. Scand. J. Rehab. Med. *3*:6–14, 1971.

47. Hartley-O'Brien, S.J.: Six mobilization exercises for active range of hip flexion. Res. Quart. Exer. Sport. *51*:625–635, 1980.

48. Haymes, E.M.: Iron supplementation. In Encyclopedia of Physical Education, Fitness, and Sports. Vol. 2. Edited by G.A. Stull. Salt Lake City: Brighton, 1980, pp. 335–343.

49. Haymes, E.M., and C.L. Wells: Environment and Human Performance. Champaign, Ill.: Human Kinetics, 1986.

50. Heaney, R.P., R.R. Recker, and P.D. Saville: Menopausal changes in calcium balance performance. J Lab. Clin. Med. *92*:953–963, 1978.

51. Herbert, V.: Nutrition Cultism: Facts and Fictions. Philadelphia: G.F. Stickley, 1980, pp. 121–150.

52. Hermansen, L., E. Hultman, and B. Saltin: Muscle glycogen during prolonged severe exercise. Acta Physiol. Scand. *71*:129–139, 1967.

53. Holloszy, J.O., and E.F. Coyle: Adaptations of skeletal muscle to endurance exercise and their metabolic consequences. J. Appl. Physiol. 56:831–838, 1984.

54. Holmer, I.: Oxygen uptake during swimming in man. J. Appl. Physiol. 33:502–509, 1972.

55. Houston, M.E., H. Bentzen, and H. Larsen: Interrelationships between skeletal muscle adaptations and performance as studied by detraining and retraining. Acta Physiol. Scand. *105*:163–170, 1979.

56. Howley, E.T., and M.E. Glover: The caloric cost of running and walking one mile for men and women. Med. Sci. Sports. *6*:235–237, 1974.

57. Ikai, M., and T. Fukunaga: Calculation of muscle strength per unit cross-sectional area of human muscle by means of ultrasonic measurement. Int. Z. Angew. Physiol. *26*:26–32, 1968.

58. Jansson, E., and L. Kaijser: Muscle adaptation to extreme endurance training in man. Acta Physiol. Scand. *100*:315–324, 1977.

59. Jensen, D.: The Principles of Physiology. 2nd ed. New York: Appleton-Century-Crofts, 1980.

60. Johnson, F.L.: The association of oral androgenic-anabolic steroids and life-threatening disease. Med. Sci. Sports. *7*:284–286, 1975.

61. Karlsson, J., B. Diamant, and B. Saltin: Muscle metabolites during submaximal and maximal exercise in man. Scand. J. Clin. Lab. Invest. 26:385–394, 1971.

62. Karvonen, M.J., E. Kentala, and O. Mustala: The effects of training on heart rate. A longitudinal study. Ann. Med. Experiment. et Biol. Fenniae. 35:305–315, 1957.

63. Kochan, R.G., et al: Glycogen synthase activation in human skeletal muscle: effects of diet and exercise. Am. J. Physiol. 236:E660–E666, 1979.

64. Komi, P.V., and J. Karlsson: Skeletal muscle fiber types, enzyme activities and physical performance in young males and females. Acta Physiol. Scand. 103:210–218, 1978.

65. Krolner, B., B. Toft, S.P. Nielsen, and E. Tondevold: Physical exercise as a prophylaxis against involutional vertebral bone loss: a controlled trial. Clin. Sci. 64:541–546, 1983.

66. Lamb, D.R.: Physiology of Exercise: Responses and Adaptations. 2nd ed. New York: Macmillan, 1984.

67. Lamb, D.R., and G.R. Brodowicz: Optimal use of fluids of varying formulations to minimise exercise-induced disturbances in homeostasis. Sports Med. 3:247–274, 1986.

68. Larsson, L., G. Grimby, and J. Karlsson: Muscle strength and speed of movement in relation to age and muscle morphology. J. Appl. Physiol. 46:451–456, 1979.

69. Laties, V.G., and B. Weiss: The amphetamine margin in sports. Fed. Proceed. 40:2689–2692, 1980.

70. Lavoie, J.-M., A.W. Taylor, and R.R. Montpetit: Skeletal muscle fibre size adaptation to an eight-week swimming programme. Eur. J. Appl. Physiol. 44:161–165, 1980.

71. Lee, C.J., G.S. Lawler, and G.H. Johnson: Effects of supplementation of the diets with calcium and calcium-rich foods on bone density of elderly females with osteoporosis. Am. J. Clin. Nutr. 34:819–823, 1981.

72. MacDougall, J.D., G.R. Ward, D.G. Sale, and J.R. Sutton: Biochemical adaptation of human skeletal muscle to heavy resistance training and immobilization. J. Appl. Physiol. 43:700–703, 1977.

73. Magel, J.R., et al.: Specificity of swim training on maximum oxygen uptake. J. Appl. Physiol. 38:151–155, 1975.

74. McArdle, W.D., F.I. Katch, and V.L. Katch: Exercise Physiology: Energy, Nutrition, and Human Performance. 3rd ed. Philadelphia: Lea & Febiger, 1991.

75. Monster, A.W., H.C. Chan, and D. O'Connor: Activity patterns of human skeletal muscles: relation to muscle fiber type composition. Science. 200:314–317, 1978.

76. Morgan, W.P.: Ergogenic Aids and Muscular Performance. New York: Academic Press, 1972.

77. Murphy, R.J., and W.F. Ashe: Prevention of heat illness in football players. JAMA. 194:180–184, 1965.

78. Newsholme, E.A.: Application of principles of metabolic control to the problem of metabolic limitations in sprinting, middle-distance, and marathon running. Int. J. Sports Med. 7 (Suppl): 66–70, 1986.

79. Nose, H., G.W. Mack, X. Shi, and E.R. Nadel: Role of osmolality and plasma volume during rehydration in humans. J. Appl. Physiol. 65:325–331, 1988.

80. Park, Y.S., et al.: Time course of deacclimatization to cold water immersion in Korean women divers. J. Appl. Physiol. 54:1708–1716, 1983.

81. Parkhouse, W.S., and D.C. McKenzie: Possible contribution of skeletal muscle buffers to enhanced anaerobic performance: a brief review. Med. Sci. Sports Exer. 16:328–338, 1984.

82. Percy, E.C.: Ergogenic aids in athletics. Med. Sci. Sports. 10:298–303, 1978.

83. Peterson, G.E., and T.D. Fahey: HDL-C in five elite athletes using anabolic-androgenic steroids. Physician Sportsmed. 12(6):120–130, 1984.

84. Pollock, M.L.: The quantification of endurance training programs. In Exercise and Sport Sciences Reviews. Vol. 1. Edited by J.H. Wilmore. New York: Academic, 1973, pp. 155–188.

85. Porter, R., and J. Whelan, editors: Human Muscle Fatigue: Physiological Mechanisms. Ciba Foundation Symposium 82. London: Pitman Medical, 1981.

86. Powers, S.K., and S. Dodd: Caffeine and endurance performance. Sports Med. 2:165–174, 1985.

87. Raven, P.B., et al.: Effect of carbon monoxide and peroxyacetyl nitrate on man's maximal aerobic capacity. J. Appl. Physiol. 36:288–293, 1974.

88. Robertson, R.J., et al.: Effect of induced erythrocythemia on hypoxia tolerance during physical exercise. J. Appl. Physiol. 53:490–495, 1982.

89. Saltin, B.: Physiological effects of physical conditioning. Med. Sci. Sports. 1:50–56, 1969.

90. Sanchez-Medal, L., A. Gomez-Leal, L. Duarte, and M.G. Rico: Anabolic androgenic steroids in the treatment of acquired aplastic anemia. Blood. 34:283–300, 1969.

91. Sapega, A.A., T.C. Quedenfeld, R.A. Moyer, and R.A. Butler: Biophysical factors in range-of-motion exercise. Physician Sportsmed. 9(12):57–65, 1981.

92. Schelegle, E.S., and W.C. Adams: Reduced exercise time in competitive simulations consequent to low level ozone exposure. Med. Sci. Sports Exer. 18:408–414, 1986.

93. Sherman, W.M., and D.L. Costill: The marathon: dietary manipulation to optimize performance. Am. J. Sports Med. 12:44–51, 1984.

94. Shibolet, S., M.C. Lancaster, and Y. Danon: Heat

stroke: a review. Aviation, Space, Environ. Med. 47:280–301, 1976.

95. Sidney, K.H., R.J. Shephard, and J. Harrison: Endurance training and body composition of the elderly. Am. J. Clin. Nutr. 30:326–333, 1977.

96. Singer, R.N.: Motor Learning and Human Performance. New York: Macmillan, 1968.

97. Smith, E.L.: Bone changes in the exercising older adult. In Exercise and Aging: The Scientific Basis. Edited by E.L. Smith and R.C. Serfass. Hillside, N.J.: Enslow, 1981, pp. 179–186.

98. Spriet, L.L., et al.: The effect of induced erythrocythemia on central circulation and oxygen transport during maximal exercise. Med. Sci. Sports Exei. 12:122, 1980 (abstract).

99. Stephens, J.A., and A. Taylor: Fatigue of maintained voluntary muscle contraction in man. J. Physiol. (London), 220:1–18, 1973.

100. Stone, J.: Steroids. Natl. Strength Condition. Assoc. J. 5:13, 1983.

101. Thorstensson, A.: Muscle strength, fiber types and enzyme activities in man. Acta Physiol Scand. Suppl. 443:1–45, 1976.

102. Tipton, C.M., R.D. Matthes, J.A. Maynard, and R.A. Carey: The influence of physical activity on ligaments and tendons. Med. Sci. Sports. 7:165–175, 1975.

103. Vander, A.J., J.H. Sherman, and D.S. Luciano: Human Physiology: The Mechanisms of Body Function. 3rd ed. New York: McGraw-Hill, 1980.

104. Warren, C.G., J.F. Lehmann, and J.N. Koblanski: Heat and stretch procedures: an evaluation using rat tail tendon. Arch. Phys. Med. Rehabil. 57:122–126, 1976.

105. Weltman, A.L., B.A. Stamford, R.J. Moffatt, and V.L. Katch: Exercise recovery, lactate removal, and subsequent high intensity exercise performance. Res. Quart. 48:786–796, 1977.

106. Wilkes, D., N. Gledhill, and R. Smyth: Effect of acute induced metabolic alkalosis on 800-m racing time. Med. Sci. Sports Exer. 15:277–280, 1983.

107. Williams, M.H.: Drugs and Athletic Performance. Springfield: Charles C Thomas, 1974.

108. Williams, M.H.: Nutritional Aspects of Human Physical and Athletic Performance. Springfield: Charles C Thomas, 1976.

109. Wright, J.E.: Anabolic steroids and athletics. In Exer. Sport Sci. Rev. Vol. 8. Edited by R.S. Hutton and D.I. Miller. Philadelphia: Franklin Institute, 1980, pp. 149–202.

BIBLIOGRAPHY

1. Astrand, P.-O., and K. Rodahl: Textbook of Work Physiology. 3rd ed. New York: McGraw-Hill, 1986.

2. Brooks, G.A., and T.D. Fahey: Exercise Physiology: Human Bioenergetics and Its Applications. New York: Macmillan, 1985.

3. Brooks, G.A., and T.D. Fahey: Fundamentals of Human Performance. New York: Macmillan, 1987.

4. de Vries, H.A.: Physiology of Exercise for Physical Education and Athletics. 4th ed. Dubuque, Iowa: William C. Brown, 1986.

5. Fox, E.L., R.W. Bowers, and M.L. Foss: The Physiological Basis of Physical Education and Athletics. 4th ed. Philadelphia: Saunders, 1988.

6. Jensen, D.: The Principles of Physiology. 2nd ed. New York: Appleton-Century-Crofts, 1980.

7. Lamb, D.R.: Physiology of Exercise: Responses and Adaptations. 2nd ed. New York: Macmillan, 1984.

8. McArdle, W.D., F.I. Katch, and V.L. Katch: Exercise Physiology: Energy, Nutrition, and Human Performance. 3rd ed. Philadelphia: Lea & Febiger, 1991.

9. Noble, B.J.: Physiology of Exercise and Sport. St. Louis: Times Mirror/Mosby, 1986.

10. Vander, A.J., J.H. Sherman, and D.S. Luciano: Human Physiology: The Mechanisms of Body Function. 3rd ed. New York: McGraw-Hill, 1980.

4

PSYCHOLOGIC FOUNDATIONS: MOTOR LEARNING, EXERCISE, AND SPORT PSYCHOLOGY

INTRODUCTION

Physical activity elicits neurophysiologic responses, which have clear overlap in biomechanics, exercise physiology, and to those who seek an effective understanding of the psychology of exercise and sport. In essence, this is a simple resultant of the fact that psychology, the science of behavior, emerged in part from the biologic sciences. The main focus of psychology, however, is on how living organisms respond to and adjust to their environment, both physical and social. As in other sciences, psychology attempts to theorize (or explain in general terms) from specific sets of observations which, however, represents a particularly difficult task when analyzing human behavior. This is so because measurement of human behavior is subject to numerous potentially confounding effects.

Significant recent advances have been made in the scientific study of human behavior in exercise and sport contexts. Current primary areas of study are: (1) motor learning, including how man produces, learns, and retains proficiency in motor performance; (2) psychosocial influences on physical performance, which includes the study of factors in one's social environment that affect the ability to produce maximum performance; (3) psychologic effects of exercise training and sports participation; and (4) motivation for engaging in organized physical activity programs, including identification and study of factors which impel man to become active and those factors which are likely to inhibit elective physical activity participation.

MOTOR CONTROL AND SKILL ACQUISITION

The terms motor control and skill acquisition represent an expansion for emphasis of what constitutes the field of motor learning. Motor control refers to the internal neuromuscular processes inherent in human motor response, while motor skill acquisition emphasizes other factors affecting the development of efficient, reproducible movements. Motor learning, then, consists of an interrelation of a neurophysiologic component (motor control) and a behavioral component (motor skill acquisition). It represents a relatively permanent change in motor behavior as a result of practice. (How long does it take to "relearn" typing or riding a bicycle, once well learned, after some years of no practice?) However, the learning is not directly observable, but is an inference based on change in performance following repeated trials (practice). For example, with appropriate instruction and practice for basketball, one increases the number of baskets he/she can make from the free-throw line for a given number of attempts. The improved performance in this set of conditions is termed motor learning. However, we can then create conditions that interfere with performance (e.g., random distractions), but which do not change the amount of motor learning that has taken place. Further, one's performance may change as a result of improved muscular strength, endurance, or both, but this is not learning. Indeed, motor learning can occur without a parallel change in performance.

HISTORIC DEVELOPMENT OF MOTOR LEARNING IN PHYSICAL EDUCATION

Motor learning has been the subject of scientific investigation by psychologists, physiologists, and more recently by physical educators. One of the earliest studies of motor skill development in this country (done in the late 1890s) was concerned with how men learned to transmit Morse Code on a telegraph key.[71] The development of extensive assembly line production during the first quarter of this century resulted in numerous studies by industrial psychologists of machine control features and the organization of assembly line tasks. The military's requirement for human's rapid learning of motor tasks associated with skilled performance of gunnery and control manipulation for numerous devices on ships, aircraft, and tanks resulted in an unparalleled period of motor learning research during WWII. Some largely descriptive research of how various factors influenced the rate at which students learned sports skills was initiated in physical education during the 1930s and continued into the 1950s. Henry, a trained psychologist working in the Physical Education Department at the University of California, Berkeley, made two particularly significant contributions to the field of motor learning during the 1950s and 1960s. The first involved recognition of the influence of individual differences in prior experience on learning rates in sports skill development, and the use of unique laboratory motor performance tasks. The second was the development of the memory drum theory to explain motor memory, and which constituted the first physical educator's use of a model to account for behavioral differences specific to motor performance.[71] This emphasis on the study of mechanisms underlying motor control and

learning has gained great emphasis in the past 15 years. There has been a shift in research by both psychologists and physical educators from a product-performance orientation to the study of processes underlying motor performance and learning.[71]

THEORIES OF MOTOR CONTROL AND SKILL ACQUISITION

Numerous theories have been advanced to explain the basic nature of motor control and skill acquisition, but no single model has been developed which can definitively explain these phenomena. In this section, several prominent theories will be developed briefly, though one should recognize that they present ideas in the form of psychologic constructs, rather than in terms of specific anatomic and functional characteristics of the CNS. Obviously, they are subject to modification with future research.

MOTOR CONTROL. Two models of motor control have been developed: (1) open-loop control, and (2) closed-loop control. Figure 4–1 is a schematic representation of the two models. A motor program is an abstract plan of movement from which the movement commands are developed, using information about the environment, desired outcome and other relevant input. The primary difference between the two theories involves the use of feedback, which provides the brain with information about some response which can be used to alter movement commands for effecting improved performance. In the open-loop control theory, movement commands are issued providing the specifications of the movement. These commands travel nerve pathways to the muscles and movement occurs. The commands are then carried out in full, and feedback can only be used after *completion* of the movement.[39] This theory can explain rapid ballistic movements, but what about slow movements in which an individual can correct the movement before its completion?

The closed-loop theory of motor control is basically the same as the open-loop theory, except that feedback is used through-

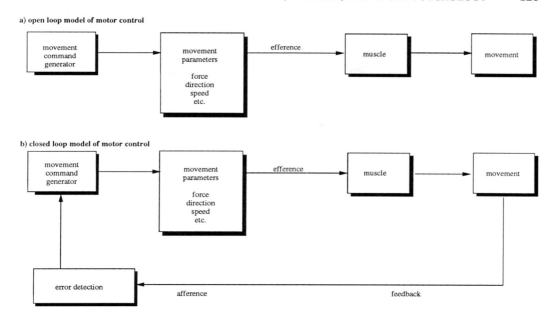

FIG. 4–1. Open- and closed-loop models of motor control. Part a) depicts an open-loop system and part b) depicts a closed-loop system. (Modified from Sage, G.H.: Motor Learning and Control: A Neurophysical Approach. Dubuque, Iowa: Wm. C. Brown, 1984, p. 232.)

out the movement to ensure correctness of the individual's response. The feedback is used to change the motor command mid-movement; thus this theory can be used to explain slow, precision movements. Rapid movements, however, cannot be explained by the closed-loop model because the entire movement time is too quick for feedback to reach the brain and correct movement commands to be sent back to the working muscles.[64] Recent research suggests that an integration of the two models may be more accurate, since both types of control can probably occur, depending on the characteristics of the movement.[64]

MOTOR LEARNING. The process of motor learning involves a relatively permanent change in behavior, which implies that changes have been made in the motor program for a given movement. This would involve the use of the structures and functions of memory as tools to achieve, retain, and recall these changes in the motor program.

Psychologists have identified two basic storage structures of memory which are termed short- and long-term memory. The functional characteristics of short- and long-term memory can be viewed as points along a continuum. Short-term (also referred to as the shallow level of processing) memory has both a relatively limited capacity for storing information, and limited, time dependent storage as well. Long-term memory (a deeper level of processing) seems to have an unlimited capacity, and duration of information storage is indefinite. The mechanism by which motor skill information moves from short- to long-term memory is still unclear,[39] but may occur in somewhat the same manner as in verbal learning, where information is grouped and categorized and often associated with past knowledge.

Two important aspects of memory are retention and forgetting. Retention is evidenced by the persistence of a learned task, while forgetting refers to a loss in performance.[58] Time seems to be the major factor for information retention in short-term memory, in that the information will be lost due to the limited storage duration characteristic of short-term memory. Retention and forgetting in long-term memory, however, are less well understood, though two basic ideas predominate. One suggests that loss of information over time is due simply to decay, while the other explains losses by the interference of new learning and experiences (i.e., information overload). However, some[39] believe that forgetting in long-term memory is perhaps a problem of relocation and retrieval of information from storage rather than a "loss" of information. Either way, however, motor skills seem to be resistant to forgetting, and the more well-learned the task, the less loss over time will occur.[58]

In the early 1970s, Adams[1] developed a closed loop theory of motor learning, in which comparison of feedback to a memory "perceptual trace" of the correct responses of the movement is used to guide its subsequent accomplishment. While this theory has been largely substantiated by results from subsequent research on slow, linear positioning movements, it is lacking in explaining how many other skills, such as ballistic and rapid tracking movements, are learned.

Subsequently, Schmidt[65] developed the schema theory of motor learning, using the work of Adams and others as a basis, while trying to eliminate their limitations. Schmidt's theory hypothesized that after a movement is made, four types of information are used to develop a relationship which can later be used to plan similar movements. They include: (1) the initial conditions before movement started (limb position, environmental conditions, etc.); (2) the response specifications or parameters of the movement (force, direction, speed, etc.); (3) the movement outcome (was it successful?); and (4) the sensory consequences of the movement (sensory feedback from proprioceptors, visual feedback, etc.). The relationship formed using these pieces of information is termed the recall schema (a rule, or set of rules, for a general type of movement). This schema is then used in future trials to select the appropriate parameters of the movement which will come closest to producing the desired outcome in light of the initial conditions. Schmidt also proposed the existence of a recognition schema which is analogous to the recall schema, but instead of selecting the parameters, it estimates the

sensory consequences of the movement and can thus be used to determine correctness.[65]

In both fast and slow movements, the parameters and expected sensory consequences are used to produce the motor commands, but in slow movements the recognition schema is also used during the movement to assure correctness via sensory feedback in comparison to the expected sensory consequences. Learning thus develops both schema more fully, such that the motor program can be modified for the specific conditions encountered.[66]

MOTOR PERFORMANCE CLASSIFICATIONS

Those who wish to develop efficient strategies for teaching motor skills have found it helpful to classify them according to several apparently dichotomous categories. They actually exist on a continuum, but this effort is still useful because it enables one to make general statements about how to teach a broad range of skills, rather than having to develop a virtually unlimited number of specific statements about how to teach each skill. The objective is to focus on what skills have in common, even when they might appear to be quite unalike, so that one can make effective use of efficient instructional techniques developed for common elements of previously well studied skills. The most frequently used motor skill classification categories are: (1) bodily involvement and precision of movement; (2) distinctiveness of beginning and end points; and (3) stability of the environment.

Bodily involvement and precision of movement evaluation of skills enables one to classify them as being more representative of gross or fine movement skills. Gross motor skills, such as running, jumping, and throwing, involve the large body musculature in coordinated movement patterns. However, elements of muscular strength, power, and endurance are also required for successful performance of these skills, while precision of movement is of less importance. Fine motor skills, such as violin playing, writing, and watch-making necessitate excellent hand-eye coordination and precision of movement.

When a skill has a distinct beginning and end, such as a basketball free throw or a golf putt, it is termed a discrete task. Some skills, such as throwing a javelin, performing a dance routine, or serving a tennis ball, require that a certain number of discrete skills be accomplished in a prescribed sequence. These are called serial tasks and usually involve a proper timing of the ordered sequence of discrete elements. If a skill has no distinct beginning or ending other than that dictated by the performer and/or external forces, such as in steering an automobile or going on a training run, it is referred to as a continuous task.

When attempting to improve certain motor skills, it is helpful to determine if they require an emphasis on previously programmed automatic response or upon the ability to perceive and interpret cues in a changing environment. In the first condition, the environmental situation is predictable and constant, and the automatic, single response is referred to as a closed skill. An example is the shooting of a basketball free throw. The physical environment in which the shot is performed remains relatively constant and unchanged each time it is attempted. The shooter is always 15 feet from the basket; the basket is 10 feet high; the net is the same length and attached to the basket in the same manner; the backboard is, for the most part, stable, made of the same materials, and stationary; the players on either side of the shooter are at least the same minimum distance away and restricted in their movement; and finally, the ball is the same circumference and weight, and is generally made of the same material. In essence, the player does not have to worry about a changing environment (i.e., an opponent jumping in front of him, the basket moving, etc.). Thus, the emphasis is placed upon technique and conformity to a prescribed standard of performance. Once the free shot has been taken and the basketball game continues, individual players are confronted by a multiple response, open skill environment, in which it is not enough to be able to perform certain parts of the game well. One must be able to integrate them in response to a complex, dynamic environment. The ability to run, cut, pivot, dribble, block and shoot, for example, is only as useful as one's ability to integrate the acts into a movement pattern which is capable of being appropriately manipulated and altered as cues are perceived, identified, and interpreted.

Bowling, archery, target shooting, and skills in gymnastics and diving are thought to be more closed than open skills, and require a great deal of standardized practice and habit formation in order for the desired results to accrue. Games such as football, basketball, soccer, and handball are examples of activities thought to be more on the "open" end of the skill continuum.

Another potentially useful motor performance evaluative procedure is the analysis of the complexity of each of four subcomponents: (1) perception; (2) decision making; (3) the motor act itself; and (4) feedback availability. This task analysis procedure, developed by Billing,[6] is summarized in schematic form in Figure 4–2.

PHASES OF MOTOR LEARNING

It appears that there is a general sequence involving several phases during the course of motor skill learning. Fitts[21] identified three phases: (1) early, cognitive; (2) intermediate, associative; and (3) final, autonomous. In the first phase, the learner must understand the goal of the motor task, the movements that will bring about accomplishment of the goal, and the strategy that will work best to produce the desired movements. Sage[64] correctly contends that effective learning of a skill does not necessarily begin when practice starts, but before with a cognitive understanding of the task. In the second, associative phase, movements become fused into well-coordinated patterns. This involves reduction in gross errors and elimination of extraneous movements, as spatial and temporal organization are achieved. The basic motor program nears full development as various components of the movement pattern, independent at first, become effectively integrated.

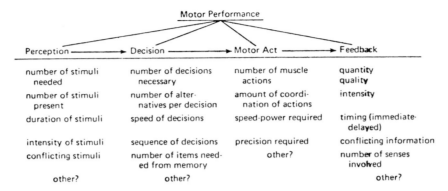

FIG. 4–2. Motor acts analyzed according to the complexity of each subcomponent. (From Billing, J.: An overview of task complexity. Motor Skills: Theory Into Practice. 4:18–23, 1980.)

The final, autonomous phase involves increasingly effective evidence of spatial and temporal aspects. This appears to be the result of motor programs of enhanced length and integration. Further, if the movement pattern is interfered with by conscious thought, the effective autonomous integration becomes partially disrupted. As a final caveat, Sage[64] contends that it is not accurate to assume that there are independent and distinct phases in motor skill learning. Rather, the process entails gradual, complex changes in movement patterns and in the involved processes.

FACTORS AFFECTING MOTOR LEARNING

Seemingly enumerable factors influence how one most effectively learns motor skills. In this section, the most prominent will be identified and briefly discussed.

Rather striking differences amongst individuals in their initial performance of a motor skill is a common observation. Evidence suggests that this is due to differences in basic motor abilities which underlie or contribute to success in one or more motor skills. Motor skills are learned, while motor abilities are theoretically personal traits or characteristics which are affected primarily by genetics, but also by previous experience. They include perceptual-motor abilities, such as multi-limb coordination, control precision, reaction time, and speed of arm movement, as well

as the physical proficiency abilities of static strength, dynamic strength, dynamic flexibility, gross body coordination, and stamina (endurance).[39] To minimize the effect of prior experience on motor performance and learning, the experimenter frequently utilizes rather unique tasks that simulate a general motor ability (e.g., coordinated movement of both hands, as is being measured in Figure 4–3).

It is surprising to many how poorly related apparently similar motor abilities are. For example, Henry[28] found a low correlation (r = 0.02) between subjects' reaction time (time from auditory tone stimulus until start of movement) and movement time of their finger through a target 30 inches away; thus these two perceptual motor abilities are clearly distinct. A similar observation was made by Drowatzky and Zucatto,[17] who found that performance on three different tests of static balance did not correlate significantly with any of three different dynamic balance tests.

It appears that it is the existence of a large number of motor abilities that each individual has different quantities of which accounts for their different levels of performance upon initial trial of a motor skill. Further, it has been observed that their ability to learn, i.e., improve performance with the same amount of practice, differs and is not related in a systematic way to their initial performance.[39] Again, this appears to be due to different levels of basic motor abilities, which have been found to influence learning to different degrees at

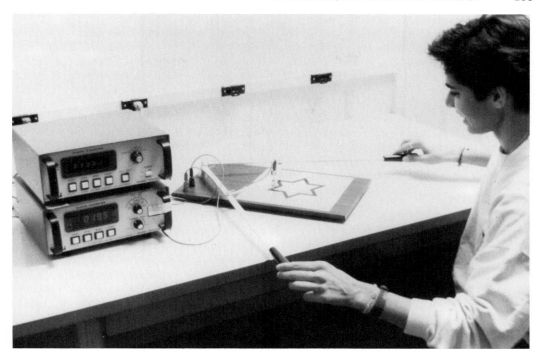

FIG. 4–3. Subject performing a star-tracing task. The goal is to trace the pattern of the star as quickly as possible while contacting the side boundaries of the star's path as little as possible. One timer measures elapsed time from start to finish, while the other records error time.

early, middle and late stages of the learning process. That is, the abilities which are important to high initial performance during the cognitive stage are not the same as the abilities which account for high levels of performance during the associative or autonomous stages.[39]

All of us are aware of the "all-around" athlete who seemingly excels in all sports and presumably any motor performance. Careful examination of this phenomenon, however, reveals that it is, in many ways a myth, especially with respect to the actual limited range of activities in which it is evidenced for any single individual.[68] When it does occur, it is in part because the particular sports necessitate a few motor abilities in common, such as dynamic strength, fast reaction time, speed of movement, and agility. The individual has uncommonly high levels in these few motor abilities, but may be below average in many others. Further, there is also evidence suggesting that these individuals are successful in several

sports because they have an unusually rich practice time in each sport than do the vast majority of individuals with whom they are compared.[66]

Learning a motor skill necessitates effective provision of information relevant to the task in a number of ways, including: (1) verbal and written directives; (2) visual and auditory perception; (3) actually performing the task and utilizing various forms of feedback available; and (4) any combination of the above. However, the best choice of one or all of these informational cue sources, together with the intensity and/or serial order of each, is not yet resolved. In addition to this perceptual input, one must match it with an effector mechanism (information processor) and decision mechanism capability in order to realize skilled performance. This distinction is a potentially fruitful intuition for identifying where critical deficiencies in skilled performance exist. For example, if one suspects a perception deficiency in being able to hit a pitched baseball, this could be determined via identification as a strike or ball, curve or fast ball, etc. on a video laboratory experimental setup. Identifying informational processing capability is difficult to distinguish from decision making time. It seems clear, however, that the most successful batters are those who can wait late to make the decision to swing or not. The pitch takes about 0.6 seconds to arrive, while the batter's reaction time and movement time entail 0.2 and 0.1 seconds, respectively. Thus, the batter must decide to swing, or not, at a time only half of that following delivery of the pitch and its arrival.

A great amount of information that is sensed is not recognized internally by the learner and thus, is not processed. For sensed information to be processed, it must be perceived. Perception is a process that requires detection and recognition. Comparison to previous experience in long-term memory facilitates the process. If the learner has little relevant experience, perception will take longer. Also, until the perception is correct, there is low probability of the response being right.

Perception is enhanced when the process of attention is functioning properly. Attention refers to the individual's readiness to receive and interpret selectively information from a variety of environmental sources. It also includes the ability to concentrate on blocking out irrelevant information, or cues, as well as anticipation to permit better positioning and timing of the response to the situational demand. This is crucial to skilled performance, as is the development of selective attention in recognizing the most important cues, since only a limited amount of information can be processed at one time. The more complex the situation, the more cues one will have to interpret.

The highly skilled performer is able to recognize and correctly interpret the most relevant cues quicker than can the novice. As the result of experience, and often by trial and error, the skilled performer is able to identify certain cues as being irrelevant to successful performance. During the early stages of learning, one reacts to a variety of cues, some of which either ad-

versely affect or contribute little to the performance of the task. After performing the task several times, one becomes better able to make decisions about the value of the various cues received. However, in some instances an individual may recognize that movement patterns are incorrect but fail to realize what should be done to bring about the correct movement pattern. Conversely, some individuals would be capable of effecting a change in behavior if they knew what they were doing wrong. The skilled performer has also learned to match the correct amount of arousal to attend optimally to the cues presented. The beginner may not be sufficiently aroused, but in many instances may become too anxious to attend to the appropriate cues that might otherwise be properly processed.

In addition to the obvious importance of providing appropriate information prior to the learner attempting a motor task, feedback, i.e., sensory information about one's performance, has been shown to affect the rate of learning. Feedback comes from two sources: (1) that which is self-generated via sensory perception, primarily occurring during the performance; and (2) supplemental feedback, termed knowledge of results (KR) following performance. Feedback can be obtained via visual and auditory stimuli, as well as by processing muscle, tendon, and joint sensory input. Knowledge of results is obtained via direct observation or through some external source, such as a teacher or more experienced performer. It appears that learning occurs as one internalizes a model of correct performance, which is formulated by the individual matching his own sensory feedback information with the KR information concerning his performance. As shown in Figure 4–4, the type of KR is of importance in facilitating learning, especially in the early stages. In this comparison, the number of errors for each block of ten trials is seen to be a function of the preciseness of KR. That is, quantitative information (e.g., how far you missed the target) generally facilitates learning more than qualitative information (e.g., you're off to the right, getting closer, etc.). However, it has been observed that too detailed KR can confuse the beginner and actually

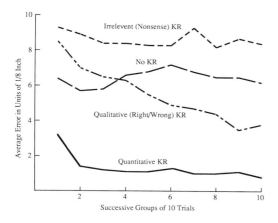

FIG. 4–4. Results of the effect of various levels of precision of knowledge of results (KR) on a line drawing task. (From Trowbridge, M.H., and H. Carson: An experimental study of Thorndike's theory of learning. J. General Psych. 7:245–260, 1932.)

deter learning. It appears that with practice the learner becomes less dependent on the KR information and is able to depend more on information stored in his own internal model of correct performance.[39]

One's motivation to learn is of vital importance, in that it affects the initiation, maintenance, and intensity of behavior.[39] Motivation to initiate learning and to persist in what may become intensive practice sessions is accomplished via internal (intrinsic) and extrinsic sources. The former includes doing something for fun, to develop skills, or to become fulfilled. Extrinsic motivation includes rewards or recognition.[69] It is important to realize that a high level of intrinsic motivation may not be present for effective learning to take place. For example, a person may be in attendance due to extrinsic factors, such as a requirement or because a friend wanted him to be. Following instruction, initial practice, and learning, the individual may become intrinsically motivated to continue practice and increase its intensity.[39]

Reinforcement is an extrinsic motivational tool which is used to increase the probability of a response occurring again. It consists of providing a tangible or intangible reward upon the individual's improved performance of a task. To be most

effective, the reinforcement must be important to the performer, and given at a time in close association with the response.[39]

Setting of meaningful performance goals that are realistic for the skill levels and capabilities of a group has been found to facilitate learning. In the classic study by Locke and Bryan[38] learning, as reflected in the correct performance of a complex motor task (Fig. 4–5), was faster and greater in a condition employing a hard but attainable goal, compared to the other group who were merely asked to do their best on each trial. Goals should be specific to the task and used before each practice attempt, as well as for each practice session. Further, they should be regularly monitored and modified as appropriate.[69]

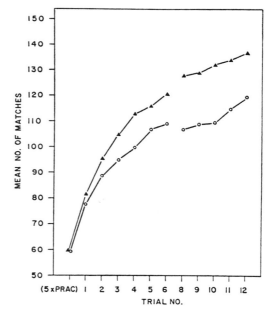

FIG. 4–5. Performance curves for two groups provided with different incentive goals for performing a complex motor task (open circles, "do your best" group; darkened triangles, group given a hard but attainable goal). (From Locke, E.A., and J.F. Bryan: Cognitive aspects of psychomotor performance: The effects of performance goals on level of performance. J. Appl. Psych. 50:286–291, 1966.)

PRACTICE CONDITIONS AFFECTING MOTOR LEARNING

There is a steadily increasing body of knowledge detailing practice methods for enhancing motor learning. First, practice should be meaningful, both in terms of adhering to general guidelines attendant to the factors affecting motor learning discussed in the immediately preceding section, as well as those which follow in this section. For example, the learner should understand the purpose of the practice session. After each attempt, some feedback should be received about the results to enable interpretations for altering subsequent execution. The quantity and quality of the information received, along with one's ability to interpret and apply it, will to a large extent govern the value of the practice and ultimately the level of skill attained.

Meaningful practice also entails ensuring that it utilizes movements in temporal and spatial relationship as close to those characteristic of highly skilled performance. For example, if both speed and accuracy are of near equal importance in skilled performance, both should be stressed, rather than to work on accuracy and then increase speed, or vice versa.[79] Solley[70] has observed that when accuracy is achieved at relatively slow speeds, it is lost quite rapidly when the performer increases the tempo of the movement pattern. It appears that when practicing at low speeds, one develops habits of coordination which may be quite different from those needed at high speeds in skilled performance. Not only is the learned coordination different, but it may actually interfere with the proper performance of the skill as it must ultimately be used.

The total amount of practice until learning shows a definite plateau represents an optimal level in terms of time efficiency. However, overlearning, i.e., practicing at the same intensity beyond that point, may lead to only slight improvements in performance, but can aid significantly in retention with reduction or cessation of practice. Further practice to achieve a greater overlearning effect is not productive, especially when one considers time limitations and the increased learning to practice time ratio that could be achieved in other aspects of a complex sport.[39]

The use of whole or part practice depends for best results on correct evaluation of the motor task with regard to its organization and complexity. If the task is highly organized (where the parts are intimately related) and of low complexity, practicing the task as a whole has been found to yield enhanced learning relative to the part method.[69] The latter method entails breaking up the whole task into a number of parts, practicing each separately until all parts are well learned, and then practicing all parts together until the whole task is well learned. This procedure has been advantageous in learning tasks that are highly complex but which have low organization, i.e., consisting of parts which are not highly interdependent. Serial tasks, such as dance or gymnastics free exercise routines, are examples of this type of motor performance. When using the part method, it is best to ensure that components of the skill which are significantly associated be practiced together as a unit. Parts of the skill that are relatively independent can be practiced separately.[39]

Mental practice occurs when one consciously visualizes the motor task to be performed in the absence of overt physical performance. It entails concentration and is concerned with accurate imagery production and "visual" rehearsal of correct performance of the skill. Research results have been rather equivocal, in that mental practice sometimes produces no greater learning than that evidenced by a control group's performance. This has been explained by Ryan and Simons[63] to be the result of mental practice affecting learning only in motor tasks with a high cognitive element. If the task is relatively simple, e.g., limb movement speed or accuracy, mental practice has no appreciable effect. It also appears that it is most productive in the early cognitive stage of complex tasks without the learner being pressured simultaneously to perform the skill. In the later stages of learning, mental practice appears to have benefit in assisting the learner to consolidate strategies, as well as to correct errors.[39]

Investigations regarding distribution of

practice effects on motor learning which compare one practice session of equivalent time to several sessions (distributed), have yielded results which suggest that distributed practice is better. However, careful analysis indicates that distributed schedule superiority is a performance attribute rather than a learning one.[39] Performance is reduced during a prolonged massed practice session due to boredom and/or fatigue. Practicing while fatigued, at least up to moderately heavy levels, appears to affect performance as shown in the first 20 trials in Figure 4–6. However, learning results were similar for both the fatigued and nonfatigued groups when retested for 10 trials 3 days later (neither group received the fatigue pretreatment on the retest day).[24] With continued practice, advanced learners appear to profit by intensive massed practice more than do inexperienced beginners. Nonetheless, caution in some events, when fatigue induces enhanced risk of injury, precludes extending practice sessions.[39]

TRANSFER OF LEARNING

This occurs as a function of the effect of a previously learned motor skill on the initial performance and/or learning of another task. In general, laboratory research indicates, as summarized in Figure 4–7, that motor skill transfer to performance of another skill occurs as a function of the degree of stimulus similarity and the degree of response similarity. When both are similar, there is highly positive transfer (performance is better); when the stimuli are dissimilar and the responses similar, there is slight positive transfer; when both the stimuli and responses are dissimilar, there is no transfer; and when the stimuli are similar, but the responses different, there can be negative transfer (i.e., performance is worse on the second task than for a control group with no practice on the first task).[15] It appears that greater positive transfer occurs when learning of the first skill is advanced and during the initial stage of learning the second task. Achievement of advanced skill in the second task comes only with continued practice in that activity.[69]

Transfer in real-world sports skills has not been studied systematically. However, there is some evidence suggesting that apparently similar skills, but with rather subtle dissimilarities (for example, the badminton and tennis stroking actions), can

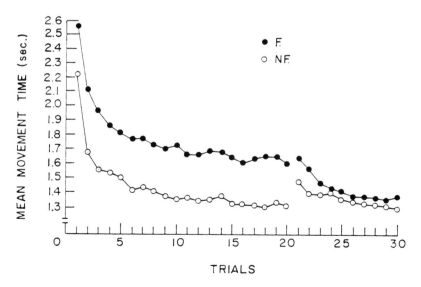

FIG. 4–6. Performance curves of mean movement time for the fatigue (darkened circles) and the no-fatigue (open circles) groups. (From Godwin, M.A. and R.A. Schmidt: Muscular fatigue and learning a discrete motor skill. Res. Quart. 42:374–382, 1971.)

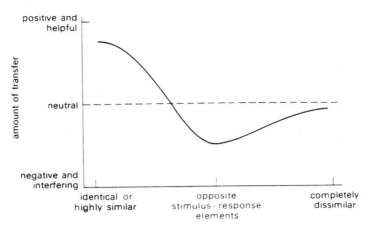

similarity between task 1 and task 2

FIG. 4–7. Effects of task similarity on transfer. When tasks 1 and 2 are identical or highly similar, performance on task 2 is facilitated. When the tasks have opposite stimulus-response elements, performance on task 2 is hindered. When the tasks are completely dissimilar, performance on task 2 is unaffected. (From Sage, G.H.: Motor Learning and Control: A Neurophysiological Approach. Dubuque, Iowa: Wm. C. Brown, 1984, p. 330.)

interfere with effective learning of the second skill.[69] In general, the degree to which one is able to transfer the knowledge and skill learned in one activity to another depends on: (1) the existence of general factors common to both activities (such factors might include rules of play, equipment involved, and strategy); (2) identical elements common to both (similar stimulus conditions and responses, including movement patterns); and (3) one's ability to recognize and utilize elements common to both tasks, as well as an awareness of those elements essential to one but not necessary to the other.

PSYCHOSOCIAL EFFECTS ON PHYSICAL PERFORMANCE

There is great public awareness of the presumed preeminent effect of the psychologic edge to achieve athletic success. This notion is enhanced by persistent media accounts from coaches and athletes to provide revelations as to what gave them the "winning edge." Nonetheless, there seems to be little of substance that one can identify with consistency. It seems likely that this situation will persist for some time, as there is undoubtedly an important psychologic dimension to all athletic performance which, however, is not yet well documented. This is due, in part, to the fact that sport psychology only emerged as a recognized subdiscipline of physical education during the late 1960s and relatively little research occurred before then. Also, there have been persistent research methodologic problems, including use of readily available but imprecise measurement techniques, lack of appropriate theoretical models, and difficulties in controlling potentially confounding factors.

PERSONALITY AND ATHLETIC PERFORMANCE

One's personality consists of a relatively stable set of characteristics or traits, which influence one's behavior. These traits were originally thought to represent reasonably accurate predictive tendencies of a person's response in a variety of environmental situations. The relationship between personality and athletic performance was the first research area to be studied persistently by sport psychologists. Ryan[60] contends that this was due largely to a prevalent belief from empirical observation that individual differences in personality distinguished between athletes and non-athletes, individual sport and team sport athletes, and between good performers and poor performers. After more than a decade of persistent research examining the credibility of this prevalent notion, it was concluded that personality traits were a poor predictor of physical abilities, accounting for only 10 to 20% of the variance in predicting performance.[20,47]

Part of the reason for this discrepancy between empirical observation and research findings is due to the fact that many individuals demonstrate behavior in a given situation, e.g., aggressiveness by a football player during a contest, which may represent only a temporary mood or state, which is at variance with a persistent personality trait measured as normal or below average in aggressiveness.[20] Thus, athletic performance may well represent a special environment that depends on more narrow personality traits than previously identified in academic psychology.[47]

More recent research in sport personology reflects a significant change, which now includes examination of competitive anxiety, achievement motivation, assessment of cognitive processes of athletes during performance (via various recall procedures), and perceptual characteristics of athletes. The latter approach is of interest, in that initial investigations of athletes and nonathletes reveal a consistent difference in perception that mirrors a previously developed theory. That is, some individuals consistently perceive stimuli as being less than they actually are (reducers), while others perceive stimuli as greater (augmentors). Contact athletes (football players and wrestlers) were found to have significantly reduced perception of pain, as well as time and kinesthetic figural after effect, compared to noncontact athletes (golf, tennis, and track), with nonathletes significantly different from both groups.[59] It is not clear how much of this perceptual behavior difference might be due to self-selectivity into contact and noncontact sports, and how much may have developed with athletic participation.

MOTIVATION AND ATHLETIC PERFORMANCE

Motivation deals with factors which energize performance. With regard to motivation for achieving excellence in athletic performance, the concern is with identifying why, when the stimulus is apparently the same, the response (behavior) is notably different.

Research results indicate that goal setting enhanced elbow flexion, strength, and middle distance run time in college non-athletes.[39] Goal setting appears effective because of its probable influence on psychologic states, such as more direct attention to important aspects of the task and intensity of effort.[25] Realistic goal setting may also increase self-confidence, a factor identified with a general psychologic profile for achieving peak performance. Other factors include: (1) self-regulation of arousal, (2) concentration (i.e., being appropriately focused), (3) positive thoughts and imagery, and (4) determination and commitment.[78]

Level of aspiration refers to the goal or standard by which a person judges his performance as a success or failure, or as being up to what is expected. Numerous factors have been found to influence one's level of aspiration. Those individuals who have a low "need for achievement" tend to set rather low, easily attainable goals that have little impact on performance. Those with high need achievement tend to set high, but attainable goals which appear to act as an incentive.[61] A more important factor seems to be one's past experiences in achieving his levels of aspiration. It has been found that successful experiences usually lead to an increased level of aspiration. However, expectation of failure has been found to develop more quickly when failure followed uninterrupted success than when it followed intermittent success and failure.[20]

Failure usually results in a lowering of one's level of aspiration. However, if the individual experiences a performance below his original level of aspiration, and sees it as a severe threat to self-esteem, he may keep his level of aspiration low to prevent such a situation from arising a second time.

On the other hand, he may set his level of aspiration so high that reaching it would be almost impossible; thus, no one could blame him for failing. In either case, the effective incentive from challenging goal setting is compromised. It may be that in competitive sports, the motive to avoid failure is often at least as strong as the achievement motive. Thus, desire for an outstanding performance may be overshadowed by fear of an inferior one. An average performance is therefore a satisfying one.[20] Zander[82] has examined achievement motivation in groups, and has speculated that groups with high motives to succeed will choose moderately challenging goals, while those high in motives to avoid failure will choose extreme goals. Goal setting seems to be a compromise between these two motives for groups, just as it is for individuals. One likely way for a group (team) to develop strong fear of failure is to have failed often in the past.[20]

Level of aspiration is also related to the difficulty of the task and the accompanying chance to succeed. If the task is too difficult and the chance of succeeding is less than 10%, then no performance is likely to be seen as unsuccessful. Atkinson[3] theorized that when there is a 50:50 chance of succeeding, the individual will raise his level of expectation and will work harder to achieve his goal. Intermediate probabilities of success promote enhanced expectation, whereas extreme probabilities (10:90 or 90:10) decrease levels of expectation.

Arousal is that aspect of motivation which energizes the body for the intensity dimension of behavior. It is important to understand that activation and the development of emotional arousal depends on the individual's perception of the situation, particularly regarding its importance and uncertainty.[39] This perception involves the cerebral cortex, reticular formation, hypothalamus, and the limbic system, which interact with the adrenal medulla and the somatic and autonomic nervous systems to produce the arousal state.[36] Resultant feelings prior to competition may include rapid heart rate, increased muscular tension, an empty feeling in the stomach, and dryness of the mouth and throat. Sometimes these sensations are so intense that they interfere with the upcoming performance. These physiologic effects of human emotion can distort behavior, inhibit finely coordinated and complex sport skills, and hamper performance.[20] Indeed, this reaction is found in a number of other performance situations, including examinations and public speaking. While abnormally high emotional arousal can disrupt performance, low arousal inhibits the transmission of impulses because sensory input is not fully processed at the cerebral cortex.[64] This suggests a continuum of arousal from low to high, which should be expected to have varied effects on an individual's performance.

There are two hypotheses which have been advanced to explain varied performance as a function of arousal: (1) the drive theory, and (2) the inverted U theory. Drive theory predicts that performance (P) is directly related to the product of habit formation (H) and drive (D). In essence, this means that with increased drive (arousal), the "habit," or dominant response, will be enhanced. Thus, with increased arousal in the early stages of learning the dominant responses are likely to be incorrect and performance will be impaired. Conversely, once the task is well learned, the dominant response is correct and increased arousal should continually enhance performance. Indeed, Oxendine[53] has suggested the notion that strength, endurance, and speed performance of highly conditioned athletes should all be facilitated by continuously enhanced arousal levels. However, others[36] have cited numerous instances of a point of diminishing returns in highly skilled strength and sprint athletes who were unable to perform well at high arousal levels because of apparent disorientation.

The inverted-U hypothesis, as described in Figure 4–8, predicts that any motor performance is enhanced with increased arousal up to a point (optimum), whereupon performance deteriorates with further increase in arousal. However, this hypothesis also has apparent deficiencies regarding task difficulty. That is, even after skills are well learned, it appears that performance of complex motor tasks is compromised by the same arousal level that is still somewhat below the optimal level for

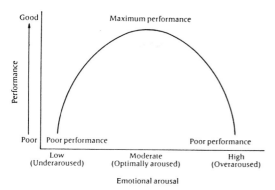

FIG. 4–8. The inverted-U relationship between arousal and performance. (From Landers, D.M. and S.H. Boutcher: Arousal-performance relationships. *In* Applied Sport Psychology. Edited by J.M. Williams. Palo Alto, CA: Mayfield Publ., 1986, p. 172.)

a more simple, well-learned task.[36] These observations have been extrapolated to identify the relative effects of arousal level in sports skills identified as either of low complexity (e.g., football blocking, running 400 meters) or high complexity (e.g., archery, golf), but there are virtually no data on actual sports performance.[54] Further, none of these studies have examined the effects of immediate pre-performance arousal on activities extending over prolonged periods of time, such as in marathon running or over the course of an entire soccer game.

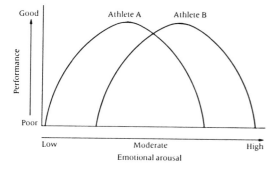

FIG. 4–9. Athlete-specific optimal levels of arousal. (From Landers, D.M. and S.H. Boutcher: Arousal-performance relationships. *In* Applied Sport Psychology. Edited by J.M. Williams. Palo Alto, CA: Mayfield Publ., 1986, p. 177.)

Another confounding factor in identifying the optimal arousal level for maximum performance is identifying individual differences in emotional arousal and performance relationships (Fig. 4–9). It appears that certain individuals with high trait anxiety levels (athlete A) can be expected to experience decrements in performance at a lower emotional arousal level than one with a lower trait anxiety level (athlete B). This means that the use of group "pep talks" to motivate a team are likely to result in disparate individual results, as suggested in Figure 4–10.

An area relative to emotional arousal and maximum performance currently receiving substantial attention is that of immediate pre-competitive anxiety/stress reduction. This interest in applied sport psychology arises from interest in why athletes perform notably worse than expected, often in competition at the highest level. The theoretical construct to explain this phenomenon is emotional over-arousal. A procedure for identifying the overaroused athlete in competition, utilizing cognitive, physiologic and behavioral responses, has been advanced by Landers and Boutcher.[36] Physiologic measurement techniques include monitoring brain wave patterns, electrical properties of the skin, heart rate, blood pressure, and muscle activity. Several questionnaires are also available to assess different effects of increased arousal. In many instances, simple observation of unusual behavior, such as flushed face, sweaty palms, hyperactivity (pacing and fidgeting), or unusually rapid speech, can be used as effective indication of competitive overarousal.

Numerous intervention techniques for decreasing arousal levels have been developed, but they all fall into one of two major categories: (1) relaxation techniques, and (2) cognitive strategies. It is important to understand, however, that the efficacy of these procedures has been established almost totally from clinical studies. Experimental studies, with appropriate control of confounding factors, including the placebo effect, are of recent origin and meager in number. A basic description of the major arousal intervention techniques in current

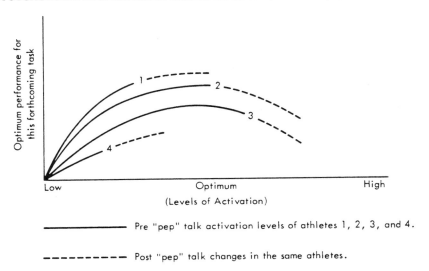

FIG. 4–10. Effects of a "pep" talk on the levels of activation and performance of four athletes. (From Cratty, B.J.: Psychology in Contemporary Sport. Englewood Cliffs, N.J.: Prentice Hall, 1973, p. 178.)

use, together with brief rationale as to how they are presumed to work, follows.

The principal relaxation techniques currently in use include: (1) progressive relaxation, (2) autogenic training, (3) transcendental meditation, and (4) biofeedback. They all are designed to facilitate reduced sympathetic nervous system tone induced by emotional overarousal. These include reduced heart rate, blood pressure, respiratory rate and muscle tension, as well as increased skin resistance and alpha brain waves, which have been collectively identified as the relaxation response.[5]

The progressive relaxation procedure, developed by Jacobson in 1930,[34] entails teaching one to gradually tighten a muscle group and then to let go; first one muscle group, then another; contract, and then relax. One becomes more aware of what muscular tension feels like, while during the relaxation phase, one gradually learns what the absence of tension feels like and that it can be voluntarily induced by passively reducing muscle tension.[20] Autogenic training is based on six psychophysiologic exercises, which are done in a quiet environment with the subject in a horizontal position and with the eyes closed. Emphasis is placed on how various parts of the body feel and learning to affect one's

perception, mental state, and muscular tension.[10]

Transcendental meditation is a relaxation procedure with religious, mystical connotations that originated in India several thousand years ago. The person begins while sitting in a quiet place by thinking of a sound (mantra) given by an instructor. The sound eventually disappears as the mind experiences subtler levels of thought and finally, by transcending, arrives at the source of the thought. Following 15 to 20 minutes of this procedure, the participant usually experiences the classic relaxation response.[9] Biofeedback is a relatively recent technique which works on the principle that one can voluntarily influence autonomic nervous system functions.[5] A machine is used to monitor heart rate, brain waves, muscle tension, or blood pressure. By feeling one's physiologic states and seeing the response displayed by the machine simultaneously, the relaxation state can be identified and produced consciously on a repeated basis. This response is learned, and upon removal of the machine, the subject is still able to reproduce the relaxed state.[9]

Principal cognitive strategies employed to reduce arousal levels include: (1) cognitive restructuring; (2) thought stopping;

(3) mental imagery; and (4) hypnosis, including self-hypnosis. These techniques have also been used to enhance self-confidence. Cognitive restructuring strategies assume that faulty cognition results in both deleterious emotional reaction and inappropriate behavior.[29] In essence, according to Ellis,[19] it is necessary to help one realize that the event does not necessarily cause the unpleasant feelings experienced, but rather that incorrect assumptions made by the individual about the event are the primary cause. This procedure, properly utilized, has been shown to reduce anxiety, though its value in sports performance has yet to be demonstrated. There is suggestive evidence, however, that cognitive restructuring can enhance performance via successful replacement of negative perceptions with positive ones. Thought stopping is a closely related strategy, which attempts to teach athletes how to stop negative thoughts about a performance situation and replace them with positive ones. The key is to recognize the negative feeling and to use this cue to stop this input and revert to prerehearsed positive thoughts, a procedure that bas been described as self-talk.[78] Nideffer[52] has provided a progression of four techniques in thought stopping and refocusing, as well as evidence from case studies to attest to the procedure's effectiveness.

The use of mental imagery to enhance motor skill learning has been discussed earlier. This technique has also been used by athletes in an attempt to focus on successful performance of a task in a high-pressure situation where self-doubt is an easily prevalent thought. If successful in enhancing performance, it obviously would aid the athlete in subsequent situations where undue self-doubt would increase anxiety and emotional arousal to a level that would interfere with maximum performance. It is thought that imagery may enhance performance via inducing innervation in the muscles associated with the imagined actions or by helping individuals encoding their movements into symbolic components which become more familiar and perhaps automatic.[77]

Mahoney and Avener[41] have classified imagery as either internal (one feels the action from a position within his body) or external (visualization of the activity from a movie camera perspective), and observed that elite gymnasts utilized internal imaging more frequently than did less skilled gymnasts. It appears that prior relaxation, when combined with imagery, is more effective than imagery alone in enhancing athletic performance.[77] A recent extension of imagery in an attempt to enhance performance in emotionally charged competition, is the use of stress inoculation. This approach assumes that it is possible to develop coping skills using imagery that gradually approximates the anticipated threatening situation.[29] For example, the basketball player might use this technique in an attempt to duplicate the anxiety and fear associated with actual competition while shooting free throws or executing other game skills during normally less anxiety-producing practice sessions. While imagery is widely used by athletes to influence arousal and enhance performance, limited experimental evidence is not consistent in showing such an effect, either in highly skilled or less skilled performers.[29,62]

Of all cognitive intervention strategies, probably the most talked about and least understood is hypnosis. Psychologists have yet to agree on what causes hypnosis or how it differs from the waking state, though it is agreed that uncritical acceptance of suggestion characterizes hypnosis.[74] The process of inducing hypnosis involves relaxation and produces similar physiologic responses characteristic of reduced arousal achieved with other cognitive interventions.[5] However, the latter encourage the development of problem solving strategy by the individual, while in hypnosis the individual is usually passive and dependent on the hypnotist. Following the induction of hypnosis, the hypnotist can effect posthypnotic suggestion to induce deep relaxation while the individual is in the hypnotic state, a procedure that has been used in the management of pre-competitive anxiety.[12]

Early studies revealed enhanced strength and endurance performance following posthypnotic suggestion in nonathletic subjects. However, consistent results in strength and endurance performance under similar conditions in highly trained athletes have not been observed.[12] Further, it appears that suggestion of increased strength and endurance performance in the nonhypnotic state may be as effective as posthypnotic suggestion.[4] These observations are in accord with the classic work of Steinhaus on the relationship of one's all-out effort (effected by his psychologic limit) to his physiologic capacity, a summary of which follows:

We pulled against a scale to measure strength of forearm flexors. Whenever the second sweep hand came to the one o'clock position the individual was to pull as hard as he could. So we registered a maximal contraction every minute. Then without warning to the individual we shot a gun at various times before the second hand came to the pulling position. Invariably, we found the individual had more strength after the shot. We found that the shot about 4 seconds before the pull got the greatest increase. We found the increase was sometimes as much as 30%. Then we tried yelling. When they yelled their strength was also more than usual. Then we tried hypnosis. Under hypnosis it is possible to do away with inhibitions. We found up to 50% improvement in strength . . . We had found three ways of crashing the psychologic barrier that stops us in the execution of strength. The psychologic limit is always short of the physiologic one . . . one of the big differences between the athlete and nonathlete is that the athlete has learned to close the gap between the psychologic and physiologic limits. He drives himself closer to the physiologic limit.[72:304]

It is important to understand that these procedures, which appear far less effective with the highly trained athlete than the non-athlete, do not effect changes in strength or endurance capacity but, instead, improve the expression of these abilities, probably via deinhibiting CNS mechanisms. It appears, then, that use of hypnosis to enhance athletic performance is of limited value, especially since only about 15% of subjects can reach a deep hypnotic trance.[18]

An experienced athlete, who has a low trait anxiety level and anticipates performing against presumed inferior competition, may well be in an under-aroused state and a prime candidate for an upset. Several of the cognitive interventions for curbing overarousal, discussed earlier, can also be used to enhance arousal. The critical issue in this effort is to avoid bypassing the optimal level of arousal. Attention to the athlete's past history in similar competition and to the type of activity will aid in this endeavor. In general, large-muscle, low complexity tasks can profit by high arousal levels, while fine, coordinated high complexity movements may be compromised even by moderate arousal levels. There is little research in this area, especially on the effects of specified "psych-up" techniques on performance with athletes using appropriate controls.

SOCIAL-PSYCHOLOGIC EFFECTS ON PHYSICAL PERFORMANCE

Social psychology is concerned with the influence of the presence and behavior of other humans, individually and collectively, on individual behavior. Study of the social psychology of physical activity is of relatively recent origin, the first textbook being published in 1975.[43] Our concern will be limited to the effect on individual performance of the presence of other humans, including passive onlookers, co-actors, and interactive audience effects. The effects of competition on individual performance, compared to noncompetitive conditions will also be examined briefly.

Social facilitation is concerned with the noninteractive influence of the presence of others as a passive audience or as co-actors. The latter term refers to a group of individuals performing the same task but with no interaction. Until 1965, studies on social facilitation appeared to give equivocal results. However, Zajonc[81] formulated a theory which appeared to identify a subtle consistency in prior research, and is summarized graphically in Figure 4–11. Basically, the theory holds that the presence of an audience impairs initial learning of a complex task but facilitates performance of a well-learned task. Subsequent studies using motor tasks and measuring emotional arousal confirmed the theory's validity.[37] Evidence also clearly indicates that the mere presence of others is not the principal source producing social facilitation, but is

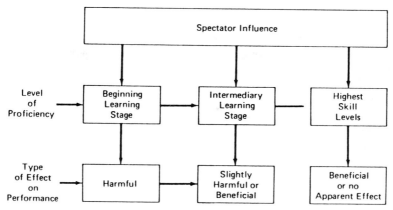

FIG. 4–11. The effect of spectators on performance. (From Singer, R.N.: Myths and Truths in Sports Psychology. New York: Harper & Row, 1975, p. 19.)

due to the evaluation apprehension associated with the presence of individuals who have the potential to evaluate the performer positively or negatively.

Interactive audience effects on physical performance have not been well studied in controlled conditions. Zajonc's social facilitation theory predicts that an audience should enhance the performance of a highly skilled athlete. However, the audience effect, shown clearly in the controlled laboratory setting, has not been consistently replicated in initial field studies of spectator or crowd effects at sports events.[56] There is clear documentation of a home court advantage in many team sports, though the reasons for its existence are unclear. Audience effects, particularly if hostile behavior is manifested, appear to be a primary factor.[9] It has been hypothesized that home basketball teams play more aggressively and the visiting team less aggressively, in part, due to the audience effect.[76] The audience's influence on the officials' judgment and its potential effect on outcome of the contest, was not evaluated.

The study of competition in controlled laboratory conditions (e.g., as depicted in Fig. 4–12) has yielded similar effects on performance as social facilitation. That is, like social facilitation, competition is a social evaluation situation that creates arousal and facilitates performance on simple or well-learned tasks, and impairs performance of complex tasks that are not well learned.[23] An interesting, consistent exception to these findings is the leveling effect in subjects engaged in competitive coaction. That is, when co-actors of unequal ability compete with each other, there is a tendency for the performance level of the co-actors to become more alike. The performance of the less skilled subjects improves, while the performance of the more skilled subjects declines. Thus, competition does not always result in enhanced performance. However, if co-actors are of equal ability, competition should enhance motivation, and results should be generally consistent with the predictions of drive theory.[9]

PSYCHOLOGIC EFFECTS OF EXERCISE TRAINING AND SPORTS PARTICIPATION

In an earlier section, the widely held notion that personality differences exist between various groups of athletes and nonathletes, was shown to lack any consistent support from a decade of persistent research effort. Most of the research investigations were cross-sectional, and usually demonstrated one or two personality trait differences between groups.[68] However, no consistent pattern was evidenced and, indeed, with a battery of 10 or more personality traits, a few isolated differences of borderline statistical significance could be expected on the basis of chance alone.

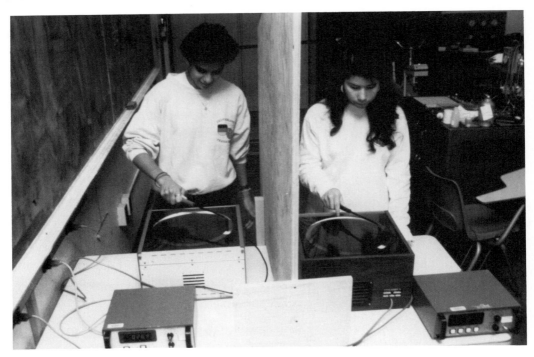

FIG. 4–12. The effects of competition in a controlled laboratory condition are being studied while utilizing the pursuit rotor tracking task. The subjects attempt to maintain contact of the stylus on the disc as the turntable moves. The timer records contact time over a specified period of competition.

Although the research results are equivocal, one should not conclude that they necessarily indicate no important personality differences associated with prolonged athletic participation. This is because there have been numerous methodologic problems associated with research in this area. First, there have been numerous personality inventories utilized which do not necessarily measure the same traits. Further, they have usually been chosen for convenience, rather than by predesigned theory, to "snoop" for possible differences revealed amongst the subject population groups.[9] Second, groups studied have not been well enough identified. That is, what is considered a highly selected, trained group of athletes at one university may actually consist mostly of individuals who would not make the team at many other institutions.[35,61] Third, studies have been done on many different age groups varying in the level of athletic competitive demand and experience. Finally, it is only recently

that personality tests incorporating second-order traits, most amenable to change induced by significant environmental input, have been used.[9]

Even if there were consistent personality trait differences identified between elite and less gifted performers in a given sport, various groups of athletes, and between athletes and nonathletes, the cross-sectional research designs used predominantly heretofore would not evidence cause and effect. That is, one cannot definitively identify whether these differences (1) existed before athletic participation, (2) were caused by athletic participation, or (3) that both factors interact.[68] Accordingly, more longitudinal investigations have been conducted in recent years. However, it should be realized that first-order personality traits and strong tendencies to exhibit second-order traits in many different situations appear to be inherent, or at least largely determined early in one's lifetime.[2] Several longitudinal studies done on pre-pubescent and adolescent males suggest some existent personality differences between athletes and nonathletes, but no change during one to several years of athletic participation.[45,68] Studies of adult athletes either indicate initial personality differences that are not altered with continued athletic participation, or reveal no significant differences from nonathletes.[13]

It has been suggested that athletic competition places unusually stressful emotional and behavioral demands on participants, thus perhaps predisposing them to possible significant long-term negative psychologic consequences.[40] Dishman[13] cites evidence that fewer than half of young high-level athletes report subjective symptoms of competitive stress. Though there are reports of youth athletes experiencing significant elevation in anxiety following competitive failure (losing), the magnitude of anxiety is no greater than that accompanying non-athletic performance when important evaluative outcomes are perceived by the participant.[13] In any case, there is no consistent research evidence indicating a persistent negative impact on personality traits of athletes. Indeed, elite athletes of both sexes are characteristically neither above average in anxiety nor depression, and collectively evidence a positive mental health profile. Further, it appears that an athletic career during youth and young adulthood exerts little generalizable impact on life adjustment and mental health, in that psychologic adjustment problems in later years appear to be no different in athletes than nonathletes of similar age and education.[13]

While future research may reveal a significant influence of athletic participation on personality, an alternate hypothesis should be considered. That is, life presents a seemingly endless array of challenging demands which each of us may well have the ability and developed desire to master. Further, few are likely to demand particularly high levels of a single personality trait, but more likely a composite of several characteristics. Hence, while the media and our own prevalent notion strongly suggest there are "obvious" differences in personality characteristics of excellence in athletics, it may well be that they constitute a weak, "random noise" relationship potential when compared to other successful achievement oriented individuals or groups.

A large majority of health professionals have for some time prescribed exercise in the adult population for its alleged psychologic benefits.[7] Further, in one survey of primarily noncompetitive runners, the following mental and emotional benefits were ascribed by the participants as resulting from their training programs: (1) relieves tension, 86%; (2) better self-image, 77%; (3) better mood, 66%; (4) more self-confident, 64%; (5) more alert, 58%; (6) relieves depression, 56%; (7) more content, 54%; and (8) think more clearly, 53%.[8] Experimental research, however, has yielded few consistent results of the psychologic effects of exercise training, although there are data suggesting probable alleviation of symptoms associated with mild or moderate depression and improvement of self-image.[73]

Several principal research methodologic flaws have slowed progress in elucidating the psychologic effects of exercise training, though the longitudinal method has been used in a significant portion of research studies. One problem has been the persistent reliance on psychometric tests without adequate attention to potentially better, more objective and theoretically based measurement techniques. Experimenter demand and subject expectancy biases are especially likely to occur in this area of research, in that many research workers and subjects possess an a priori belief that exercise produces psychologic benefits. Thus, lack of rather sophisticated experimental control procedures—especially in accounting for the placebo effect—has been a persistent problem. Morgan[48] has summarized a particularly perceptive example of these problems in the assessment of acute treatment effects on reducing anxiety. Twenty minutes of either transcendental meditation, biofeedback, or exercise have all been shown to reduce anxiety. However, it seems that 20 minutes of quiet rest in a noise-filtered room is just as effective as the other, more sophisticated procedures. With more attention now being given to important experimental design and measurement procedures, a clearer picture of the psychologic effects of exercise training should be forthcoming.

Depression is a major mental health problem, and there is strong evidence that exercise training probably alleviates mild to moderate levels.[73] In an early study,[50] for example, no significant effect of 6 weeks vigorous aerobic training on depression levels of middle-age males was seen in subjects within the normal range. However, 11 subjects who had depression of clinical significance upon initiation of training experienced a significant decrease with training. A subsequent study[26] demonstrated that aerobic exercise training, performed for 12 weeks by 10 patients who sought treatment for neurotic or reactive depression, was just as effective in its antidepressant effect as two forms of traditional psychotherapy. Further, all but one of the patients in the running group were free of depressive symptoms at 12-months' follow-up, whereas half of the psychotherapy patients had returned for treatment.[49]

Cardiac patients scoring within the normal range on psychometric tests of depression upon initiating aerobic training showed no change following training for 6 months to 2 years.[13] Reduction in depression levels consequent to exercise training, when present, have been attributed to diversion, social reinforcement, improved self-concept, and increased neurotransmission of catecholamines and/or endogenous opiates.[32]

Surprisingly, there have been no experimental studies of exercise effects on patients with clinically documented anxiety disorder. Further, there is no consistent evidence that exercise training evokes a change in trait anxiety amongst clinically normal subjects.[73] However, relatively small but statistically significant reductions in state anxiety following training have been reported.[13] Perhaps more important is the consistently observed temporary reduction of state anxiety in clinically normal individuals who undertake vigorous exercise. It appears that this acute effect persists for 4 to 6 hours, though there may be a return to baseline within 24 hours. Thus, a major benefit of exercise on state anxiety

may be as a method for intermittent coping with daily events which could prevent the onset of chronic anxiety.[49] Means by which exercise may affect state anxiety levels are not clear, but have been attributed to diversion, social reinforcement, enhanced self-concept, and reduced physiologic response to stress (i.e., lower muscle tension and catecholamine levels).[13,49]

It appears that exercise training may produce improvements in physiologic responses to mental-emotional stress beyond that induced by several relaxation techniques.[73] However, mechanisms are unclear, in that heart rate and subjective anxiety responses were similar to a mental stress stimulus, though recovery was faster in one study, while reduced heart demand for oxygen during mental stress was observed in a more recent study.[13]

Exercise training has been shown to result in consistently enhanced self-concept in children and young adults with low pretraining self-esteem.[32] However, the effect of exercise training on self-concept in middle-age adults, including cardiac patients, is not well defined.[73]

An interesting and prevalent psychologic phenomenon associated with exercise training is that participants report "feeling better." This general perception occurs sometimes in accord with decreased depression and anxiety, but also without measurable changes in these moods.[49] Since major population surveys confirm an enhanced "feel better" response amongst those who engage in systematic exercise, this aspect of the psychologic effect of exercise training merits careful investigation.[73]

The occurrence of the presumed euphoric state termed "runner's high," has been reported variously by from 10 to 78% of habitual runners sampled.[13] The improved mood reported has been hypothesized as a resultant of enhanced exercise induced endogenous opiates—particularly beta-endorphins. However, increases in beta-endorphins during heavy exercise are not directly related to exercise induced positive mood changes.[13] Also administration of the opiate antagonist naloxone did not block psychometric mood elevations reported during long distance runs.[42] None-

Table 4–1.   Proposed Psychological Harms of Exercise Overindulgence*

Addiction to exercise
Compulsiveness
Decreased involvement in job, marriage, and so on
Escape or avoidance of problems
Exacerbation of anorexia nervosa
Exercise deprivation effects
Fatigue
Overcompetitiveness
Overexertion
Poor eating habits
Preoccupation with fitness, diet, and body image
Self-centeredness

*From Taylor, C.B. et al.: The relation of physical activity and exercise to mental health. Public Health Rep. *100*:199, 1985.

theless, high opiate levels do appear associated with lower levels of fatigue and exercise induced pain sensitivity.[32] "Runner's high," though, still remains a subjective phenomenon of undefined origin.[13]

There have been several anecdotal reports that persistent exercise training may elicit harmful psychologic effects, a number of which are listed in Table 4–1. However, little is known of the true health and social impact of excessive exercise involvement, its etiology, diagnosis, and treatment.[13] Morgan[46] described eight individuals with "running addiction" in whom commitment to running had assumed higher priority than commitments to family, interpersonal relationships, work, and medical advice. This was accompanied in some cases with apparent withdrawal symptoms under enforced exercise deprivation. Reports from two experimental studies suggest evidence of depressed mood, elevated anxiety, and altered sleep pattern following exercise abstention. However, it is not known whether voluntary abstinence elicits the same response patterns as enforced cessation due to injury, illness, or attending to other unavoidable personal commitments.[13] While as yet ill-defined, obsession with exercise involvement, and the inability or unwillingness to reduce training and to attend adequately to medical, vocational, and familial concerns, may be indicative of underlying personality problems of clinical importance.[13] This appears to be the case

with only about one-fourth of anorexic women who train compulsively.[80] Anorexics typically demonstrate symptoms of depression, paranoia, and borderline personality disorder.[13] Thus, it is not clear that persistent exercise training causes negative behavior, but rather that certain personalities are predisposed to abuse exercise involvement as a way of coping with, or even avoiding other problems.[73]

MOTIVATION FOR VOLUNTARY EXERCISE PARTICIPATION

Modern man's need for regular vigorous physical activity was discussed in Chapter 1. It was emphasized that exercise must be a continuing lifetime habit, as the training effect is transient. For example, former college athletes have been found just as likely to have coronary heart disease as nonathletes, unless they continue regular exercise beyond college athletics.[55] However, surveys indicate that about 50% of U.S. adults are sedentary, and that only one-third of all adults participate in exercise on a weekly basis.[57] While most states have physical education requirements from elementary through tenth grade, it is estimated that only about one-third of children and adolescents, ages 10 to 17, participate in daily school physical education programs.[75] The U.S. Office of Disease Prevention and Health Promotion[11] has set a goal for participation in regular, vigorous physical activity by 90% of youth and 60% of adults by 1990. A principal barrier to developing effective methods to increase the number of individuals engaged in regular physical activity is the present poor understanding of behavioral determinants of participation.[14] That is, what are the factors that motivate, or enhance the likelihood of initiating and adhering to a program of regular, vigorous physical activity, and what are those which act to inhibit, or decrease the likelihood of participation?

Motivation is the conceptual term used to explain the causes of one initiating and sustaining action, as well as the intensity at which it is pursued. It consists of the sum of determinants that impel one to action, or inaction, in various situations. De-

Table 4–2. Maslow's Hierarchy of Needs*

Needs Category	Examples of Needs
1. Physiologic	Body homeostatic needs for air, food, and water; also sleepiness and activity.
2. Safety	Security, freedom from harm, and reasonable constancy of environment.
3. Love and Acceptance	Social and physical contact, including care, affection and belonging.
4. Self-Esteem	Personal achievement and recognition, feeling of success, and a sense of self-worth.
5. Self-Actualization	Opportunity for self-fulfillment and attainment of personal potential.

*Modified from Maslow, A.: Motivation and Personality. New York: Harper & Row, 1970, pp. 35–47.

terminants of activity include physiologic drives and psychologic motives which are acquired in response to our social and physical environments. Drives and motives develop from basic needs, both physiologic and psychologic, which compel us to fulfill them.

Maslow[44] has developed a theory of motivation which is useful in its categorization of basic human needs. It includes the notion of a hierarchy, ranging from physiologic needs, which must be sufficiently satisfied before attention can be directed to other categories of more mature needs. Table 4–2 summarizes pertinent descriptive aspects of the five major categories. Physiologic needs, which for Maslow include not only body homeostatic needs for food, water, air, etc., but also sexual desire, sleepiness, and activity (at least in the young), are pre-potent. Provided one has little problem satisfying these needs, attention can be effectively directed to needs at a higher level. However, if one is unable to fulfill a preeminent physiologic need such as hunger, then higher level needs may be pushed into the background or become simply nonexistent. Conversely, one may develop an unwillingness to acknowledge the basic physiologic need for hunger as in the case of individuals who have

starved to the point of death for a particular cause.

The second level of Maslow's needs hierarchy concerns safety, which, when adequately achieved, enables one to deal with needs for belongingness and love. It seems clear that the infant's behavioral development exemplifies this progression, which as the child grows, leads to concern for and realization of self-esteem needs. Harris[27] contends that there is little scientific knowledge about self-esteem needs, but that ineffective attention to them appears to be a primary contribution to psychologic maladjustment states. Further, physical activity and sports participation appear to provide an excellent opportunity for many to achieve various aspects of this category of needs on a regular basis, including self perception of mastery and competence that is readily recognized by esteem provided from others. It is this self-esteem need which provides principal credibility to the achievement motive theory advanced by Murray and colleagues.[51] They contend that need achievement is rooted in an individual's interest, whether it be the desire for social prestige, intellectual distinction, or athletic success.

The final category of needs in Maslow's hierarchy, and the most mature, is that of self-actualization. This entails man's need for freedom to achieve his fullest potential. Unfortunately for many of us, our concern is almost always directed to unsatisfied needs at lower levels which predispose the individual to conform to the cultural standards around him. However, when basic needs for safety, comfort, love, belongingness, and respect are achieved, it then becomes possible for one to live on a "self-actualizing" level. At this level, one does not strive in one area, e.g., sports, to compensate for inadequacies or tensions in another area. Instead, he participates in the activities for fun, or as ends in themselves, rather than as a means to an end. The self-actualized man, then, is motivated by personal goals arising from his own growth. He pursues them without anxiety, and at these times, conforms only superficially to society's conventions and restraints. While Maslow describes the self-actualization level as the needs of a musician to play music, an artist to paint, and a poet to write, as if realization of one's extraordinary talent was the only means to achieve this end,[44] this need not be the case, as illustrated in the following example developed by Harris:

A "peak experience" can be achieved at any level of skill, and may well be the motivation behind the duffer who goes to the golf course every weekend and continues to hit the divots farther than the ball. He may be there on the chance that maybe, just maybe today, he will hit that one good shot. There are probably enough good shots scattered throughout his weekends where everything seems to go together that he has a sense of really being totally involved. That provides the incentive to get him back again and again. Frequently, only the good athlete senses this feeling, but the less skilled can also share in these experiences. These peak experiences are very individualized and cannot be planned for; they are not a means to an end, but an end in themselves.[27:46]

In such situations, the performer is not concerned with other's evaluation of his performance, but intent on enjoyment of the activity in his own individualized terms.

It is important to understand that participation in physical activity can fulfill achievement of needs at all levels of Maslow's hierarchy. Many mistakenly conclude that activity is not a primary drive in humans, since many adults lead a sedentary existence. However, if one accepts the notion that motivation to engage in most human behavior involves an interaction of numerous determinants affecting drives and motives—some positively, others in an inhibitory manner—then it is possible to conceptualize that man has a primary physical activity drive, perhaps under the control of an activity center located in the hypothalamus, as has been demonstrated in rats.[31] Hill[30] found that immobilization of animals, provided adequate food and water was supplied, resulted in the development for an activity need. Animals confined for 24 and $46\frac{1}{2}$ hours demonstrated significantly greater activity during the $1\frac{1}{2}$ hour free period that followed than did those immobilized for 5 hours and those who were not confined. Hill concluded that the differences in running activity following confinement were explicable only by postulating a genuine activity drive that is built up by the enforced deprivation of activity. It is important to recall that all young of mammalian species are inherently active in what many times appears purposeless play, but which may facilitate the developmental process.[33] Indeed, it would appear the human's primary drive for physical activity is strongest in the infant and growing child, and that it serves to promote optimum bodily function and development, as well as the development of other more mature needs in Maslow's hierarchy. For example, the movements of an infant during the first few months of life may well be based on an attempt to satisfy the dominant physiologic needs and to establish a sense of security through experiencing the sensations of the surrounding environment. As the child matures, play becomes a dominant feature of life and serves as a means of gaining approval, friendships, and developing a sense of esteem and self-worth.[16]

It should be apparent also that an adult's participation in an exercise training program can represent an interaction of behavioral determinants that meet needs at several levels on the Maslow hierarchy scheme. For example, regular exercise promotes more optimum bodily function (physiologic needs) and provides a group camaraderie that increases one's feeling of acceptance and sense of identification with a group. Also, the success experienced with improved performance can lead to a better self-concept.[73] Self-actualization opportunities become more likely the longer the individual adheres to the program, as he feels increased freedom from attending to other needs and loses himself in the fun of the activity.

While the human may indeed possess a primary drive for physical activity, it is vital to realize that if one's immediate physical environment is not conducive to regular physical activity and the prevailing sociocultural attitudes do not attribute much importance to this behavior, then the primary drive is overridden for many adults who then follow a sedentary lifestyle. However, it should be realized that almost no adult is totally inactive. In fact, in view of the increasing hypokinetic disease accompanying our present decreasing activity pattern, the consequences of total inactivity in man's present evolutionary state would be virtually disastrous. If one considers that the human's primary physical activity drive may well decrease with age, identifying and maximizing positive sociocultural determinants of initiating and adhering to regular, vigorous physical activity, as well as minimizing negative (inhibitory) ones, becomes crucial.

Only recently have a number of factors which may enhance or hinder initiation of and adherence to a vigorous physical activity program been identified. Research is especially limited in the area of individual participation in unsupervised activity programs, but research involving supervised exercise programs has yielded some interesting and informative data.

There appear to be a rather large number of factors which act as determinants for the initiation of and adherence to vigorous physical activity programs. They appear to work interactively to determine the likelihood of an individual's action. These determinants have been classified into categories, including personal characteristics, environmental factors (social and physical), and program characteristics.[14]

Personal characteristics of adults which are positively related to participation in vigorous physical activity include: (1) upper socioeconomic status, as indicated by income, education, and occupation; (2) young age; and (3) being male. Conversely, the individual who smokes, is a blue collar worker, or suffers from obesity, is less likely to adhere to an organized exercise program.[14]

One's social and physical environments can also have strong influence on exercise program initiation and adherence. Research indicates that individuals who receive strong social support and encouragement from their spouse, friends, and program leader are far less likely to drop out.[67] Workouts in group settings are especially motivating to many people. Program participants are also characterized as being in the middle and upper income levels, which may also be related to the importance of the physical environment of the individual. A person who lives in the suburbs generally has ready access to safer conditions in which to exercise (for example, urban streets may be so congested that bicycling becomes a dangerous activity choice). The presence of par courses, jogging, cycling, and walking trails, lockers and showers (at the worksite), public pools and sports courts, etc. are also important in determining the likelihood of participation.[14]

Both the personal and environmental factors discussed above are important when planning supervised exercise programs. There are, however, several other characteristics of programs which influence initiation and adherence rates. Initial screening and subsequent assessment to monitor progress are extremely important tools to enhance program participation; for many individuals, feedback in terms of measurable progress, can serve as an incentive to continue. Well-trained, motivated leaders are also important, both for protection from exercise related injuries, and to provide recognition of participants' achievements. Many participants also cite convenience, in terms of time and location of exercise classes, as a primary factor in their decision to adhere to an exercise program. It is important to realize that a successful program leader is not one who merely educates the participants in the hows and whys of exercise but, more importantly, who motivates them. In this connection, Steinhaus states:

> The educator who undertakes to help people to form and reform habits of living cannot content himself with facts and their dissemination. He must dig deeply into the mechanism of man to discover the mainsprings that drive his actions, to learn what really makes him "tick." Understanding this, he may influence the harnessing of these driving forces to new action patterns. When he is able to do this, he now guides the development of attitudes, of readiness to act.[72:219]

Franklin[22] has summarized many of the major factors affecting adherence to exercise training programs. Figure 4–13 depicts the potentially negative and positive forces. If the negative forces outweigh the positive, adherence is likely to be poor. On the other hand, if the effect of the negative forces can be reduced so that the positive forces are predominant, good adherence is likely.

Despite the above-mentioned approaches to exercise programming which can positively influence initiation and adherence, there are several prevalent negative societal influences which inhibit participation. Their overall impact is significant, as reflected in the relatively large proportion of adults in the U.S. who still remain sedentary despite the current "fitness boom." They include:

Superiority of Mental Over Physical. This impression denies the accepted psychologic principle of the unity of mind and body. Nevertheless, it does exist to a marked degree. As technologic advances increase in America, there is more knowledge to be mastered. This knowledge aids greatly in making our standard of living the highest the world has ever known. Indeed, the forces of our formal educative process have been geared to developing the intellect necessary to continue this advance. As a consequence, many tend to treat the body as a second class entity giving it limited attention, and then only when the atrophy of inactivity and stagnation of organic function causes pain and literally demands our concern.

Vestige of Puritanical Attitude. There remains a remnant of the Puritanical attitude in our society that participation in physical activity for fun, or play, is wasteful of the serious minded adult's time. This view appears to be much less prevalent than it was a decade ago.

Glorification of the Winner. In our society, the winner is praised and the loser ignored, at best. This is difficult for the loser and too often leads to a feeling of failure and dejection, and ultimately to avoidance of participation. Even the winner can become bored with the lack of challenge in activity. Not infrequently this predisposes one to association with a winner as a spectator. When this happens, one has forgotten two things: First, that it is more fun to participate than watch, even though it requires effort; and secondly, that the physiologic values of participation are virtually the same, whether you win or lose. Thus, it is the participation that is most important, not the score.

Perceived Time Pressure. Our lives are complex, being impacted by work, spouse, family, community, and personal concerns. Organizing one's day to meet perceived demands in all areas is difficult, especially considering that all things affecting one's daily life are not always routine. Time pressures arise and make it difficult for one to find the "window" in his day's activity for exercise.

Facilities for Physical Activity. Much im-

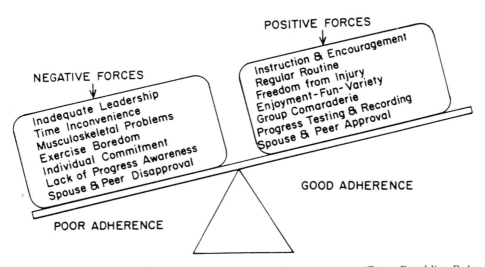

FIG. 4–13. Factors affecting adherence to exercise training programs. (From Franklin, B.A.: Motivating and educating adults to exercise. JOPER. 49(6):13–17, 1978.)

provement has been made in this area during the past two decades, with increased community attention to planned open space and sports facilities. In addition, there are now many business and industrial concerns with in-house exercise facilities, and even some in larger motels and hotels. Nonetheless, getting to the facility when open (and available) with a partner or competitor, often presents difficulties which act as a deterrent to regular activity participation.

SUMMARY

1. The scientific study of human behavior in exercise and sport includes four primary areas: (1) motor learning, (2) psychosocial effects on performance, (3) psychologic effects of exercise training and sports participation, and (4) motivation for electing to participate in vigorous physical activity.

2. Motor control refers to the internal neuromuscular processes inherent in human motor response, while motor skill acquisition emphasizes other factors affecting the development of efficient, reproducible movements.

3. The open-loop model of motor control accounts for the generation and performance of rapid movements, while the closed-loop model entails an error detection mechanism that accounts for the use of feedback in altering the course of slower movements after their initiation.

4. Motor skill classification categories include (a) whether it involves fine or gross movement, (b) distinctiveness of beginning and end points, and (c) stability of the environment. Each category provides useful orientation to develop more effective motor learning.

5. There are three phases of motor learning: (a) early, cognitive, (b) intermediate, and (c) final, autonomous, which permits skilled performance without conscious thought of the details involved.

6. One's initial performance in a new motor task is not well related to the rate and amount of subsequent learning and improvement in performance.

7. Effective motor learning entails re-ceiving appropriate amounts of information from a variety of sources about what is to be done and how well one does in successive trials. The latter is facilitated by quantitative information that is not too detailed.

8. Motor learning proceeds more rapidly when practice is meaningful and challenging, yet not overly fatiguing. In skills which utilize movements with specific temporal and spatial relationship, practice should emphasize them together, rather than emphasizing accuracy first, then speed, and then attempting to integrate the two.

9. Mental practice (imagery) occurs when one consciously visualizes the motor task to be performed in the absence of overt physical performance. It has been found to facilitate initial stages of motor learning in tasks with a complex cognitive element. While imagery is widely used by athletes to influence arousal and enhance self-confidence, limited experimental evidence is not consistent in showing such an effect in highly skilled performers.

10. Transfer of learning from one skill to another occurs most readily when important elements of each are identical or highly similar, and the performer recognizes and utilizes them.

11. Realistic goal setting, including one's level of aspiration, i.e., the standard by which a person judges his performance as a success or failure, affects one's intensity of effort and quality of motor performance.

12. Performance is improved with increased arousal up to a point, whereupon additional arousal has a disorienting, adverse effect. Relatively simple skills are facilitated by higher levels of arousal, while complex skill performance will become poorer.

13. Pre-competitive anxiety/stress reduction techniques currently employed with some success are (1) progressive relaxation, (2) autogenic training, (3) transcendental meditation, and (4) biofeedback.

14. Evidence suggests that athletes learn how to make their actual performance (limited by psychologic inhibitions) more closely match their physiologic capacity.

15. Social facilitation is concerned with the noninteractive influence of the pres-

ence of others as a passive audience. Initial learning of complex tasks is impaired by presence of an audience, while performance of a well-learned task is enhanced.

16. Only limited evidence suggests personality trait differences between athletes and nonathletes. Moreover, the cross-sectional experimental designs used in previous research studies precludes evidence of cause and effect. That is, one cannot definitively conclude whether any differences (a) existed before athletic participation, (b) were caused by athletic participation, or (c) that both factors interact.

17. Experimental research has yielded few consistent results of the psychologic effects of exercise training, although there are data suggesting probable alleviation of symptoms associated with mild or moderate depression and improvement of self-image.

18. A bout of vigorous exercise has been observed to reduce state anxiety for 4 to 6 hours, and may be an effective method for intermittent coping with daily events which could allay the onset of chronic anxiety.

19. Motivation is the conceptual term used to explain the causes of one initiating and sustaining action, as well as the intensity at which it is pursued. It consists of determinants—physiologic drives and psychologic motives which are acquired in response to our social and physical environment.

20. There is evidence that the human has a physiologic drive for physical activity, which is probably strongest in pre-adult years. However, numerous factors in one's social and physical environment interact to strengthen or weaken this drive.

21. Programs are being developed which attempt to enhance the influence of factors which impel one to initiate and adhere to exercise training while also seeking to attenuate the effects of factors which have an inhibitory influence.

REFERENCES

1. Adams, J.A.: A closed-loop theory of motor learning. J. Motor Behav. 3:111–149, 1971.
2. Allport, G.W.: Pattern and Growth in Personality. New York: Holt, Rinehart & Winston, 1961.
3. Atkinson, J.W.: Motivational determinants of risk-taking behavior. Psychol. Rev. 64:359–372, 1957.
4. Barber, T.X.: The effects of hypnosis and motivational suggestions on strength and endurance: a critical review of research studies. Br. J. Soc. Clin. Psych. 5:42–50, 1966.
5. Benson, H., J.F. Beary, and M.P. Carol: The relaxation response. Psychiatry. 37:37–46, 1974.
6. Billing, J.: An overview of task complexity. Motor Skills: Theory Into Practice. 4:18–23, 1980.
7. Byrd, O.E.: A survey of beliefs and practices of psychiatrists on the relief of tension by moderate exercise. J. Sch. Health. 33:426–427, 1963.
8. Callen, K.E.: Mental and emotional aspects of long-distance running. Psychosomatics. 24:133–151, 1983.
9. Cox, R.H.: Sport Psychology: Concepts and Applications. Dubuque, Iowa: Wm. C. Brown, 1985.
10. Cratty, B.J.: Psychology in Contemporary Sport: Guidelines for Coaches and Athletes. Englewood Cliffs, N.J.: Prentice-Hall, 1973.
11. Department of Health and Human Services, Office of Disease Prevention and Health Promotion: Prevention '82. DHHS Publication No. (PHS) 82–50157. U.S. Government Printing Office, Washington, D.C., 1982.
12. Dishman, R.K.: Overview of ergogenic properties of hypnosis. JOPER. 51(2):53–54, 1980.
13. Dishman, R.K.: Medical psychology in exercise and sport. Med. Clin. N. Am. 69:123–143, 1985.
14. Dishman, R.K., J.F. Sallis, and D.R. Orenstein: The determinants of physical activity and exercise. Pub. Health Rep. 100:158–171, 1985.
15. Drowatzsky, J.N.: Motor Learning: Principles and Practices. (2nd ed.) Minneapolis, Minn.: Burgess, 1981.
16. Drowatzsky, J.N., and C.W. Armstrong: Physical Education: Career Perspectives and Professional Foundations. Englewood Cliffs, N.J.: Prentice-Hall, 1984.
17. Drowatzsky, J.N., and F.C. Zuccato: Interrelationships between selected measures of static and dynamic balance. Res. Quart. 38:509–510, 1967.
18. Edmonston, W.E., Jr: Hypnosis and Relaxation: Modern Verification of an Old Equation. New York: Wiley, 1981.
19. Ellis, A.: Reason and Emotion in Psychotherapy. New York: Lyle Stuart, 1962.
20. Fisher, A.C.: Psychology of Sport: Issues & Insights. Palo Alto, Calif.: Mayfield, 1976.
21. Fitts, P.M.: Factors in complex skill training. In Training Research and Education. Edited by R. Glasser. New York: Wiley, 1965.
22. Franklin, B.A.: Motivation and educating adults to exercise. JOPER. 49(6):13–17, 1978.
23. Gill, D.L.: Current research and future prospects

in sport psychology. *In* Perspectives on the Academic Discipline of Physical Education. Edited by G.A. Brooks. Champaign, Ill.: Human Kinetics, 1981, pp. 342–378.

24. Godwin, M.A., and R.A. Schmidt: Muscular fatigue and discrete motor learning. Res. Quart. 42:374–383, 1971.

25. Gould, D.: Developing psychological skills in young athletes. *In* Coaching Science Update. Edited by N.L. Wood. Ottawa, Ontario: Coaching Assn. of Canada, 1983.

26. Greist, J.H., et al.: Running as treatment for depression. Comprehensive Psychiatry. 20:41–53, 1979.

27. Harris, D.V.: Involvement in Sport: A Somatopsychic Rationale for Physical Activity. Philadelphia: Lea & Febiger, 1973.

28. Henry, F.M.: Reaction time-movement time correlations. Perceptual and Motor Skills. 12:63–66, 1961.

29. Heyman, S.R.: Cognitive interventions: theories, applications, and precautions. *In* Cognitive Sport Psychology. Edited by W.F. Straub and J.M. Williams. New York: Lansing, 1984, pp. 289–303.

30. Hill, W.F.: Activity as an autonomous drive. J. Comp. Physiol. Psychol. 49:15–19, 1956.

31. Horvath, S.M.: The physiological factors in human performance. A paper presented at the 14th annual meeting of the American College of Sports Medicine, Las Vegas, Nevada, March 10, 1967.

32. Hughes, J.R.: Psychological effects of habitual aerobic exercise: a critical review. Prevent. Med. 13:66–78, 1984.

33. Huizinga, J.: Homo ludens: A Study of the Play Element in Culture. Boston: Beacon, 1950.

34. Jacobson, E.: Progressive Relaxation. Chicago: University of Chicago Press, 1930.

35. Kroll, W.: Sixteen personality factor profiles of collegiate wrestlers. Res. Quart. 38:49–56, 1967.

36. Landers, D.M., and S.H. Boutcher: Arousal-performance relationships. *In* Applied Sport Psychology. Edited by J.M. Williams. Palo Alto, Calif.: Mayfield, 1986, pp. 163–184.

37. Landers, D.M., and P.D. McCullagh: Social facilitation of motor performance. *In* Exercise and Sport Sciences Reviews. Vol. 4. Edited by J.E. Keogh and R.S. Hutton. Santa Barbara, Calif.: Journal Publishing Affiliates, 1976, pp. 125–162.

38. Locke, E.A., and J.F. Bryan: Cognitive aspects of psychomotor performance: The effects of performance goals on levels of performance. J. Appl. Psychol. 50:286–291, 1966.

39. Magill, R.A.: Motor Learning: Concepts and Applications. Dubuque, Iowa: Wm. C. Brown, 1980.

40. Magill, R.A., M.J. Ash, and F.C. Smoll (eds.): Children in Sport. Edition 2. Champaign, Ill.: Human Kinetics, 1982.

41. Mahoney, M.J., and M. Avener: Psychology of the elite athlete: an exploratory study. Cognitive Therapy and Research. 1:135–141, 1977.

42. Markoff, R.A., P. Ryan, and T. Young: Endorphins and mood changes in long distance running. Med. Sci. Sports. 14:11–15, 1982.

43. Martens, R.: Social Psychology and Physical Activity. New York: Harper & Row, 1975.

44. Maslow, A.: Motivation and Personality. New York: Harper & Row, 1970.

45. Morgan, W.P.: Psychological consequences of vigorous physical activity and sport. *In* Beyond Research—Solutions to Human Problems. Amer. Acad. of P.E. Papers No. 10, Edited by M.G. Scott. Iowa City, Iowa: Amer. Acad. of P.E., 1976, pp. 15–35.

46. Morgan, W.P.: Negative addiction in runners. Physician Sportsmed. 7(1):57–70, 1979.

47. Morgan, W.P.: The trait psychology controversy. Res. Quart. 51:50–76, 1980.

48. Morgan, W.P.: Psychological benefits of physical activity. *In* Exercise in Health and Disease. Edited by F.J. Nagle and H.J. Montoye. Springfield: Charles C Thomas, 1981, pp. 299–314.

49. Morgan, W.P.: Physical activity and mental health. *In* Exercise and Health. Amer. Acad. of P.E. Papers No. 17. Edited by H.M. Eckert and H.J. Montoye. Champaign, Ill.: Human Kinetics Publ., 1984, pp. 132–145.

50. Morgan, W.P., J.A. Roberts, F.R. Brand, and A.D. Feinerman: Psychological effect of chronic physical activity. Med. Sci. Sports. 2:213–217, 1970.

51. Murray, H.A., et al.: Explorations in Personality: A Clinical and Experimental Study of 50 Men of College Age. New York: Oxford Press, 1938.

52. Nideffer, R.M.: The Ethics and Practice of Applied Sport Psychology. Ithaca, N.Y.: Mouvement Publications, 1981.

53. Oxendine, J.B.: Emotional arousal and motor performance. Quest. 13:23–30, 1970.

54. Oxendine, J.B.: Psychology of Motor Learning. Englewood Cliffs, N.J.: Prentice-Hall, 1984.

55. Paffenbarger, R.S., Jr., A.L. Wing, and R.T. Hyde: Physical activity as an index of heart attack risk in college alumni. Amer. J. Epidemiol. 108:161–175, 1978.

56. Paulus, P.B., B.B. Judd, and I.H. Bernstein: Social facilitation and sports. *In* Psychology of Motor Behavior and Sport—Vol. II. Edited by R.W. Christina and D.M. Landers. Champaign, Ill.: Human Kinetics, 1977.

57. Perrier study: fitness in America. Perrier-Great Waters of France, Inc., New York, 1979.

58. Rivenes, R.S.: Foundations of Physical Education: A Scientific Approach. Boston: Houghton Mifflin, 1978.

59. Ryan, E.D.: Perceptual characteristics of vigorous people. *In* New Perspectives of Man in Action. Edited by R.C. Brown and B.J. Cratty. Englewood Cliffs, N.J.: Prentice-Hall, 1969, pp. 88–101.

60. Ryan, E.D.: The emergence of psychological research as related to performance in physical activity. *In* Perspectives on the Academic Discipline of Physical Education. Edited by G.A. Brooks. Champaign, Ill.: Human Kinetics, 1981, pp. 327–341.
61. Ryan, E.D., and W.L. Lakie: Competitive and noncompetitive performance in relation to achievement motivation and manifest anxiety. J. Personality and Soc. Psychol. *1*:342–345, 1965.
62. Ryan, E.D., and J. Simons: Efficacy of mental imagery in enhancing mental rehearsal of motor skills. J. Sport Psych. *4*:41–51, 1982.
63. Ryan, E.D., and J. Simons: What is learned in mental practice of motor skills: a test of the cognitive-motor hypothesis. J. Sport Psych. *5*:419–426, 1983.
64. Sage, G.H.: Motor Learning and Control: A Neuropsychological Approach. Dubuque, Iowa: Wm. C. Brown, 1984.
65. Schmaidt, R.A.: A schema theory of discrete motor skill learning. Psychol. Rev. *82*:225–260, 1975.
66. Schmidt, R.A.: Motor Control and Learning: A Behavioral Emphasis. Champaign, Ill.: Human Kinetics, 1982.
67. Serfass, R.C., and S.G. Gerberich: Exercise for optimal health: strategies and motivational considerations. Prevent. Med. *13*:79–99, 1984.
68. Singer, R.N.: Myths and Truths in Sports Psychology. New York: Harper & Row, 1975.
69. Singer, R.N.: The Learning of Motor Skills. New York: Macmillan, 1982.
70. Solley, W.H.: The effects of verbal instruction of speed and accuracy upon the learning of a motor skill. Res. Quart. *23*:231–240, 1952.
71. Spirduso, W.W.: The emergence of research in motor control and learning. *In* Perspectives on the Academic Discipline of Physical Education. Edited by G.A. Brooks. Champaign, Ill.: Human Kinetics, 1981, pp. 257–272.
72. Steinhaus, A.H.: Toward an Understanding of Health and Physical Education. Dubuque, Iowa: Wm. C. Brown, 1963.
73. Taylor, C.B., J.F. Sallis, and R. Needle: The relation of physical activity and exercise to mental health. Pub. Health Rep. *100*:195–202, 1985.
74. Ulett, G.A., and D.B. Peterson: Applied Hypnosis and Positive Suggestion. St. Louis: Mosby, 1965.
75. U.S. Department of Health and Human Services. Promoting Health/Preventing Disease: Objectives for the Nation. Washington, D.C.: U.S. Government Printing Office, 1980.
76. Varca, P.E.: An analysis of home and away game performance of male college basketball teams. J. Sport Psychol. *2*:245–257, 1980.
77. Vealey, R.S.: Imagery training for performance enhancements. *In* Applied Sport Psychology. Edited by J.M. Williams. Palo Alto, Calif.: Mayfield, 1986, pp. 209–231.
78. Williams, J.M.: Psychological characteristics of peak performance. *In* Applied Sport Psychology. Edited by J.M. Williams. Palo Alto, Calif.: Mayfield, 1986, pp. 123–132.
79. Woods, J.B.: The effect of varied instructional emphasis upon the development of a motor skill. Res. Quart. *38*:132–141, 1967.
80. Yates, A., K. Leehey, and C. Shisslak: Running—an analog of anorexia? New England J. Med. *308*:251–255, 1983.
81. Zajonc, R.B.: Social facilitation. Science. *149*(1):269–274, 1965.
82. Zander, A.F.: Productivity and group success: team sport vs. the individual achiever. Psychol. Today. *8*(11):64–68, 1974.

BIBLIOGRAPHY

1. Cox, R.H.: Sport Psychology: Concepts and Applications. Dubuque, Iowa: Wm. C. Brown, 1985.
2. Fisher, A.C.: Psychology of Sport: Issues and Insights. Palo Alto, Calif.: Mayfield, 1976.
3. Harris, D.V.: Involvement in Sport: A Somatopsychic Rationale for Physical Activity. Philadelphia: Lea & Febiger, 1973.
4. Magill, R.A.: Motor Learning: Concepts and Applications. Dubuque, Iowa: Wm. C. Brown, 1980.
5. Sage, G.H.: Motor Learning and Control: A Neuropsychological Approach. Dubuque, Iowa: Wm. C. Brown, 1984.
6. Schmidt, R.A.: Motor Control and Learning: A Behavioral Emphasis. Champaign, Ill.: Human Kinetics, 1982.
7. Singer, R.N.: The Learning of Motor Skills. New York: Macmillan, 1982.
8. Williams, J.M. (ed.): Applied Sport Psychology. Palo Alto, Calif.: Mayfield, 1986.

SOCIOLOGY OF SPORT AND PHYSICAL EDUCATION

INTRODUCTION

The historic development of sport in American society was examined in Chapter 1. It was mentioned that sport has been the predominant component of school and college instructional physical education programs since the 1930s. Further, in part because of their presumed potential for positive development of desired attitudes, values, and beliefs, athletic programs have been supported in educational institutions through most of the 20th century. However, it was stressed that sport in America has grown rapidly in the last 30 years, and has a much greater societal impact than that evidenced in educational institutions alone. This includes the large professional sports phenomenon, sports and politics (e.g., the Olympic Games boycotts), the economic impact of sports, and sports participation during leisure-time. Before examining the societal impact of sport in detail, it is useful to review some basic terminology and concepts regarding society and its systematic study.

THE SOCIOLOGIC PERSPECTIVE

Sociology is the behavioral science concerned with the study of society's structure, function, and processes as they affect human social behavior. It is through society's major institutions and its many groups that various elements of its culture (including all mental, physical, and social skills necessary to function effectively) are trans-mitted. This process of acquiring the culture of a society is termed socialization.

Sociologists examine major societal institutions, such as family, government, religion, economics, and education in terms of the factors that cause them to persist, as well as their interdependence and the factors that cause them to change. They are also concerned with the forms of organization of social groups, the relationships among them, patterns of individual and group interaction, attitudes within groups, and group influences on behavior. The sociologist seeks to isolate underlying regularities of human social behavior by careful observation and analysis of the most important structural and functional characteristics of a particular social system.[74]

The sociologists' basic thrust is not directly concerned with why something malfunctions from the point of view of societal officials or authorities, and how to make it better. Rather, it is in developing generalizations of how and why the social system works as it does, and in better understanding and prediction of human behavior in specified conditions. Since factors influencing human behavior are complex, these predictions can only be in terms of probabilities.

As a scientist, the sociologist attempts to be objective, to control personal preferences and prejudices, and to perceive clearly rather than to judge against preconceived normative behavior.[6] Eitzen and Sage[27] contend that, while sociologists must be objective in their observations, a value-neutral approach (i.e., not good or bad) supports the status quo. Hence, they encourage the utilization of the normative approach in problem formulation (e.g., racism exists in sports) and interpretation of whether the evidence supports or fails to support their hypothesis.

SPORT AS A SUBJECT OF STUDY BY SOCIOLOGISTS

With the increasing importance of sport in American society, it would seem a particularly attractive realm of study by the sociologist. Snyder and Spreitzer,[88] however, contended that the sociology of sport had yet to become a mainline specialty in sociology by the mid-70s, and that some in the discipline might question whether it ever should. They went on to develop a convincing case for the systematic study of sport, as follows:

We suggest that sport as a substantive topic has as much claim on the sociologists' attention as the more conventional specialties of family, religion, political, and industrial sociology. Sports and games are cultural universals and basic institutions in societies, and are some of the most pervasive aspects of culture in industrial societies . . . the sociology of sport is of value to the larger discipline primarily in terms of its capacity to serve as a fertile testing ground for the generating and examination of theoretical frameworks.

The phenomenon of sport represents one of the most pervasive social institutions in the United States. Sports permeate all levels of social reality from the societal down to the social phychological. The salience of sports can be documented in terms of news coverage, financial expenditures, number of participants and spectators, hours consumed, and time samplings of conversations. Given the salience of sports as a social institution, a sociology of sport has emerged that attempts to go beyond the descriptive level by providing theoretically informed analyses and explanations of sports activity.[88:467-8]

Given that sport is a major phenomenon in contemporary society, one might legitimately wonder why it has only recently become the subject of systematic study by social scientists. Snyder and Spreitzer[88] contend that this has been due to a number of factors, including: (1) the ubiquitous presence of sport in American society—outside educational institutions—is a rather recent, post-World War II development; (2) many sociologists considered sport as involving physical rather than social interaction, and that it represents essentially a frivolous children's pastime undeserving of serious scholarly study; (3) many scholars envisioned sport as a reflection of a lower level of human nature, and inferior to other cultural forms such as art, literature, and music; and (4) until recently, the availability of publication outlets for scholarly studies has been sparse.

BRIEF HISTORIC OVERVIEW OF THE SOCIOLOGY OF SPORT

Social development as a cornerstone of physical education program justification was effectively summarized by Williams as early as 1927,[103] although the presumed social outcomes of physical education and interscholastic athletic programs were not subjected to systematic investigation. In 1953, Cozens and Stumpf[19] published a pioneering treatise on the effect of sports in American life. However, it was not until 1965 that Kenyon and Loy's seminal article, entitled "Toward a Sociology of Sport,"[42] effectively challenged the profession to consider the importance of this area of scholarly study. Simultaneously, the UNESCO sponsored formation of the International Committee for Sport Sociology, which was comprised of scholars from physical education and sociology. The *International Review of Sport Sociology*, published in Poland continuously since 1966, was a direct outgrowth of this action.

During the next decade, there was significant growth in higher education and fragmentation of knowledge in disciplines to emerging subdisciplines. Sport sociology became one of over 20 subfields identified in sociology.[81] Concurrently, physical education experienced a shift in perspective from teacher preparation to the development of an academic discipline. By 1978, the sport sociology literature in North America included over 650 publications from 100 authors, but Loy and colleagues[52] concluded that sport sociology had yet to be perceived as a legitimate subfield within either physical education or sociology, owing to factors associated with lack of a critical mass of faculty, academic status, and ideologic orientations. However, sport sociology continued to grow during the 1980s, with an increasing number of courses at the undergraduate and graduate levels offered in both physical education and sociology departments.[41,81] Research publication outlets have increased, with the appointment in December 1978 of a sociology of sport associate editor to the *Research Quarterly for Exercise and Sport*, representing recognition of the subdiscipline by research colleagues in other subdiscipline areas of physical education. Similarly, the American College of Sports Medicine has had a sport sociologist since 1981 on the editorial board for its annual publication of *Exercise and Sport Sciences Reviews*. Professional organizations in physical education and sociology sponsor regular research sessions on the sociology of sport, and sport sociologists have formed their own organization, the North American Society for the Sociology of Sport. Nonetheless, Coakley maintains that there remains a need for high-quality empirical research coupled with efforts to build a body of useful theory. He further asserts that research and theory in sport sociology must extend well beyond concern with athletes to discover more about the nature of sport as a social institution and how it effects people generally and society as a whole.[14] Before examining these issues of concern to sport sociologists, it is necessary to examine the definition of sport in its several forms and clearly distinguish it from the associated terms of games, play and recreation.

SPORT DEFINED

Defining sport seems almost ludicrous in that it is so pervasive in our society. However, a few questions follow that should convince one that a more precise definition is needed by sport sociologists than that commonly accepted by the laity. Most of us would agree that baseball, football, basketball, volleyball, and track and field are sports, but what about chess, hiking, hunting and fishing? Does how the "sport" activity is organized have an important bearing on whether it is properly categorized as sport? For example, is a spontaneous half-court basketball game between friends similar to a scheduled basketball game in the NBA? Are professional wrestling and the Roller Derby properly categorized as sport? Is one who participates in the latter contest playing a sport, or working in an occupation demanding physical work in a game atmosphere?

There are elements of play and games in sport, but distinction between the primary focus of each can be made clearly apparent. Play is among the cultural universals of humankind, though it occurs in widely variant forms dependent in part upon the particular culture's attitude toward physical activity.[61] Caillois[11] characterizes play as activity that is (1) engaged in solely by choice, (2) separate in time and space from other activity, (3) uncertain with regard to end result or outcome, (4) unproductive in terms of material gain, (5) non-utilitarian in the sense that the purpose of the activity is inherent, (6) governed by rules that evolve as activity progresses, and (7) contains make-believe roles that one does not necessarily identify with when the play activity ends.

Loy and colleagues[54] contend that games are playful, in that they generally have one or more of the seven elements of play, but that they are distinguished from play by the element of competition. They define competition as a struggle for supremacy between two or more opposing sides, whether between humans and other objects of nature, both animate and inanimate. Roberts and Sutton-Smith[73] have classified games according to three primary outcome attributes: (1) those in which physical skill is paramount; (2) games of strategy in which one exercises rational choices in electing courses of action; and (3) games of chance. Games, then, are any form of playful competition in which the outcome is determined by physical skill, strategy, or chance, singly or in combination.[54]

Most sport sociologists contend that sport entails elements characteristic of games, but that it differs primarily in terms of required use of highly developed physical skills and abilities acquired through training.[54] Thus, since playing cards or chess require predominantly cognitive skills and not complex physical skills or vigorous physical exertion, they are games. On the other hand, auto racing is a sport in that it requires considerable physical practice for the driver to develop the skill and timing to effectively handle the racing car.

Another important characteristic distinguishes sport from games, in that participation in a competitive physical activity as a single occurrence, primarily for the enjoyment of the participants, is properly categorized as a game.[54] Examples include a horseshoe pitching contest among friends or an impromptu neighborhood basketball game. However when games requiring physical prowess become formally organized and sponsored contests (i.e., institutionalized), they are properly categorized as organized sport.[27] Coakley[14] lists several elements of institutionalization that usually occur in this transformation: (1) rules are carefully standardized; (2) rule enforcement is taken over by official regulatory agencies; (3) organizational and technical aspects become important; and (4) emphasis is on formalized physical skill development.

Snyder and Spreitzer[91] have devised a play-sport continuum (Fig. 5–1) in identifying where physical activity participation that demonstrates characteristics of both play and sport should most appropriately be placed. For example, if one participates in community recreation, it would most likely be in the form of play or a game. On the other hand, if one plays on a basketball team in an adult industrial league, it would represent informal sport, while practicing and playing on a professional team represents formal sport. An added dimension to Snyder and Spreitzer's continuum is the growing contention among sport sociologists that participants in big-time college and professional athletics experience increasing connotations of work in their formal sport participation. This notion is apparent in Figure 5–2, in which athletics is seen on the far end as a subset of occupations, and occupations as a subset of

work. On the near end, sport is depicted as a subset of games, and games as a subset of play. Loy and colleagues[54] conclude that modern sport, in its numerous forms, may be best conceived as located on a continuum between work and play.

This somewhat extended examination of what the term sport means may prove disconcerting to students who have a more global perspective of its definition. However, if one wishes to examine how sport relates to other social institutions, how sport participation affects social values, whether sport participation has affected the social mobility of blacks, or whether sport participation represents an especially important socialization instrument in school children, it is essential that one define sport in the context of interest.

SPORT AS A MICROCOSM OF SOCIETY: LINKAGES WITH MAJOR SOCIAL INSTITUTIONS

Sport has a complex interrelationship with other essential elements of society. This is expressed both at the micro level in small groups and in its macro level relationship with other major societal institutions, such as education, religion, government, economic order, and more recently, science. These relationships, together with the notion that sport reflects a microcosm of society, will now be examined.

Luschen[56] examined questions regarding how sport as a social institution was related to other institutions, particularly in terms of what social values they promoted in common. This notion may have emanated from the early, perceptive analysis of American sport by Boyle,[8] who concluded that sport is a mirror of society involving elements of social life, such as clothing design, commerce, concepts of law, ethical values, language, race relations, and stratification. Indeed, Robertson,[74] the author of a leading introductory sociology textbook contends that sport, as competitive physical activity guided by established rules, provides in some respects a microcosm of society. That is, "by understanding crucial aspects of sport—the kinds of games that are popular, the social groups

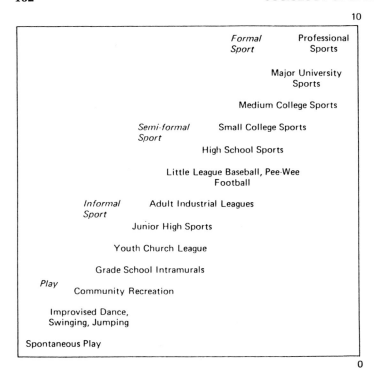

FIG. 5–1. Summary of physical activities from play to formal sport. (Modified from Snyder, E.E., and E. Spreitzer: Social Aspects of Sport. 2nd ed. Englewood Cliffs, N.J.: Prentice-Hall, 1989, p. 121.)

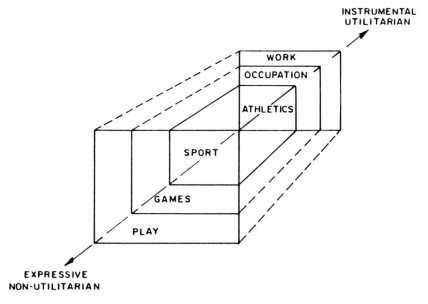

FIG. 5–2. Sport on a play-work continuum. (From Loy, J.W., B.D. McPherson, and G. Kenyon: Sport and Social Systems: A Guide to the Analysis, Problems, and Literature. Reading, MA: Addison-Wesley, 1978, p. 23.)

that participate, the statuses and roles of these involved, the distribution of power and wealth within this institution, the linkages of sport with other institutions, and the values sport represents—we can learn much about American society as a whole."[74:85] Eitzen and Sage[27] support this contention, briefly discussing six qualities in sport that are also present in the larger society. These include: (1) a high degree of competitiveness, with strong emphasis on winning; (2) emphasis on materialism in the rapid growth of corporate sport; (3) prevalence of racist attitude and actions; (4) the domination of individuals by conservative bureaucratic organizations; (5) the unequal distribution of power amongst the wealthy in securing and maintaining control of corporate sport; and (6) the use of conflict, via strikes, boycotts, and demonstrations, by the less powerful to gain advantage in sport and society.

Snyder[86] studied the use of high school athletic dressing room slogans by coaches in Ohio, as exemplifying characteristics supported by values inherent in the Protestant Ethic. He was able to categorize these slogans used by coaches in an attempt to model athletic behavior to enhance players' performance as follows: (1) mental and physical fitness, (2) aggressiveness and competitive spirit, (3) basic skills must be painfully learned, (4) perseverance, (5) self-discipline, and (6) subordination of self to the group. Similarly, Edwards[23] examined newspapers, magazines, and a prominent coaching journal for statements of social values attributed to sport. He identified seven central themes as constituting what he termed the "American Sports Creed." They bear considerable resemblance to Snyder's analysis of coaches' identification of desirable qualities in athletic endeavor, but also include religiosity, in terms of sports achievement relating to traditional American Christianity, and nationalism, in terms of relating sport to patriotism and love of country.

These notions were examined by Spreitzer and Snyder,[92] who surveyed over 500 adults in a large midwestern U.S. metropolitan area regarding their value orientations of the functions and consequences of sport. Both males and females agreed in near equal percentages that sports: (1) are valuable because they teach self-discipline (89%); (2) promote the development of fair play (81%); (3) are important for the well-being of society (75%); (4) are valuable because they teach children respect for authority (72%); (5) are valuable because they teach children to become good citizens (71%); and (6) present emphasis on competition for children effects more good than harm (68%). However, less than 50% agreed that sports are valuable because they provide an opportunity for individuals to get ahead in the world, and that sports are valuable because they contribute to the development of patriotism.

In a more recent survey of 525 undergraduate students attending either a liberal arts college or a state university, examining acceptance of the American "sports creed," Nixon[64] observed that over 80% of the students felt that sports participation developed better self-discipline, promoted better physical health, built "character" and made better citizens, and developed leadership qualities. However, only 23% of the students affirmed that "in the long run you learn more about life and success in the sports arena than in the classroom or anywhere else" (i.e., sports as preparation for life), and less than 15% felt that "athletes tend to be stronger believers in God and country than nonathletes."

In this section, evidence has been presented which supports the contention that sport is a microcosm of society, in that it reflects many aspects of society as a whole. One aspect, that sport is a "value-receptacle" for dominant social values, has been examined in some depth. Sport also interacts with other social institutions, reflecting not only persistent social values, but also elements of societal strain and change. Sport, then, is not an isolated social institution, but one that interacts with other institutions. The linkages and resultant interactions of sport and several major societal institutions will now be examined.

SPORT AND EDUCATION

In the United States, much of sport takes place within educational institutions in physical education classes, intramurals, and athletics. Organized athletics in educational institutions is almost universal, and is peculiar to this country. Snyder and Spreitzer underline this contention:

Organized sport in Western European countries is more closely linked to the community within a nexus of clubs. In communist countries, sport tends to be closely linked with governmental and political units. The peculiarly close relationship between sport and educational institutions in the United States represents a sociologically intriguing connection.[91:105]

Education, as a fundamental institution of society, is charged with the systematic, formalized transmission of knowledge, skills, and values. As discussed in the previous section, sport is widely perceived as an effective means of reinforcing values and norms of behavior held in esteem by society in general. The institution of sport entails definition of the values of participation as well as specifications of how sport is socially organized.[3] Within the formal educational context, this involves a complex interaction which involves elements of the community, the economy and government. Some contend that the present conduct of athletics at the collegiate and secondary school levels is not effectively compatible with the primary mission of the educational institution.[14,27,91] There is a limited but growing body of scientific literature concerning this question, which will now be examined.

"BIG-TIME" COLLEGIATE ATHLETICS. The principal concern of athletics at the collegiate level is directed at those institutions sponsoring "big-time" programs in football and/or basketball. At this level, sport becomes, in essence corporate, essentially exemplifying elements of professional sport.[27] Page[66] used a bureaucratic model to analyze the structure of "big-time" athletic departments, and found them to exemplify many elements of big business concerns. Snyder and Spreitzer[91] contend that success in the big business/bureaucratic model of social organization is determined by the output or product. In corporate sport oriented collegiate programs, this means winning teams must be produced so that the athletic department can compete successfully for the public's entertainment dollar. The usual social system inputs, organizational characteristics, and the usual outputs are depicted in Figure 5–3. Social system inputs include university alumni and community support, as well as presumed favorable social values. The organizational structure is highly organized, hierarchical, and more committed to organizational autonomy than are programs without pressures of similar magnitude to win and maintain financial solvency. Snyder and Spreitzer[91] maintain that this social context is helpful in explaining increasingly more prevalent unethical practices, such as illegal recruiting of athletes, illegal subsidies to athletes, manipulation of eligibility standards, and exploitation of athletes.

It appears clear that "big-time" collegiate athletics are no longer primarily sponsored to accomplish educational goals for the participant. Though there is an obviously strong institutional support for this type of program, the evidence substantiating espoused benefits in terms of creating increased resources for the entire university is not strong. Nonetheless, most collegiate administrators apparently feel that the "big-time" athletics high publicity profile increases alumni support and funds coming from the state legislature, even to the extent of providing funds to make up for the shortfall in athletics income versus expenses. Lopiano[49] surveyed intercollegiate athletic programs and found that almost 70% were not self-supporting. Ullrich[100] observed a positive correlation between "big-time" football success and the award of doctoral degrees and the receipt of federal funding for University programs and research between 1948 and 1968 in emerging land grant universities, but not in established universities. Springer[94] surveyed schools that dropped intercollegiate football teams between 1939 and 1974, and found no change in alumni support and funding from the state legislature. Further, a number of academically prestigious universities, such as Ivy League institutions, the University of Chicago, Johns Hopkins University, and Massachusetts Institute of Technology have not experienced dimin-

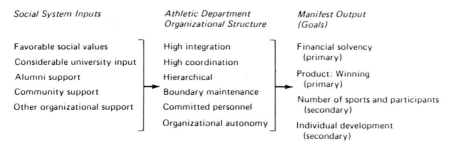

Social System Inputs

Favorable social values
Considerable university input
Alumni support
Community support
Other organizational support

Athletic Department Organizational Structure

High integration
High coordination
Hierarchical
Boundary maintenance
Committed personnel
Organizational autonomy

Manifest Output (Goals)

Financial solvency (primary)
Product: Winning (primary)
Number of sports and participants (secondary)
Individual development (secondary)

FIG. 5–3. Organizational characteristics of the sport subsystem within the university. (From Snyder, E.E. and E. Spreitzer: Social Aspects of Sport. 2nd ed. Englewood Cliffs, N.J.: Prentice-Hall, 1983, p. 108.)

ished support because they dropped intercollegiate athletic programs or maintained them on a small-time basis.[14] However, these institutions have created strong public relations images using programs other than sports, which takes much longer to achieve than the "big-time" athletics public relations image emanating from media generated national rankings.[32] Roper and Snow[75] studied the relation of two measures of academic excellence with rankings of "big-time" football and basketball programs, between 1968 and 1972, and observed that good students and excellence in academic programs were not significantly correlated with "big-time" athletic program success.

ATHLETICS IN THE SECONDARY SCHOOL. In his classic study of the adolescent and the school, Coleman described the image of an American high school likely to be observed by an outside visitor:

A visitor entering a school would likely be confronted, first of all, with a trophy case. His examination of the trophies would reveal a curious fact: the gold and silver cups, with rare exception, symbolize victory in athletic contests, not scholastic ones. The figures adorning these trophies represent men passing footballs, shooting basketballs, holding out batons; they are not replicas of "The Thinker." The concrete symbols of victory are old footballs, basketballs, and baseballs, not works of art or first editions of books won as literary prizes. Altogether, the trophy case would suggest to the innocent visitor that he was entering an athletic club, not an educational institution.

Walking further, this visitor would encounter teenagers bursting from classrooms. Listening to their conversations, he would hear both casual and serious discussions of the Friday football game, confirming his initial impression. Attending a school assembly that morning, he would probably find a large segment of the program devoted to a practice of school cheers for the athletic game and the announcement of a pep rally before the game. At lunch hour, he would be likely to find more boys shooting baskets in the gymnasium than reading in the library. Browsing through a school yearbook, he would be impressed, in his innocence, with the number of pages devoted to athletics.

Altogether, this visitor would find, wherever he turned, a great deal more attention devoted to athletics by teenagers, both as athletes and as spectators, than to scholastic matters. He might even conclude, with good reason, that the school was essentially organized around athletic contests and that scholastic matters were of lesser importance to all involved.[16:35–6]

One consequence of the extraordinary popularity of athletics in American secondary schools is the high status of athletes among their peers. Coleman's classic study[15] of ten mid-Western secondary schools revealed a number of interesting values and attitudes that held regardless of school size, location, or socioeconomic composition. Belonging to the schools' "leading crowd" was based on achievements (especially in athletics for boys), but girls were included because of ascribed characteristics, such as parents' achievement, good looks, and possessions. In response to the question of how he would like to be remembered at school, 44% of the boys chose as an athletic star, 31% as a brilliant student, and 25% as being most popular. In contrast, almost 75% of the boys' parents wanted their sons to be remembered as brilliant students. This suggests an adolescent subculture, in which values and norms vary from the larger society. Since this and other studies of adolescent attitudes and athletics had been done in the early 1960s, prior to significant social changes in America, Eitzen[26] replicated some of Coleman's research. Students in 14 secondary schools, which ranged in student population from 92 to 2,937, and in communities ranging in population from 400 to over 600,000, were surveyed. The questionnaire included an item ranking (from 1 to 5) of the various criteria necessary for status among boys, and an item in which girls ranked the criteria that "makes a guy popular with girls." Mean rankings are given in Table 5–1. The comparison of boys' rankings from the two studies is strikingly similar, and indicates athletics remains an important element of adolescent male status. Contrary to Coleman's observations, Eitzen[26] found significant differences in individual factors including (1) nonwhite boys were more interested in sport than whites, (2) that more importance was attached to athletics by boys in smaller schools, and (3) that the more rural the community, the greater the importance of athletics.

A persistent concern of the importance placed on athletics in the secondary school is the effect of athletic participation on academic orientation and performance. Coleman[15] suggested that the inordinate amount of attention focused on athletics in

high school resulted in a depreciation of academic pursuits. However, in most of the schools he surveyed, star athletes had a higher grade point average (GPA) than did nonathletes. Subsequently, numerous studies have been done, almost all showing that male high school athletes have a higher GPA than nonathletes.[27] However, problems in interpretation remain. For example, athletes may have a higher GPA because they must meet a minimum level to be eligible to participate. Thus, some students with poor academic performance may not ever attempt to participate in athletics. Finally, all of these studies have been cross-sectional, so the relationship cannot be considered a causal one. Coakley[14] contends that the most logical explanation is that interscholastic athletic programs tend to attract students with self-confidence, above average academic abilities, and favorable attitudes toward school. A summary of how this selection process could be responsible for the relationship between interscholastic athletic participation and academic success is depicted in Figure 5–4.

It appears that the association between athletic participation and higher educational expectations is strongest among high school boys from lower socioeconomic status. Buhrman[10] studied a group of adolescent boys over 6 years, and observed that academic performance is more closely related to athletic participation among boys from poorer socioeconomic status. He concluded that athletics may be the most im-

Table 5–1.   Ranking of Criteria Boys and Girls Use to Rate the Popularity of Boys*

Criteria for Status	Eitzen (1976)	Coleman (1961)
Boys' Ranking of Criteria to Be Popular with Boys		
Be an athlete	2.2	2.2
Be in leading crowd	2.15	2.6
Leader in activities	2.77	2.9
High grades, honor roll	3.66	3.5
Come from right family	3.93	4.5
Girls' Ranking of Criteria for Boys to Be Popular with Girls		
Be in leading crowd	2.17	
Be an athlete	2.38	
Have a nice car	3.03	
Come from right family	3.32	
High grades, honor roll	3.80	

*Modified from Eitzen, D.S.: Sport and social status in American public secondary education. Review of Sport and Leisure. *1*:139–155, 1976.

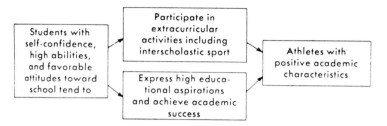

FIG. 5–4. Illustration of how the selection process could be responsible for the relationship between interscholastic sport participation and academic success. Sport does not create the positive characteristics but merely attracts many students who already possess them. (From: Coakey, J.J.: Sport in Society: Issues and Controversies. 2nd ed. St Louis: Times Mirror/Mosby, 1982, p. 115.)

portant means for lower socioeconomic status boys to gain social recognition and acceptance and, through it, higher academic aspiration and scholarship.

Interscholastic athletic programs are supported by secondary school administrators for numerous reasons. Eitzen and Sage[27] suggest that, aside from athletic contests, schools have few, if any, collective goals that tend to provide cohesiveness for the institution. In addition to this envisioned unifying effect, interscholastic athletics are considered by many administrators to facilitate social control, incubate societal values, and enhance student interest in physical activity participation.[14,27] Coleman[16] contends that interscholastic athletics provide an important community cohesiveness function, both in small towns and city neighborhoods, that is apart from that provided the school itself. Whether the interest created amongst alumni and community translates into concern for academic programs and educational concerns of the school—other than athletics—is unknown.[14] While some evidence relative to the relationship of interscholastic athletics and educational goals has been reviewed, there are many unresolved issues. A summary of arguments for and against interscholastic sports programs is given in Table 5–2.

PREADOLESCENT SPORT PARTICIPATION. Snyder and Spreitzer have astutely summarized the role of sport among preadolescents. They observe that preadolescent participation in sport:

Has not received the scholarly attention that is evident at the high school and collegiate levels. One of the reasons for this relative and unfortunate neglect is the fact that most sport activity for children is organized outside the context of the elementary school. Sports activities for children should be a serious topic for scientific study because the organizers of such community activities are largely untrained volunteers who organize and coach the activities. The impact of the formal physical education curriculum in the elementary school is substantially less potent than the energy surrounding Little League and Pop Warner teams . . . furthermore, although participation in sport affects people of all ages and educational levels, its influence is likely to be greatest on younger, more impressionable people.[91:117]

Coakley[14] concludes that though organized sport for children has come under attack in the 1970s and 1980s, programs for boys have continued to grow and are now complemented by a rapidly increasing number of similar programs for girls. Dowell[21] reviewed the literature concerning reasons advanced in support of these programs: (1) enhanced physical fitness, (2) emotional development, (3) social adjustment, (4) development of competitive attitude, and (5) insulation against delinquency. Potential deleterious effects advanced were: (1) overemphasis on winning, (2) increased risk of injury, (3) emotional strain, in part due to psychologic unreadiness, (4) premature athletic specialization, (5) elitism, with participation by only the most skilled, and (6) adult dominance. At present, there are only limited experimental data, with no clear evidence

Table 5–2. Traditional Arguments For and Against Interscholastic Sport Programs*

Arguments For	Arguments Against
1. Involves students in school activities and increases interest in academic activities	1. Distracts the attention of students away from academic activities
2. Builds the character and vigor required for adult participation in society	2. Focuses the attention of students on a set of values no longer appropriate in society
3. Stimulates interests in physical activities among all students in the school	3. Relegates most students to the role of spectator rather than active participant
4. Generates the spirit and unity necessary to maintain the school as a viable organization	4. Creates a superficial, transitory spirit subverting the educational goals of the school
5. Promotes parental, alumni, and community support for all school programs	5. Deprives educational programs of resources, facilities, staff, and community support

*From Coakley, J.J.: Sport in Society: Issues and Controversies. 4th ed, St. Louis, MO: Times Mirror/Mosby, 1990, p. 323.

of the overall physical and psychologic effects of organized sports on children.[14,91]

From a combined observational and interview study, Coakley[14] reports the contrasting essential elements of children's behavior and perceptions when involved in (1) informally organized, player-controlled games in parks and school playgrounds, or (2) in league organized sports. In the former, players indicated that their primary concern was in initiating and maintaining action and personal involvement, reaffirmation of personal friendships, and in playing in a close contest. Their activity was characterized by an impromptu initiation with little organization time. Rules were generally based on popular game models, but were modified to maximize action and personal involvement. In contrast, the organized league games resulted in adult control of action and involvement, with the players' behavior strictly patterned by specialized rules and roles. Actual play of the game was governed by time schedules and players never left the playing field without permission of the adult coach or referee. While Coakley's study did not deal directly with developmental factors, he concluded that the implications of involvement in organized sport programs were considerably different from what they might be in informal games.

SPORT AND RELIGION

As discussed in Chapter 1, the Puritans and other early American church leaders disapproved of play and sport, and advised their members not to participate in such activities. Numerous changes in living conditions and in prevalent societal attitudes have occurred, such that there is now a facilitative interaction between American sport and religion as basic social institutions.[27]

Religion in society fulfills important functions, including social integration, serving as an effective instrument of social control by reinforcing society's norms, values and beliefs, and generally tends to legitimize secular social structures.[27] Common values advanced by religion, sport, education, and other societal institutions include moral development, self-discipline, work ethic, meritocracy, loyalty, sociability, and social order.[91]

Numerous religious congregations in urban areas have church playgrounds and recreation centers with facilities, equipment, and instruction that substitute for, or complement those provided by municipal governments.[27] Church related organizations, such as the Young Men's Christian Association (YMCA), the YWCA, and the Catholic Youth Organization, have utilized sports as part of their social service mission. Churches and church related organizations have become attracted to the moral development dimensions espoused in the American Sports Creed, i.e., clean living, self-discipline, and respect for authority.[23,91] This has helped produce several associations specifically for athletes, including the Fellowship of Christian Athletes (FCA), Athletes in Action (AIA), and Pro Athletes Outreach. The FCA publishes a periodical, *The Christian Athlete,* which contains on its title page its intended purpose—"to confront athletes and coaches and through them the youth of the nation, with the challenge and adventure of following Christ and serving him through the fellowship of the Church . . ."[27:145] The Campus Crusade for Christ sponsors the sport missionary group, AIA, which consists primarily of former collegiate athletes. With dispensation from the NCAA, the AIA teams compete against collegiate and other amateur teams. As part of each appearance they make brief testimonial statements to the assembled crowds and distribute religious materials without cost. Eitzen and Sage[27] conclude that the increased utilization of sport by churches corresponds with the increasing secularization of North American society in an effort to accommodate activities that may solidify and integrate church membership.

As alluded to earlier, a strong case can be made for a congruence between predominant values of the Protestant work-ethic and the ideology of the dedicated athlete; viz., commitment to success, self-discipline, and hard work. Many coaches routinely admonish athletes to adhere to this basic belief system in maximizing development of their athletic talent. However, even after the most intelligent and dedicated preparation, there is a strong element of inherent unpredictability in athletic competition which results in many coaches and athletes employing religious and magical practices to cope with this stress. Eitzen and Sage[27] describe the use of prayer and the employment of magical practices, including rituals, taboos, and fetishism, by athletes and coaches.

SPORT AND POLITICS

The linkage between sport and politics in terms of the U.S. government's impact on sports during the last two decades has been profound. It has included: (1) antitrust legislation affecting control of televising collegiate and professional football; (2) legislation restructuring amateur athletic competition, (3) legislation reducing discrimination against women from access to sports (Title IX); (4) legislation establishing federal agencies for physical fitness, health promotion, and sports medicine; and (5) the successful pressure brought by President Carter in 1980 on the U.S. Olympic Committee to boycott the Moscow summer Olympic Games in retaliation for the Soviet invasion of Afghanistan.[13]

From an international perspective, the area of principal interest amongst sport sociologists has been the greatly increased use of sport for nationalism and as a political propaganda vehicle.[14,27] Many national governments have moved from the role of sport supporter to one of sport controller, charging central government agencies with responsibility for funding, organizing, and controlling sport at both the mass and elite levels.[54] The Communist nations, particularly the Soviet Union and East Germany, have developed elaborate, massive national sports programs which feature testing of children at age 7 to identify individuals with the most promising potential, and special sports training schools for the best athletes. The success of this system was apparent at the 1976 Montreal Olympic Games when athletes from the eight Communist Eastern bloc countries won 53% of the medals, though they represented less than 15% of the total number of contestants.[27] These nations see sport as an effective vehicle for achieving greater national fervor and unity, but primarily to illustrate that the Communist way of life is superior. However, worldwide, the developing nations may be attempting to use sport even more for enhancement of nationalism and for political purposes. Goodhue[34] reported that only 35 of 133 (26%) members of the United Nations in 1973 had a cabinet-level position related to sport, while 87% of the developing countries had such a post. Though the United States government has no such position, there is no lack of increasing concern for the importance of doing well in international sports competition. This is evidenced by federal funding provided in 1976 to the U.S. Olympic Committee for the establishment of permanent training sites, which have been in continuous operation since.

While some have espoused diffidence between sport and politics in connection with the intended purpose of the modern Olympic Games, this was not a rationale understood by Baron de Coubertin of France. His concern in initiating the Modern Games was both to enhance the physical fitness of French youth and to promote international goodwill and peaceful coexistence by bringing together the youth of all countries periodically for amicable trials of muscular strength and agility.[50] There have been numerous examples of political involvement in the modern Olympic Games, beginning notably with the 1936 Berlin Olympics staged to advance the notion of Arian supremacy. Following World War II and the banning of participants from Germany, Italy, and Japan in the 1948 London Olympics, other examples of political "interference" with the Games' "espoused original purpose" have occurred. Most notably from the United States' perspective is the 1968 black athletes' clenched fist and bowed head protest during the national anthem medal awarding ceremony. While these athletes were later required to return their medals and barred from future Olympic competition, subsequent affirmative actions of national "attachment" have not been reprimanded by the Olympic Committee.[91]

In 1980, President Carter wrote a letter to the United States Olympic Committee to explain his administration's purpose in proposing a boycott of the Moscow Summer Olympic Games. It acknowledged the significant sacrifice that American athletes would make in not participating at Moscow, and he affirmed a desire to keep Government policy out of the Olympics, but that deeper issues were at stake. Access to a major part of the world's oil supplies and Soviet military aggression were the major issues of concern. Since the head of the Moscow Olympic Organizing Committee was a high Soviet Government official, boycotting of the Games by countries of the "free world" would send a powerful signal of outrage that could not be hidden from the Soviet people and might deter future Soviet aggression.[91]

It seems clearly apparent that the Olympics have always been political, but Sugden and Yiannakas[98] contend that it is only when the vast world-wide notoriety of the Olympics is used to bar participation of certain countries, or attempts are made to coerce a nation to alter its internal or political/military activities, that the Olympic movement is seriously jeopardized.

Loy, et al.[54] contend that a second basis for a close relationship between politics and sport exists in terms of the social structure of sport organizations. That is, sport organizations are little different from any other organization in which internal politics play a role in policy making, recruitment of new members, succession to executive roles, and evaluation of performances. Eitzen and Sage elaborate:

As sport has become increasingly organized, a plethora of teams, leagues, players' associations, and ruling bodies have been created. These groups acquire certain powers that by their very creation are distributed unequally. Thus, there may be a power struggle between players and owners (e.g., the major league baseball player strike in 1985), or between competing leagues (e.g., NFL vs. USFL in professional football), or between various sanctioning bodies (AAU vs. NCAA in amateur athletics).[27:167]

SPORT AND ECONOMICS

Nixon and Jewett contend that ideally, sport in America reflects the values of democratic capitalism:

The payoff (the winning of the game or the earning of a corporate profit) depends upon the individual and collective effort of the workers (or the players), striving for a common goal, being rewarded for a successful performance, displaying habits of compliance to orders, perseverance, fighting or working hard even during times of difficulty, and being a contributing member of the "team."[65:136]

The interrelationship of sport and the economy has grown in parallel with the technologic advance attendant to the Industrial Revolution, which resulted in a vastly increased urban society, with a higher standard of living, and substantially greater leisure time.[18] Increased discretionary income has provided impetus for expanded leisure and fitness activity expenditures. It has also facilitated growth in spectator sports, aided primarily by programming and attendant advertising in the mass media, especially television. Spectator sport is now much more than a form of public entertainment. It is big business, appropriately referred to as corporate sport.[27,46]

Corporate sport in America is epitomized by the teams of the four major professional sports—baseball, basketball, football, and hockey. They are similar in many respects to other business organizations, and thus are subject to analysis in conventional structural and functional contexts, including exchange of goods and services, productivity, division of labor, job dissatisfaction, unions, strikes, franchises, and monopolies.[54] Professional sports leagues operate as a monopoly and, for the most part, as an unregulated one. This means that the teams within a league operate as a cartel, arranging agreements on matters of mutual interest (such as rules, schedules, expansion, and media contracts) with essentially no direct competition or federal regulation. In essence, this means that in a given city, only the owner of the team has the right to sell tickets to the games for that professional sport, to offer broadcasts of games, and to sell concessions at the games.[91] Many of the present professional sports team owners are corporate managers who utilize the unique tax advantage for depreciating the salaries of players as an investment cost to offset losses on income or to minimize taxable profits.[27] Further, as a member of the league cartel, they are in a position to restrict the addition of new franchises, which tends to increase the worth of existing franchises. The 1961 Sports Broadcast Act permits professional sports leagues to sell their national television rights as a group without being subject to the antitrust law.[27]

Another important aspect of professional sport teams' near monopoly is that players are still limited in their choices and bargaining power. While a few stars make large salaries and capitalize on product endorsement income, many professional athletes (especially if one considers those in the minor leagues of baseball and basketball) do not make large salaries and have only a few productive playing years. Other personnel directly concerned with the production of sport, such as field and business managers, coaches, scouts, trainers, maintenance workers, publicity officers, and officials receive salaries for services provided. However, it is the corporate managerial class that reaps the primary economic gain.[74]

Corporations also benefit significantly from the professional sports enterprise via direct sales of sports-related products. Numerous other corporations benefit indirectly from the effective use of advertising to sell their various products by utilization of sport and sport personalities to reach preidentified consumer categories or to enhance general visibility of their products.[27]

During the 1920s and 1930s, a rapid expansion in the coverage of sports in newspapers and on the radio paralleled the birth of professional sports and the emergence of big-time collegiate sport. A symbiotic relationship evolved, in which the media promoted sport, and sport sold the media. This marriage between sports and the mass media paralleled broader societal trends toward consumerism and the development of the advertising industry.[27] Television in the 1950s grew rapidly and proved to be an extremely powerful medium for promoting sports. The televising of sport events became an increasingly important source of low-cost entertainment for the masses and a major source of revenue for professional sport. Television effectively functioned as a middleman, collecting money from commercial sponsors, deducting their expenses and retaining a profit, and then passing on a large portion of this revenue to sport leagues or teams.[54] Currently, in the four major professional sports, about 35% of their income is obtained from television and radio contracts, with about 55% coming from ticket sales.[46] Obviously, without this television and radio income, professional sports franchises could not function as they presently do. Snyder and Spreitzer[91] point out the disruptive effect of television on the very process of sports contests, including rescheduling of sport competition dates and starting times, as well as increasing the number and length of time-outs, in order to facilitate the media's marketing emphasis of sport as a product.

Another important concern of television's impact on sport is the increasing professionalization of amateur sport, including the Olympic Games and big-time intercollegiate athletics. While television has played a primary role in enhancing public interest in intercollegiate football and basketball, those institutions sponsoring big-time programs have become increasingly dependent on television revenues.

SPORT AND SMALL GROUPS

Robertson defines a group as "a collection of people interacting together in an orderly way on the basis of shared expectations about each other's behavior."[74:155] Individuals form groups for a purpose, i.e., achievement of a goal. This involves development of an appropriate group structure and process for effective achievement of the group's goal. These include development of boundaries, norms, values, and roles and status for group members, such as leader or follower. Resolution of the latter is essential for effective communication and achievement of purpose.

However, since our society is so complex and necessitates that each of us be members of many groups—even simultaneously, why study a particular group's structure and interactive process in achieving their primary purpose? Mills[60] contends that there are several important reasons: (1) to understand what happens within such groups because their dynamics affect the way individuals lead their daily lives; (2) because social pressures and pressures from the individual meet in the small group, it is a convenient context in which to ferret out the interplay among these pressures; and (3) small groups are essentially microcosms of larger societies, in that they reflect miniature, societal features of importance, thus providing means of developing effective ways of thinking about social systems in general.

Sport groups appear to provide a particularly attractive small social group for analysis, since they usually provide roles that are clearly defined, performance measures that are reasonably straightforward (e.g., points scored for or against, or winning percentage) and situations in which observer contamination involved with artificiality and obtrusiveness of the investigator is less of a problem than with other social groups.[88] By controlling for confounding factors, such as group size, hierarchy of roles, communication networks, and rules of conduct, the effect of other social conditions on group attainment of its primary goal is more easily assessed. As an example, Eitzen[25] found that group homogeneity (as determined by socioeconomic status and religion) of high school basketball team members was related to team success. The relationship was interpreted in terms of heterogenity increasing the likelihood of cliques within the team, thus reducing cohesion and ultimately resulting in poorer team performance.

Lewin[48] defined two major elements in the sociological study of group dynamics: (1) group structure (a stabilized pattern of statuses and roles, including leadership that exists among members of groups); and (2) group functioning, i.e., the social processes that occur, such as communication, cohesiveness, and social control. Stability of team line-ups and leadership longevity (e.g., baseball managers and basketball coaches) are two elements of group structure found to be directly associated with team success. However, these empirical observations do not reveal a cause and effect, since stable line-ups and leadership longevity may be a consequence of—not a cause of—task success.[46] An aspect of group structure that has yielded interesting results is the relationship of spatial location and social interaction of team members as it effects selectivity to leadership roles. Grusky[37] contended that, within the context of organizational centrality, high interactors with others in the group are more likely to be selected for exclusive positions than are low interactors. Loy and Sage[55] found support for Grusky's centrality hypothesis, in that infielders and catchers (central positions) were more likely to be chosen as team captain. Grusky[37] found that virtually all professional baseball managers were former baseball players, and that over 75% had played high interaction (central) positions. Leonard[46] contends that, in general, other studies of the team sports of basketball, football and hockey have provided empirical substantiation that leadership tends to emerge from those having played in central (high interaction) positions. While the centrality organization hypothesis underlines the importance of one group dynamics aspect in defining leadership, it does not provide reasons for how leadership in groups develops.

Fielder[30] developed a model to explain leadership effectiveness. His contingency model involves an interrelationship of four factors: (1) the situation, (2) the task to be accomplished, (3) the leader, and (4) the characteristics of the group. One important aspect of his research entailed determination of the leader's primary orientation to the group, whether task-centered or people-centered. In other words, the leader's primary focus on task-centered or people-centered orientation appeared contingent on the specific situation. In a study of college volleyball teams, Bird[7] found that the most successful teams with highly skilled players (Division I) perceived their coach as people-oriented, whereas the most successful teams in Division II perceived their coach as task-oriented. The author suggested that the successful Division I teams had more uniform, high level ability players that permitted a more flexible playing strategy, and success of the people-oriented leadership provided by their coaches.

The effect of numerous other group dynamics factors on performance and success, including competition, conflict, cooperation and cohesion, have been studied with mixed results. As an example, the effect of group cohesiveness on team success will be examined in some detail. Cohesiveness is defined by Carron[12] as the tendency to stick together and remain united, and represents the strength of the group's social bond. It is not something that is brought to the group or is necessarily an automatic structural component.

Gill[33] analyzed the results of studies of the relationship of cohesiveness (usually measured with a questionnaire) to group performance (generally defined by season win/loss record). She found several studies that reported a positive cohesiveness-performance relationship, but also a few in which negative or no relationships were reported. In general, positive cohesiveness-performance relationships were observed when cohesiveness is defined and measured as attraction to individuals within the group. Also, the types of teams studied appear to have a significant effect on the existent cohesiveness-performance relationship. For example, Leonard[46] points out the difference in role relations among interacting groups in which team members are engaged simultaneously in a task requiring continuous adjustment and coordination (e.g., in baseball, basketball, football, and volleyball), and coacting groups in which participants perform a task independent of other team members (e.g., bowling, golf, gymnastics, swimming, and wrestling). Landers and Luschen[44] observed that cohesion is more likely to be related to team success within interacting sport groups that emphasize complementary tasks. Conversely, they observed that negative cohesion-performance relationships were most common in studies of coacting groups such as bowling and rifle teams. They suggest that in-group conflict and rivalries among team participants may be related to achievement of optimum arousal levels and thus, conducive to team success.

Nixon[63] has observed that a team's prior success tends to reinforce conditions of cohesiveness in an interactive sport (basketball), and makes future success more likely. Ruder and Gill[76] found significantly enhanced team cohesiveness among members of winning women's college intramural volleyball immediately following matches, while the losing teams' cohesiveness was adversely affected, though to a lesser degree.

SOCIALIZATION AND SPORT

Socialization is the process by which individuals acquire the culture of their society, learning its language, norms, values, and their roles in various groups with respect to socially acceptable and personally rewarding behaviors. Socialization agents include the family, school, peer group and mass media, as well as religious groups, youth organizations, and voluntary clubs.[74] Socialization effected by schools tends to be more formal and structured than that afforded by other agents.

It has generally been assumed that participation in athletics and physical education is an effective agent of socialization via development of group interaction skills, attitudes, and values that have potential for transfer to other societal situations.[3,17,18] However, until recently, there has been little systematic investigation of socialization through sport and its converse, socialization into sport. Leonard[46] had developed a model for conceptualizing socialization into sport and socialization via sport, depicted in Figure 5–5, which is useful in the ensuing discussion.

SOCIALIZATION INTO SPORT

Snyder and Spreitzer[91] state that study of socialization into sport focuses on the agents or agencies that influence children and youth into sport or physical activity involvement. It includes acquisition of the social, psychologic, and physical skills requisite to participation in sport. The latter would include play activity as a young child, in which learning to play the roles of specific persons represents a develop-

mental step for learning the behavior and attitudes of adults, and is a prelude to participation in games. Games are rule-bound and involve competition with others. Successful participation in games is evidence of appropriate maturation for socialization into sport.

The societal agents most likely to influence the child to become involved in sport include the family, school, peers, community, and the mass media.[91] The introduction to sport is most likely to occur in the family if the child has parents and/or older siblings who are interested in and participate in sports. Peer influence in the neighborhood is frequently an early socialization experience into sports participation. The school provides an instructional program with continuous professional, peer, and self-evaluation. If the latter indicates less ability than most, and the school environment is perceived as placing significant importance on this ability, the child may well place increased interest and effort in other activities providing more positive feedback.[91]

The community is likely to play a role both in whether children and youth perceive great importance in being an athlete, and in which sports are available. Sports available in a community depend on geographic and climatic factors, as well as socioeconomic factors influencing sport preferences. The latter is affected by ethnic composition of the community, its rural or urban nature, and the resultant availability

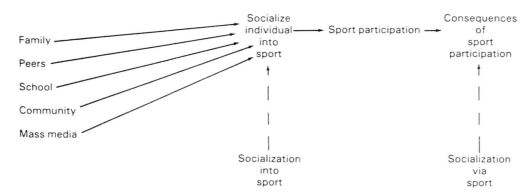

FIG. 5–5. A model for conceptualizing socialization into sport and socialization via sport. (From Leonard, W.M.: A Sociological Perspective of Sport. 2nd ed. Minneapolis, Minn.: Burgess, 1984, p. 83.)

and access to sport facilities. The mass media has provided an opportunity for youth to become acquainted with sports and to perceive role models for behavior emulation.[91] The latter has been diffused by increasing media attention to the basic individual human frailty, also existent in athletes, but which has long been largely ignored until recently.

Research substantiates the importance of the various elements identified above in affecting socialization into sport, but not in terms of equal effects. An illustration of this contention is apparent in Table 5–3, in which Smith[84] summarized results from his study of 1,000 male and female athletes, ages 12 to 19 years, involved in one of several sports. It is apparent that the school physical education teacher or coach was seen by both boys and girls as being most responsible for initiating interest in their sport. There was also a clear sex differentiation in terms of both parental and peer influence on one's first becoming interested in sport. Snyder and Spreitzer[89] observed that female interscholastic athletes received more sport participation encouragement from their mother if they competed in gymnastics or track, but more from their father if they were basketball players. Athletes in all sports received more sport participation encouragement from their girlfriends than from their boyfriends. The most striking difference between these female athletes and their nonathlete counterparts was that a much greater proportion of the athletes had participated in organized sport during their elementary school and junior high years. Kenyon and McPherson[43] observed that college athletes, Olympic athletes, and youth athletes reported varying degrees of

influence by family, teachers, coaches, and friends for certain individuals, but that all three groups showed similar collective interaction of these affecting agents.

Spreitzer and Snyder[93] surveyed middle-aged adults, and found that those who participated in some sport were much more likely to have parents who had encouraged early sport participation, to have participated in formally organized athletic programs as a youth, and to possess positive attitudes toward sport and self-perception of athletic ability. Snyder and Spreitzer[91] call attention to the fact that socialization into sport and physical activity generally occurs during one's youth, and that many individuals develop negative attitudes that socialize them away from an active lifestyle. They note particularly the increased emphasis on high-level performance in high school that is now extended to youth leagues in baseball, football, and soccer, with their potential for the less gifted majority of youth to experience failure and frustration. They have observed that such attitudes, once formed, tend to carry over to adulthood and decrease the likelihood of sport and physical activity participation in this phase of the life cycle.[91]

SOCIALIZATION VIA SPORT

In his critical examination of the effects of physical activity participation on the social development of children, Sage states:

Many believe that physical activities, especially play, games, and sports, provide an environment for acquiring culturally valued personal-social attitudes, values and behaviors, and that what is learned in these settings transfers to other spheres of life.[80:22]

Table 5–3. Summary of Responses to the Question, Who Was Responsible for You First Becoming Interested in Your Sport? (Numbers are in percent of responses.)

Sex	Father	Mother	Male Friends	Female Friends	School P.E. Teacher/Coach	Other*	Total No.
Male	10.9	9.8	24.7	1.5	25.1	28.0	275
Female	5.7	14.6	1.0	15.8	33.8	29.1	717

*Includes brothers, sisters, other relatives, classroom teachers, club or recreational agency personnel, and "other." These categories were collapsed after statistical manipulations.

Modified from Smith, M.D.: Getting involved in sport: sex differences. Internat. Rev. Sport Sociol. 14(2):93–101, 1979.

Stevenson and Nixon[97] contend that sport is generally believed to socialize participants toward such desirable social values and personality characteristics as self-discipline, leadership, cooperation, respect for rules, sportsmanship, self-control, achievement drive, and respect for opponents.

But just how effective is sport in the socialization of children and youth? Sage[80] contends that developmental scientists are virtually unanimous in agreement that play is vital to social development, but that there is little well conceived and conducted research evidence on the effects of involvement in organized sport on social development. Further, he notes that the origins of belief in the character development potential of team sports participation occurred in all-male private boarding schools in England in the mid-19th century in a situation that appears to contrast sharply with that existing in American schools today. First, the games were almost entirely governed by students themselves who organized and administered them. While the games were contested in a spirited manner, there was an emphasis on fellowship, sacrifice, cooperation, sportmanship, and a willingness to accept defeat gracefully; there was also a belief that how one played the game was a marker of how one would later behave.[58] It is apparent that there was a rational basis established between social purpose, process, and outcome, though no one appears to have attempted an empirical evaluation of the social development effects of school sports.[80] This notion has been transferred with little sensitivity to the strikingly disparate cultural conditions existent in America. Perhaps paramount is that youth and secondary school sports in America are dominated by adult control and the idea of losing a contest graciously is sometimes seen as a character flaw. Further, Sage[80] contends that youth sport has become increasingly reflective of adult authoritarian and hierarchical organization, with endorsement of the performance principle, meritocracy, and overemphasis on winning.

Webb[102] studied the attitudes of sportsmanship and winning by questionnaire responses from 1200 students in grades 3, 6,

7, 10, and 12. He found that as the years in school increased, the importance of victory and demonstration of skill became progressively more important than having fun and playing fairly. Maloney and Petrie's[57] study of Canadian youth in grades 8 through 12 revealed that males attached greater importance to the achievement aspect of sport participation (i.e., skill and victory) than did females, and that these attitudes increased progressively for the boys with grade level. Snyder and Spreitzer[90] surveyed college students who were either participants or nonparticipants in athletics during their high school years. They found that nonathletes of both sexes attached significantly greater importance to having fun and playing fair in sports than did athletes. At the college level, Richardson[72] analyzed questionnaire responses of 223 male physical education majors and found that letter winners had lower regard for sportsmanship than nonletter winners, and that scholarship recipients ranked lower in sportsmanship than those who had not been awarded athletic scholarships. Thus, the notion that sports participation develops fair play and sportsmanship seems suspect.

In 1975, Stevenson[96] examined the research evidence bearing on whether beneficial socialization effects result from participation in sports. He concluded:

Although some population differences have been shown between athletes and nonathletes, and although some positive relationships have been demonstrated between certain characteristics and participation in sport, the serious methodological inadequacies of the research effectively damns any attempt at generalization. One very clear conclusion must be, however, that to date there is no valid evidence that participation in sport causes any verifiable socialization effects. The stated educational legitimation of physical education and of athletics must, therefore, remain in the realm of "belief" and should not be treated as "fact."[96:299]

The methodologic considerations that prevent establishing a cause and effect relationship between sport participation and positive socialization effects centered primarily on the cross-sectional designs utilized in comparing athletes and nonathletes.

SPECIFICITY VS. GENERALIZED SOCIALIZATION VIA SPORT. The basic question addressed here is whether whatever socialization effects occur from sport participation are limited to playing specific roles in the sports subculture, or whether they represent generalized role skills applicable to other social scenarios. Ulrich[101] contends that physical education behavior is specific and, though it is thought that behavioral patterns can be taught in one place and used in another, any transfer of behavior would have to be emphasized in the teaching/learning process. Snyder and Spreitzer,[88] however, assert that the potency of the socialization process and its likely specific–diffuse outcome should vary according to the individual's degree of involvement in sport, and other social dimensions derived from analysis of the situational context within which physical education and athletics take place.

In this connection, Snyder[85] identified five dimensions of social interaction in the socialization process that vary with the situational context within which athletics and sport participation in physical education take place. *First* is the degree of involvement by the participants in terms of frequency, duration and intensity, which is much greater for the varsity athlete than for the average student in a physical education class. *Second* is voluntary or involuntary selection for, and participation in, an activity. Typically, physical education class participants are meeting a requirement, while athletes voluntarily participate and are likely to be much more involved with their peers and coaches, and to experience a diffuse level of socialization. A *third* dimension relates to the quality of the socialization relationship between participants and socializing agents (teacher or coach). A purely instrumental socializing relationship imparts knowledge and skills functionally specific for the achievement of a desired end. An expressive relationship is usually more personally satisfying and permits broader and deeper levels of communication. A *fourth* dimension is the prestige and power of the socializer. This varies among coaches and physical educators according to their knowledge and skill, but is generally higher for coaches because of the great school and community interest in athletics. The *fifth* dimension refers to the personal and social characteristics of the participant. Personal physical and mental abilities, as well as one's self-perception, are vital in the diffusion of behavioral outcomes. However, the interrelationships of social class, racial, and ethnic affiliations, in terms of role models and ideals for social mobility, present potentially important possibilities for enhanced socialization that seem more likely to develop in athletics.

ATHLETIC PARTICIPATION AND DELINQUENCY. A commonly held assumption regarding interscholastic athletic participation is that it helps keep youth out of trouble, presumably because through sport they are taught conventionality, traditional values, and are kept busy.[91] Cowell[17] notes that games and sports often become substitute responses which redirect behavior and satisfactorily reduce the original instigation by satisfying emotional and social needs. Ryan and Foster[77] found personality characteristics among athletes to be similar to those of juvenile delinquents studied by Petrie et al.,[68] and hypothesized that the former group has merely found a socially acceptable way of satisfying a basic need to be hyperactive. Neumeyer[62] has noted that supervised sports activities in social centers, schools, churches, and community parks tend to reduce juvenile delinquency, while unsupervised recreation and certain forms of commercial recreation apparently have deleterious effects.

Snyder and Spreitzer,[91] however, caution that there is an inherent difficulty in analyzing the consequences of sport involvement in terms of isolating the probable effects of selectivity into and out of the sport stream from the socialization that occurs within sport. This process of selectivity should be kept in mind when interpreting research that reports a lower rate of delinquency among athletes as compared to nonathletes. For example, athletes are likely to be given preferential treatment by social control agents. Moreover, nonconformist youth are likely to be screened out of organized athletics by eligibility requirements and by coaches who tend to be conservative.

SOCIAL STRATIFICATION AND SPORT

Robertson[74] asserts that societies are universal in differentiating among their members with respect to those who have certain characteristics and those who do not, including age and sex. In addition, a society may also treat its members differently on other bases such as educational achievement, physical strength, religion, or skin color. The usual result of this differentiation is social inequality. The latter exists when people's access to social rewards, such as influence, money, and respect, are determined more by group, rather than personal characteristics. In general, sport preference, both as a participant and spectator, reflects social stratification in numerous ways. The most widely studied have been social class accorded by wealth, sex discrimination, and race, both in terms of bias and social mobility.

SPORT AND SOCIAL CLASS

One's social class influences their choice of sport, both as a participant and spectator. A particularly notable study is that of Anderson and Stone,[2] in that they report comparisons of interview results of metropolitan residents from a broad range of social backgrounds in 1960 and 1975. Table 5–4 shows results of social class differences in individuals' responses to the designation of their favorite sport as either a participant or as a spectator. The upper class show a clear preference for participant over spectator sport, while the middle and lower classes seem to prefer sports spec-

tatorship. Snyder and Spreitzer[91] contend that the trend toward increased spectatorship reflects the impact of television on sports across all social classes. This notion also appears substantiated by Anderson and Stone's[2] observation that while the lower class engaged in sport conversation significantly less than did the upper class in the 1960 study, there was no significant difference in the frequency of sport conversations in the 1975 study.

Robertson[74] asserts that economic well-being is strongly related to sports participation preference, as only the upper class can afford to take part in yachting and polo. They, along with many of the middle class, can afford to participate in golf, skiing, and tennis. However, the lower classes are likely only to participate in such sports as basketball, bowling, and boxing. Robertson[74] also contends that social class biases toward particular sports tend to be passed on by parents to their children. For example, a child whose parents are country club members is likely to develop an interest in swimming, golf, or tennis. A child who lives in a city slum is more likely to play basketball, because of the availability of playground facilities and minimum equipment costs. Results of a study of the social background of 845 former athletes (all males) at UCLA, done by Loy,[51] confirms the link of participation in certain sports according to their father's occupation. About 40% of the athletes who participated in baseball, football, and wrestling came from blue-collar backgrounds, while only about 12% with similar backgrounds participated in crew, swimming, and tennis.

Table 5–4. Social Class Differences in the Designation of Spectator or Participant Sport as Favorites in 1960 and 1975*

Favorite Sport	Upper Class 1960 (%)	Upper Class 1975 (%)	Middle Class 1960 (%)	Middle Class 1975 (%)	Lower Class 1960 (%)	Lower Class 1975 (%)
Spectator	36	44	57	58	55	65
Participant	64	56	43	42	45	35

*Modified from Anderson, D.F., and G.P. Stone: A fifteen year analysis of socio-economic strata differences in the meaning given to sport by metropolitans. In The Dimensions of Sport Sociology. Edited by M.L. Krotee. West Point, N.Y.: Leisure Press, 1979, p. 174.

SOCIAL MOBILITY AND SPORT

There have been numerous media accounts of young professional star athletes, who have risen from low socioeconomic levels to fame and fortune. Thus, sport is widely perceived as an effective social escalator. This contention has been examined extensively by sport sociologists during the past 20 years.

Loy[51] suggests that participation in interscholastic athletics can stimulate higher levels of educational aspirations in order to extend one's athletic career, and thus indirectly result in higher educational achievement and acquisition of secular skills that can facilitate social mobility. Rehberg and Schafer summarized their conclusions from research directed to this issue as follows:

(Our) data have shown that a greater proportion of athletes than non-athletes expect to enroll in a four-year college, even when the potentially confounding variables of status, academic performance, and parental encouragement are controlled. This relationship is especially marked among boys not otherwise disposed toward college, that is, those from working-class homes, those in the lower half of their graduating class, and those with low parental encouragement to go to college.[71:739]

Bend[5] analyzed data of high school graduates 5 years later and found that athletic participation was associated with heightened postgraduate income.

At the college level, only a few studies comparing the occupational status and income of athletes and nonathletes after graduation have been reported. In the most complete study, which compared football players and nonathletes at a Mid-Western university over a 20-year period,[78] the athletes and nonathletes had achieved virtually equivalent incomes since graduation. However, the football players came from poorer backgrounds, with only 23% being from upper class homes and 51% from lower class origins, as compared to 53% upper class and 21% lower class for the nonathletes. They also found that football was the mechanism that permitted the players from lower class homes to attend the University.

Eitzen and Sage[27] contend that the increased corporate sport orientation of big-time athletic programs has resulted in more recruitment of academically inferior students and greater athletic focused time demands on football and basketball players. They cite evidence of less than 50% of the players receiving football scholarships from the 63 member institutions of the College Football Association in 1978 to 1979 having graduated 5 years later. The percentage of seniors playing men's basketball in 15 Division I NCAA conferences in 1983 who graduated at the end of that year ranged from 100% in the Ivy League to 17% in the Southwest Conference, with only five conferences having a graduation rate above 50%.

As alluded to earlier, professional sports offers a direct means for athletes with superior talent from lower class backgrounds to acquire wealth and enhanced social status. However, this vehicle of enhanced social mobility is extremely limited. For example, Eitzen and Sage,[27] cite evidence that there were 600,000 high school football players in 1985, with less than 7% as many college players. Of these 40,000 college players, only about 250 rookies will make a National Football League team, and then the average length of their career is only 4½ years. Durso[22] cited similar restricted opportunity for men's basketball players. While there are about 200,000 high school senior players and 5,700 college senior players each year, only about 55 rookies make a National Basketball Association team each season. Similar limitations exist for high school baseball players making it to a major league team.[91] Given these considerations, Edwards[23] has expressed concern that intense involvement in sport by lower income black youth acts as a counterproductive magnet away from higher level occupations as a more effective, broad-based avenue for social mobility.

RACISM IN SPORT: THE BLACK ATHLETE

Since winning at the big-time collegiate and professional level is so important, it has been widely believed that sport was devoid of prejudice and discrimination. This notion assumes that gifted nonwhite athletes are able to get ahead solely on the basis of their talent, and has been substantiated by the disproportionally higher representation of black athletes (than the percentage of blacks in the U.S. population) in professional baseball, basketball, boxing, and football. Eitzen and Sage[27] contend, however, that sociologic evidence indicates that corporate sport is not a meritocracy in which skin color is disregarded, but a microcosm of society where racism is both blatantly and subtly evident.

One aspect of the evidence that sport is a microcosm of society with respect to racism is that there are no black race car drivers, polo players, swimmers, or skiers, and few golfers, tennis players, and ice skaters. As previously mentioned, athletes in these sports come primarily from the upper social class. On the other hand, facilities for baseball, basketball, and football are readily available at public expense in the neighborhood school or playground.

While the proportion of black athletes in professional baseball, basketball, and football is well above their proportion in the total United States population, this has occurred primarily in the 1960s and 1970s at a time when the civil rights movement achieved similar, though less pervasive changes in other institutions.[74] In 1945, there were no black athletes in any professional sport except boxing.[27] Coakley[14] contends that intercollegiate sport was almost totally segregated until the 1954 Supreme Court desegregation decision. Even then, it was not until the 1960s that most colleges in the North had blacks on their teams, while the Southeastern Conference still had two schools without a single black athlete in 1970. Even in the 1980s, most black athletes were males in basketball and football, with a few black females in basketball and track and field. Other collegiate sports teams are disproportionately or totally white.[14]

Coakley astutely distinguishes between racial desegregation and elimination of prejudice:

It is important not to equate desegregation with the elimination of prejudice or with the achievement of true racial integration. Desegregation is marked simply by the opening of doors. The actual *elimination* of prejudice and the achievement of integration are marked by unqualified invitations to come through the doors and join *all* the activities going on inside regardless of where they are happening or who is involved.[14:212]

That elimination of prejudice has not occurred in professional athletics has been demonstrated in numerous studies, though there is increasing evidence of notable improvement. Eitzen and Yetman[29] observed that the mean batting average for major league baseball players from 1966 to 1970 and from 1971 to 1975 was 20.8 and 21.0 points higher for black than white players during both time periods. Pascal and Rapping[67] examined performance for black and white players at each position in 1967, noting better mean batting averages for blacks, as well as a better pitching record than for white pitchers. They concluded that on average, a black player must be better than a white player if he is to have an equal chance of playing in the major leagues. Phillips'[70] more recent comparison of black and white major league baseball players' performance from 1975 to 1980 shows that, while still present, the racial gap has diminished.

Professional football differential comparisons of blacks and whites have been constrained because of the lack of a prevalent common denominator for player performance, such as batting average in baseball. However, there have been several studies comparing blacks and whites in professional basketball, in which blacks represent about 70% of the NBA players. Johnson and Marple[40] found a near equal number of white rookies, while the percentage of white players was reduced to 38% in the 2 to 4 years' experience category. They interpreted this observation to mean that less skilled white players were given more opportunity to make the team than black players. Subsequently, Lapchick[45] observed that among players who had more than 5 years' experience and had averaged less than 8 points per game, whites outnumbered blacks. However, among those players with more than 5 years' experience and who have averaged more than 8 points per game, 72% were blacks. Lapchick concluded that marginal white players, with respect to points per game, have a better chance of continuing their professional basketball career than do similarly skilled black players.

The awarding of athletic scholarships in intercollegiate basketball has been found also to illustrate unequal opportunity for equal ability. Yetman and Eitzen[104] studied 246 integrated NCAA men's basketball teams in 1970 and found that 67% of the black players were starters, while only 44% of the white players were starters. These authors also observed that blacks were less likely to be recruited and awarded athletic scholarships unless they were expected to become starters. This was true when academic potential was controlled for blacks and whites. By 1975, however, Eitzen and Yetman[29] found a reduction in the proportion of blacks among the top five scorers on men's NCAA teams from 76% in 1962 to 61%. This suggests that black players who may not be starters are being recruited in increasing numbers, especially if they have adequate academic background.[91]

Another form of apparent racial discrimination in professional sport is the position allocation phenomenon referred to as stacking. This occurs when clearly disparate proportions of black and white athletes are found at various positions on a team. Loy and McElvogue[53] analyzed stacking in baseball and football, advancing the notion of centrality—in terms of spatial location and a high degree of interdependency in function—as an explanation. They argued that blacks were underrepresented in these positions, and were stacked in noncentral or peripheral positions, by team coaches or managers, thus representing a form of discrimination.

Table 5–5 summarizes the percent of blacks at ten different positions in professional football for 1960, 1975 and 1983. It is apparent that, though there is a consistent increase in the proportion of blacks at all positions, they are still significantly underrepresented at quarterback, kicker, center, and offensive guard. However, significant changes in greater proportional representation relative to their total 12% in 1960 and 50% in 1983 have occurred at linebacker (a central position)—from 4% in 1960 to 47% in 1983. Schneider and Eitzen[82] examined the evidence for stacking in an

Table 5–5. Distribution of Black Players (in % of Total Players, Black + White) by Position in Professional Football*

Position	1960	1975	1983
Quarterback	0	3	1
Kicker	0	1	2
Center	0	5	3
Offensive guard	3	27	23
Offensive tackle	28	32	32
Linebacker	4	26	47
Defensive tackle	15	48	53
Defensive back	28	67	80
Wide receiver	5	55	77
Running back	18	65	88
Total team	12	42	50

*Modified from Eitzen, D.S. and G.H. Sage: Sociology of North American Sport. Dubuque, Iowa: Wm. C. Brown, 1986, p. 273; Eitzen, D.S. and N.R. Yetman: Immune from racism. Civil Rights Digest. IX(2):5, 1977; and from Lapchick, R.: Broken Promises: Racism in American Sports. New York: St. Martin's Press, 1984, p. 228.

analysis of 9 of the top 20 college football teams in 1978. They found that blacks were underrepresented at the same central positions and concentrated in the noncentral positions at about the same proportion as in professional football.

Figure 5–6 illustrates the percentage of black players in major league baseball during the 1988 season. Blacks are concentrated in the noncentral positions (outfield and first base) and are underrepresented at other infield positions and especially at the central positions of catcher and pitcher.[14] While the percentage of black outfielders and first basemen has increased since the 1967 season analysis by Loy and McElvogue,[53] there has been no change in the percentage of black pitchers and catchers, and only a marginal increase at other infield positions.

Evidence for stacking in men's basketball was observed by Eitzen and Tessendorf[28] in their 1970 to 1971 study of 274 collegiate teams. They found underrepresentation at the center and guard positions, which up to that time were regarded as central positions, and greater representation at forward. More recently, Leonard[47] observed that stacking in men's collegiate basketball has declined, particularly at the center position. Coakley[14] attributes this to changes

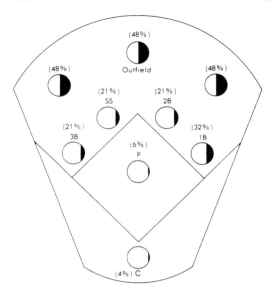

FIG. 5–6. Percentage of black players in each baseball position during the 1985 season (represented by the shaded areas). (From Coakley, J.J.: Sport in Society: Issues and Controversies. 4th ed. St. Louis: Times Mirror/Mosby, 1990, p. 214.)

in offensive strategy, such that outcome control is now more diffuse. He also maintained that professional basketball, in which about 70% of the players are black, now evidences no notable disparate representation at any position.

Several explanations for stacking have been advanced, including inherited physical and psychologic differences by race that would yield advantages for performance at certain positions in various sports. There are no substantive data to support this contention.[91] Most authors have attributed stacking to one or both of two factors. The first hypothesis entails the existent white coaches' stereotyping of blacks not possessing the requisite characteristics for playing central positions that require leadership, decision-making, highly refined techniques, and stability under pressure. Rather they tend to perceive them as having speed, aggressiveness, good hands, and instincts, which they feel are more important attributes for playing noncentral positions. The second hypothesis is based on the notion that young blacks are so-

cialized toward playing specific positions because they emulate black "role models" who are disproportionately represented in noncentral positions. Thus, the ratio of blacks and whites in specific positions, which may have originated from racial discrimination, is perpetuated through the learning of sport roles.[91]

Perhaps the most blatant example of racial discrimination in professional sport is the virtual absence of career opportunities for blacks in any role other than that of athlete. Blacks are underrepresented in proportion to their 13% of the American population in all coaching, management, and support positions in the major sports.[14] For example, in the NBA, where about 70% of the players are black, only 29 blacks were employed in a total of 544 coaching, management and administrative positions during 1982.[45] Similarly, there were only 61 blacks among the 879 coaches, administrative staff, and executives listed for all NFL teams in 1983.[45] In major league baseball, of the 913 front office positions, only 32 were held by blacks, with 26 of these being secretarial positions.[24] The underrepresentation of blacks extends beyond the professional leagues to the media covering these sports. For example, as of 1984 only 1 black has had a primary television sports coverage position.[27]

SOCIAL INEQUALITY IN SPORT FOR WOMEN

Until recently, sport in America has long been a predominantly male preserve. Robertson states:

In this respect, sport once again has paralleled such other American institutions as religion, the economy, politics, law, the military, and science, in which women were also refused access to high statuses. The reason for the exclusion of women from sport is a cultural one; namely, that the traditional role expectations for women seemed fundamentally at odds with role expectations for athletes.[74,91]

While there are numerous non-Western societies where heavy physical labor is considered a woman's job, Western culture had held for centuries that the female is biologically limited in her physical abilities.[74] Further, in America, as well as other Western cultures, the difference between masculine and feminine behavior is associated with sharp contrasts in temperament. The male is viewed as naturally aggressive and active, which are characteristics compatible with vigorous, highly competitive sport. Conversely, the female is seen as naturally nonaggressive and passive.[9] Further, Western culture has traditionally defined females as inferior and dependent on men, with their primary role responsibilities being as childbearers, rearers of children, homemakers, and otherwise facilitating their husband's achievement and success.[27] This prevailing role of a feminine woman clearly was at odds with that of a competitive athlete which was seen as demanding aggressiveness, dominance, tough mindedness, and risk taking.[38]

Robertson[74] asserts that sex roles have changed significantly in recent years in America, primarily because unprecedented numbers of women have entered economic life and have demanded equality with men, at first in the workplace, and then in other aspects of life. The women's movement has elicited numerous changes in public social and political consciousness, and has helped redefine occupational and family roles for women. Coakley[14] contends that the women's movement encouraged the dramatic increase in sports participation among girls and women since the early 1970s. Even more important, though, has been the effect of Title IX of the 1972 Education Amendments, which mandated that sex cannot serve as grounds for exclusion from participation in any educational program or activity that receives federal assistance. In 1970, there were less than 300,000 females on interscholastic and intercollegiate athletic teams, while in 1984 there were nearly 2 million. Other factors underlying increased female sports participation include the health and fitness movement and the increased visibility of athletic role models.[14] However, Eitzen and Sage caution that, although reduced inequality of female sports participation has occurred:

Prejudices are not altered by courts and legislation, and culturally conditioned responses to gender-role ideology are ubiquitous and resistant to sudden changes. Therefore, while laws may force compliance in equality of opportunity for females in the world of sport, sexism in sport will probably continue, albeit in more subtle and insidious forms.[27:288]

A factor of particular importance in continued resistance to full equality in sports participation for females are the persistent effects of several social institutions which are traditionally slow to change. One's learning of their sexual identity is initiated by their family, and is subject to significant differences in childrearing practices. Children learn parental expectations of sex-appropriate behavior, which includes sports and vigorous physical pursuits being identified with the male role and negatively associated with the female role.[27]

The school tends to reinforce and extend the traditional gender-role stereotyping initiated by the family. Sadker and Sadker[79] have observed that teachers foster an environment in which boys learn to be aggressive and physically capable, while girls learn to be submissive and passive. Further, physical education has traditionally been sex-segregated after elementary school, in part so envisioned sex-appropriate physical activities could be learned.[59] The notion of sex-appropriate sports participation for females is intensified during adolescence with negative feedback from adults (parents and teachers) and peers for girls who participate in sports involving strength, power, and contact, rather than those which emphasize balance, grace, and poise.[14] This contention is substantiated by the results summarized in Table 5–6 of a study of 500 mid-Western adults' perception of the appropriateness of certain sports for females.[87] It is clear that gymnastics, swimming and tennis are seen as more sex-appropriate for females than are basketball, softball, and track. The data summarized in Table 5–7 from Snyder et al's.[87] study of college women shows a similar hierarchy of sex-appropriateness in the degree of stigma associated with sports participation. Greendorfer[36] studied the relative impact of three social agents: (1) family, (2) peers, and (3) schools on fe-

Table 5–6.   Perceptions of the General Population Concerning the Effects of Athletic Participation on Female Characteristics*

Questionnaire Item	Percent Responding "Yes"
In your opinion, would participation in any of the following sports enhance a girl's/woman's feminine qualities?	
Swimming	67
Tennis	57
Gymnastics	54
Softball	14
Basketball	14
Track	13
In your opinion, would participation in any of the following sports detract from a girl's/woman's feminine qualities?	
Track	30
Basketball	21
Softball	20
Gymnastics	6
Tennis	2
Swimming	2

*From Snyder, E.E., J.E. Kivlin, and E.E. Spreitzer: The female athlete: An analysis of objective and subjective role conflict. In Psychology of Sport and Motor Behavior II. Penn State HPER Series No. 10, edited by D.M. Landers. Pennsylvania State University, 1975, p. 167.

Table 5–7.   Perceptions of College Women Athletes Concerning Female Participation in Athletics According to Type of Sport Participation*

Sport	Percent Responding "Yes"
Question: Do you feel there is a stigma attached to women who participate in the sport you specialize in?	
Basketball	56
Track and field	50
Swimming and diving	40
Gymnastics	31

*Modified from Snyder, E.E., J.E. Kivlin, and E.E. Spreitzer: The female athlete: An analysis of objective and subjective role conflict. In Psychology of Sport and Motor Behavior II. Edited by D.M. Landers. Penn State HPER Series No. 10. The Pennsylvania State University, 1975, p. 168.

male's socialization into sports participation during childhood, adolescence, and young adulthood. She found that parents were the most important social agent during childhood, that peers, teachers, and coaches became most important during adolescence, and that the peers became most important during young adulthood.

Another increasingly important social institution, the mass media, has rather consistently reinforced the traditional gender role stereotype.[27] There is great disparity in the amount of coverage of men's and women's sports by radio, television, and the print media, which reflects the traditional attitude of sport as predominantly a male domain. Further, while sportswriters would not think of extolling the physical "charms" of a male athlete, they often include descriptions of the shape, size, hair style, and eye color of female athletes, with proportionally less emphasis on individual athletic performance.

It should be apparent that prevalent cultural beliefs, and the impact of social agents perpetuating them, have a continuing effect on maintaining the status quo. With respect to social inequality in sport, Eitzen and Sage[27] assert that the consequences take three primary forms: (1) perpetuation of alleged biologic and psychologic weaknesses of females which affects attitudes regarding appropriate and inappropriate female behavior; (2) the resultant unequal opportunity for sports participation; and (3) unequal access to the authority and power structure.

Traditionally, justification for the lack of female need to participate in sport has been advanced on presumed physiologic and social-psychologic differences. Eitzen and Sage[27] have identified two persistent physiologic "myths" regarding female athletic participation: (1) it produces unattractive, bulging muscle definition, and (2) it is harmful to the health of females. It is true that persistent heavy resistance exercise training will induce muscle hypertrophy, but the amount is largely dependent on the individual's androgen hormone levels. Few women incur high enough androgen levels that, in combination with heavy training, will produce a masculinized physique. There is no substantive evidence that athletic competition, together with properly prescribed training and diet, entails a greater risk of injury[39] or harm to the health of females,[99] or adversely affects future pregnancy and childbirth.[105]

Eitzen and Sage[27] also have identified a social-psychologic "myth" which holds that females lack real interest and are not good at sports. Those making this point noted that there were few females involved in sport, and that their performances were inferior to men's. However, with increased participation and intensity of training, female athletes in the 1980s have closed the gap in comparable athletic performances of men to what one would expect on the basis of body size and muscle mass differences.[31] Simone de Beauvoir has aptly described the appropriate manner of comparing male and female sports performance:

In sports the end in view is not success independent of physical equipment; it is rather the attainment of perfection within the limitations of each physical type; the featherweight boxing champion is as much a champion as is the heavyweight; the woman skiing champion is not the inferior of the faster male champion; they belong to two different classes.[4:311]

Coakley[14] maintains that gender inequality in sport is still evidenced by two primary forms of discrimination: (1) against women athletes; and (2) against women coaches and administrators. Youth sports programs introduce most children to the experience of organized sport. Until the late 1970s the vast majority of youth programs were for boys, with girls representing only a small percentage of participants. This is changing in the 1980s, as Eitzen and Sage[27] state that about 150,000 girls were playing youth soccer by the early 1980s, with another 250,000 playing softball. Age-group swimming had as many girls as boys participating, and young girl gymnasts outnumbered boys by 10 to 1. The passage and implementation of Title IX significantly reduced overt sex discrimination in schools and colleges since the mid-1970s with females now having far greater sport participation opportunities than ever before. However, sex discrimination in sports remains to some degree in most institutions, in that females have fewer opportunities for participation. Further, there are frequently program discrepancies regarding facilities, equipment, and support services.[14]

Sex discrimination in intercollegiate sport is most apparent in the unequal opportunity for coaching and administrative jobs. For example, between 1977 and 1984, when there was an increase in the number of sports teams for women in NCAA member institutions from 5.6 to 6.9, there was a decline in the percentage of women coaches from 58.2 to 53.8%.[1] Table 5–8 shows comparisons for the ten most popular women's sports, all of which show a reduced percentage of women coaches in 1984. The women's athletic programs at 86% of all coeducational colleges and universities were under the control of a male athletic director in 1984; 38% of those programs had no females in any administrative position.[1] Male dominance of the administration of women's intercollegiate athletics appears to have occurred primarily because of the previously all-male NCAA's decision to offer subsidized women's championships in 1981. This resulted in women's programs being combined with men's programs at many member institutions in the early 1980s.[14] In 1984, women's representation at all major policy making levels of the NCAA ranged from 5 to 24%.[27] Coakley[14] contends that the forces creating gender inequality have now been built into the structure of intercollegiate programs and that, as long as women lack the power to define their program philosophies and to assume their roles as coaches and administrators, these inequalities will remain.

AGEISM AND SPORT

Ageism is the systematic stereotyping of and discrimination against people because they are old. It assumes that they are physically and mentally incapable of maintaining an active lifestyle.[74] Ageism sets subtle limits on the opportunities and range of behavior and, because sport participation is associated primarily with youth and young adulthood, tends to define this form of physical activity as inappropriate for the

Table 5–8. Percentage of Women Coaches for the 10 Most Popular Women's Intercollegiate Sports, 1977 and 1984*

Sport	1977 (%)	1984 (%)	Percentage Change
Basketball	79.4	64.9	−14.5
Volleyball	86.6	75.5	−11.1
Tennis	72.9	59.7	−13.2
Softball	83.5	68.6	−14.9
Cross country	35.2	19.7	−15.5
Track	52.3	26.8	−25.5
Swim/dive	53.6	33.2	−20.4
Field hockey	99.1	98.2	−.9
Golf	54.6	39.7	−14.9
Soccer	29.4	26.8	−2.6

*Modified from Acosta, R.V., and L.J. Carpenter: A. Women in athletics: a status report. B. Status of women in athletics; changes and causes. JOPERD. 56:30–37, 1985.

older person. This age-grading has a negative effect on maintenance of an active lifestyle, in that it reinforces the stereotypes of mature adulthood as a sedentary stage of life.[91]

While aging does result in a loss of basic physiologic capacities, about half of the loss in strength and endurance in the elderly appears to be due to substantially reduced activity levels.[69,83] For example, Gordon and colleagues[35] studied the leisure activities of about 1500 adults, ranging in age from 20 to 94 years, and observed a marked decrease with age. These observations are in accord with Stephens'[95] analysis of adult physical activity patterns reported in several national surveys between 1971 and 1985. In the 1985 survey, 39% of adults over age 65 reported only sedentary activity levels, while less than 15% reported vigorous activity equivalent to 2 miles per day of fast walking.

While the older person's individual initiative, as well as social characteristics of one's immediate environment have been found to be important aspects of individual motivation to elect an active lifestyle,[20] Snyder and Spreitzer[91] ascribe particular importance to general societal expectations in affecting the older person's behavior. Despite this fundamental constraint, there are now numerous examples of senior and master's sport competition, together with indications of enhanced individual physical activity levels, which suggest that societal expectations for the increasingly numerous elderly population are changing. It seems clear, also, that the subdiscipline of

sport sociology will need to be expanded to include study of the sociologic aspects of physical activities other than sport which, until recently, have been virtually ignored.[91]

SUMMARY

1. Sport in America has grown rapidly in the last 40 years, and now has a much greater societal impact than that evidenced in educational institutions alone.

2. Systematic study of the sociology of sport was initiated in the mid-1960s, with a few scholars from sociology interested in sport and a somewhat greater number of physical educators interested in the sociologic aspects of sport.

3. Sport is seen as a microcosm of society. That is, by understanding crucial aspects of sport, e.g., the social groups that participate, the statuses and roles of those involved, the distribution of power and wealth within this institution, the linkages of sport with other institutions, and the values sport represents, one can learn much about American society as a whole.

4. Sport interacts with other major social institutions, such as education, religion, politics, the economy, and the family, reflecting not only persistent social values, but also elements of societal strain and change.

5. Sport in educational institutions is widely perceived as an effective means of reinforcing values and norms of behavior held in esteem by society in general. How-

ever, social analysis indicates that "big-time" collegiate athletic programs are increasingly organized as corporate enterprises to produce a high profile public relations image and to complete for the public's entertainment dollar, rather than for social development of the participants.

6. Interscholastic athletics are supported by educational administrators and the community for a number of reasons, including (a) serving as a vehicle for institutional cohesiveness, (b) aiding in social control, (c) incubating societal values, and (d) enhancing student interest in physical activity participation.

7. While studies consistently show that high school athletes have a higher grade point average than nonathletes, this appears due to selectivity factors rather than to cause and effect.

8. The impact of the formal physical education curriculum in elementary school is much less potent than the rapidly growing preadolescent organized sports movement that has occurred outside of the school. Social analysis indicates cause for concern, in that highly organized preadolescent sport is adult controlled, with the players' behavior strictly patterned by specialized rules and roles, which are in direct social contrast to informally organized, player-controlled games in parks and school playgrounds.

9. While the Puritans and other early American church leaders disapproved of play and sport, changes in living conditions and in prevalent societal attitudes have occurred, such that there is now a facilitative interaction between American sport and religion as basic social institutions.

10. Numerous actions by the Federal government during the last 20 years have exerted a profound impact on sport. From an international perspective, the area of principal interest among sport sociologists has been the greatly increased use of sport for nationalism and as a political propaganda vehicle.

11. There is a symbiotic relationship between sport and the economy. For example, greater leisure time and increased discretionary income have provided impetus for expanded sports and fitness activity participation. Conversely, television acts as the middle-man in selling advertising to major corporations, shown during telecasts of highly popular professional sports contests.

12. Sociologists have found sports teams to be an effective model for studying small group structure and dynamics in achieving the group's primary goal.

13. Studies indicate that the family and neighborhood peer influence are important agents of a child's socialization into sports participation. Thereafter, in school, peers continue to exert an important effect, but the influence of physical education teachers and coaches becomes preeminent.

14. Many believe that sports provide an environment for acquiring culturally valued personal-social attitudes, values, and behaviors, and that what is learned in this setting transfers to other spheres of life. Research, however, provides no valid evidence that participation in sport causes any verifiable socialization effects.

15. One's social class influences their choice of sport, both as a participant and spectator. The upper class shows a clear preference for participant over spectator sport, with the middle and lower classes indicating less preference for sport participation than for spectator sport.

16. Evidence suggests that athletes from lower and middle socioeconomic status achieve a greater degree of social mobility than do nonathletes of similar background.

17. Evidence indicates that blacks are significantly underrepresented in certain positions in professional baseball and football. This appears to be due to (a) the predominantly white coaches and managers stereotyping of blacks not possessing requisite characteristics for certain positions, and (b) young blacks being socialized to certain positions because they emulate black "role models" in these positions.

18. While black athletes are disproportionally represented in professional baseball, basketball, and football—relative to the percentage of blacks in the U.S. population, blacks are underrepresented in all coaching, management, and support staff positions in these sports.

19. Federal legislation has increased compliance in equality of opportunity for

females in sport, but sexism continues, often in subtle and insidious forms. For example, traditional gender-role stereotyping, begun in the family and reinforced in the school, tends to reduce female interest and desire for participation in sports, particularly in those thought to be sex-inappropriate.

20. Sex discrimination in intercollegiate sport is most apparent in the unequal opportunity for coaching and administrative jobs. For example, at a time when the number of sports teams for women increased by 20% in NCAA member institutions, the percentage of women coaches decreased from 58 to 54%. Further, only 14% of these institutions had a female athletic director in charge of the women's athletic program.

21. Ageism is the systematic stereotyping of older people, which includes defining an active lifestyle as inappropriate. Recent evidence, however, suggests that the elderly are increasing participation in sport and other vigorous physical activities.

22. Because of the enhanced interest in participation in physical activities other than sport—particularly among middle-age and older adults—it is expected that the subdiscipline of sport sociology will expand its focus accordingly.

REFERENCES

1. Acosta, R.V., and L.J. Carpenter: A. Women in athletics: a status report. B. Status of women in athletics: changes and causes. JOPERD. 56(6):30–37, 1985.
2. Anderson, D.F., and G.P. Stone: A fifteen year analysis of socio-economic strata differences in the meaning given to sport by metropolitans. In The Dimensions of Sport Sociology. Edited by M.L. Krotee. West Point, N.Y.: Leisure Press, 1979, pp. 167–184.
3. Barrow, H.M., and J.P. Brown: Man and Movement: Principles of Physical Education. 4th ed. Philadelphia: Lea & Febiger, 1988.
4. Beauvoir, S. de: The Second Sex. New York: Bantam Books, 1952.
5. Bend, E.: The Impact of Athletic Participation on Academic and Career Aspirations and Achievement. Pittsburgh: American Institutes for Research, 1968.
6. Berger, P.L.: Introduction to Sociology. Garden City, N.Y.: Doubleday, 1963.
7. Bird, A.M.: Development of a model for pre-dicting team performance. Res. Quart. 48:24–32, 1977.
8. Boyle, R.H.: Sport: Mirror of American Life. Boston: Little, Brown, 1963.
9. Broom, L., P. Selznick, and D. Broom Darroch: Sociology. 7th ed. New York: Harper & Row, 1981.
10. Buhrman, H.: Scholarship and athletics in junior high school. Int. Rev. Sport Sociol. 7:119–131, 1972.
11. Caillois, R.: Man, Play and Games. New York: Free Press, 1961.
12. Carron, A.V.: Cohesiveness in sport groups: interpretations and considerations. J. Sport Psych. 4:124–138, 1982.
13. Clumpner, R.A.: Pragmatic coercion: the role of government in sport in the United States. In Sport and Politics. Edited by G. Redmond. Champaign, Ill.: Human Kinetics, 1984, pp. 5–12.
14. Coakley, J.J.: Sport in Society: Issues and Controversies. 4th ed. St. Louis: Times Mirror/Mosby, 1990.
15. Coleman, J.S.: The Adolescent Society. New York: Free Press, 1961.
16. Coleman, J.S.: Adolescents and the Schools. New York: Basic, 1965.
17. Cowell, C.C.: The contributions of physical activity to social development. Res. Quart. 31(Suppl.):286–306, 1960.
18. Cowell, C.C., and W.L. France: Philosophy and Principles of Physical Education. Englewood Cliffs, N.J.: Prentice-Hall, Inc., 1963.
19. Cozens, F.W., and F. Stumpf: Sports in American Life. Chicago: University of Chicago Press, 1953.
20. Dishman, R.K., J.F. Sallis, and D.R. Orenstein: The determinants of physical activity and exercise. Pub. Health Rep. 100:158–171, 1985.
21. Dowell, L.J.: Environmental factors of childhood competitive athletics. The Physical Educator. 28(3):17–21, 1971.
22. Durso, J.: The Sports Factory: An Investigation into College Sports. New York: Quadrangle Books, 1975.
23. Edwards, H.: Sociology of Sport. Homewood, Ill.: Dorsey, 1973.
24. Edwards, H.: The collegiate arms race: origins and implications of the "Rule 48" controversy. J. Sport and Soc. Issues. 8:11–12, 1984.
25. Eitzen, D.S.: The effect of group structure on the success of athletic teams. Int. Rev. Sport Sociol. 8(1):7–17, 1973.
26. Eitzen, D.S.: Sport and social status in American public secondary education. Rev. Sport Leisure. 1:139–155, 1976.
27. Eitzen, D.S., and G.H. Sage: Sociology of North American Sport. 3rd ed. Dubuque, Iowa: Wm. C. Brown, 1986.

28. Eitzen, D.S., and I. Tessendorf: Racial segregation by position in sports: the special case of basketball. Rev. Sport Leisure. 3:109–128, 1978.

29. Eitzen, D.S., and N. Yetman: Immune from racism? Civil Rights Digest. 9:3–13, 1977.

30. Fielder, F.E.: A contingency model of leadership effectiveness. In Advances in Experimental Social Psychology. Edited by L. Berkowitz. New York: Academic, 1964, pp. 149–190.

31. Fox, E.L., R.W. Bowers, and M.L. Foss: The Physiological Basis of Physical Education and Athletics. 4th ed. Philadelphia: Saunders, 1988.

32. Frey, J.H.: The place of athletics in the educational priorities of university alumni. Rev. Sport Leisure. 6(1):48–64, 1981.

33. Gill, D.L.: Current research and future prospects in sport psychology. In Perspectives on the Academic Discipline of Physical Education. Edited by G.A. Brooks. Champaign, Ill.: Human Kinetics, 1981, pp. 342–378.

34. Goodhue, R.M.: The politics of sport: An institutional focus. Proceed. N. Am. Soc. Sport Hist. 1974, pp. 34–35.

35. Gordon, C., C.M. Gaitz, and J. Scott: Leisure and lives: personal expressivity across the life span. In Handbook of Aging and the Social Sciences. Edited by R.H. Binstock and E. Shanas. New York: Van Nostrand Reinhold, 1976, pp. 310–341.

36. Greendorfer, S.L.: Socialization Into Sport. In Women and Sport: From Myth to Reality. Edited by C.A. Oglesby. Philadelphia: Lea & Febiger, 1978, pp. 115–140.

37. Grusky, O.: The effect of formal structure on managerial recruitment: a study of baseball organization. Sociometry. 26:345–353, 1963.

38. Harris, D.V.: Involvement in Sport: A Somatopsychic Rationale for Physical Activity. Philadelphia: Lea & Febiger, 1973.

39. Haycock, C.E., and J.V. Gillette: Susceptibility of women athletes to injury: myths vs reality. JAMA. 236:163–165, 1976.

40. Johnson, N.R., and D.P. Marple: Racial discrimination in professional basketball. Sociolog. Focus. 6:6–18, 1973.

41. Kenyon, G.S.: The significance of social theory in the development of sport sociology. In Sport and Social Theory. Edited by C.R. Rees and A.W. Miracle. Champaign, Ill.: Human Kinetics, 1986, pp. 3–22.

42. Kenyon, G.S., and Loy, J.W.: Toward a sociology of sport. JOHPER: 36(5):24–25, 68–69, 1965.

43. Kenyon, G.S., and B. McPherson: Becoming involved in physical activity and sport. In Sport, Culture, and Society. 2nd ed. Edited by J.G. Loy and B. McPherson. Reading, MA: Addison-Wesley, 1981, pp. 217–237.

44. Landers, D.M., and G. Luschen: Team performance outcome and cohesiveness of competitive co-acting groups. Int. Rev. Sport Sociol. 9(2):57–69, 1974.

45. Lapchick, R.: Broken Promises: Racism in American Sports. New York: St. Martin's/Marek, 1984.

46. Leonard. W.M.: A Sociological Perspective of Sport. 2nd ed. Minneapolis, Minn.: Burgess, 1984.

47. Leonard, W.M.: Stacking in college basketball: a neglected analysis. Sociol. Sport J. 4:403–409, 1987.

48. Lewin, K.: Field theory and experiment in social psychology: concepts and methods. Am. J. Sociol. 44:868–897, 1939.

49. Lopiano, D.: Solving the financial crisis in intercollegiate athletics. Ed. Record. 60(4):394–408, 1979.

50. Lowe, B., D. Kanin, and A. Strenk: Olympism. In Sport and International Relations. Edited by B. Lowe, D.B. Kanin, and A. Strenk. Champaign, Ill.: Stipes, 1978, pp. 110–117.

51. Loy, J.W.: The study of sport and social mobility. In Aspects of Contemporary Sport Sociology. Edited by G.S. Kenyon. Chicago: The Athletic Institute, 1969, pp. 101–119.

52. Loy, J.W., G.S. Kenyon, and B.D. McPherson: The emergence and development of the sociology of sport as an academic speciality. Res. Quart. Exer. Sport. 51:91–109, 1980.

53. Loy, J.W., and J.F. McElvogue: Racial segregation in American Sport. Int. Rev. Sport Sociol. 5:5–24, 1970.

54. Loy, J.W., B.D. McPherson, and G.S. Kenyon: Sport and Social Systems: A Guide to the Analysis, Problems, and Literature. Reading, MA: Addison-Wesley, 1978.

55. Loy, J.W., and J.N. Sage: The effects of formal structure on organizational leadership: an investigation of interscholastic baseball teams. In Contemporary Psychology of Sport. Edited by G.S. Kenyon and T. Grogg. Chicago: Athletic Institute, 1970, pp. 363–373.

56. Luschen, G.: Sociology of sport and the cross-cultural analysis of sport and games. In The Cross-Cultural Analysis of Sport and Games. Edited by G. Luschen. Champaign, Ill.: Stipes, 1970, pp. 6–13.

57. Maloney, T.L., and B.M. Petrie: Professionalization of attitude toward play among Canadian school pupils as a function of sex, grade, and athletic participation. J. Leisure Res. 4:184–195, 1972.

58. Mangan, J.A.: Athleticism in the Victorian and Edwardian Public School. London: Cambridge Univ. Press, 1981.

59. Metheny E.: Symbolic forms of movement: the feminine image in sports. In Connotations of Movement in Sport and Dance. Edited by E. Metheny. Dubuque, Iowa: W. C. Brown, 1965.

60. Mills, T.M.: The Sociology of Small Groups. Englewood Cliffs, N.J.: Prentice-Hall, 1967.

61. Murdock, G.P.: The common denominators of cultures. In Science of Man in the World Crisis. Edited by R. Linton. New York: Columbia Univ. Press, 1945, pp. 123–142.

62. Neumeyer, M.H.: Juvenile Delinquency in Modern Society. 3rd ed. Princeton, N.J.: D. Van Nostrand, 1961.

63. Nixon, H.L.: Reinforcement effects of sports team success cohesiveness-related factors. Int. Rev. Sport Sociol. 12(4):17–38, 1977.

64. Nixon, H.L.: Acceptance of the 'dominant American sports creed' among college students. Rev. Sport Leisure. 4:141–159, 1979.

65. Nixon, J.E., and A.E. Jewett: An Introduction to Physical Education. 9th ed. Philadelphia: Saunders, 1980.

66. Page, C.H.: The mounting interest in sport. In Sport and Society: An Anthology. Edited by J.T. Talamini and C.H. Page. Boston: Little, Brown, 1973, pp. 3–14.

67. Pascal, A., and L.A. Rapping: Racial Discrimination in Organized Baseball. Santa Monica, CA: The Rand Corp., 1970.

68. Petrie, A., R. McCulloch, and P. Kazdin: The perceptual characteristics of juvenile delinquents. J. Nervous Mental Disord. 134:415–421, 1962.

69. Petrofsky, J., and A.R. Lind: Aging, isometric strength and endurance, and cardiovascular responses to static effort. J. Appl. Physiol. 38:91–95, 1975.

70. Phillips, J.C.: Race and career opportunities in major league baseball: 1960–1980. J. Sport Soc. Issues. 7:1–17, 1983.

71. Rehberg, R.A., and W.F. Schafer: Participation in interscholastic athletics and college expectation. Am. J. Sociol. 73:732–740, 1968.

72. Richardson, D.E.: Ethical conduct in sport situations. Nat'l College Phys. E. Assn. for Men. Proceedings. 1963, pp. 98–104.

73. Roberts, J.M., and B. Sutton-Smith: Child training and game involvement. Ethnology. 1:166–185, 1962.

74. Robertson, I.: Sociology. 2nd ed. New York: Worth, 1981.

75. Roper, L.D., and K. Snow: Correlation studies of academic excellence and big-time athletics. Int. Rev. Sport Sociol. 11(3):57–68, 1976.

76. Ruder, M.K., and D.L. Gill: Immediate effects of win-loss on perceptions of cohesion in intramural and intercollegiate volleyball teams. J. Sport Psych. 4:227–234, 1982.

77. Ryan, E.D., and R. Foster: Athletic participation and perceptual augmentation and reduction. J. Pers. Soc. Psych. 6:472–476, 1967.

78. Sack, A., and R. Thiel: College football and social mobility: a case study of Notre Dame football players. Sociol. Educ. 52:60–66, 1979.

79. Sadker, M., and D. Sadker: Sexism in the schoolroom of the '80's. Psychology Today. 19(3):54–57, 1985.

80. Sage, G.H.: The effects of physical activity on the social development of children. In Effects of Physical Activity on Children. Amer. Acad. of P.E. Papers No. 19. Edited by G.A. Stull and H.M. Eckert. Champaign, Ill.: Human Kinetics, 1986, pp. 22–29.

81. Sage, G.H.: Pursuit of knowledge in sociology of sport: issues and prospects. Quest. 39:255–281, 1987.

82. Schneider, J., and D.S. Eitzen: Racial discrimination in American sport: continuity or change? J. Sport Behav. 2:136–142, 1979.

83. Smith, E.L., and C. Gilligan: Physical activity prescription for the older adult. Physician Sportsmed. 11(8):91–101, 1983.

84. Smith, M.D.: Getting involved in sport. Sex differences. Int. Rev. Sport Sociol. 14(2):93–101, 1979.

85. Snyder, E.E.: Aspects of socialization in sports and physical education. Quest. XIV:1–7, 1970.

86. Snyder, E.E.: Athletic dressing room slogans as folklore: a means of socialization. Int. Rev. Sport Sociol. 7:89–100, 1972.

87. Snyder, E.E., J. Kivlin, and E. Spreitzer: The female athlete: An analysis of objective and subjective role conflict. In Psychology of Sport and Motor Behavior. II. HPER Series No. 10. Edited by D. Landers. University Park: Penn. St. Univ., 1975, pp. 160–175.

88. Snyder, E.E., and E. Spreitzer: State of the field. Sociology of sport: an overview. Sociol. Quart. 15:467–487, 1974.

89. Snyder, E.E., and E. Spreitzer: Correlates of sport participation among adolescent girls. Research Quart. 47:804–809, 1976.

90. Snyder, E.E., and E. Spreitzer: Orientations toward sport: intrinsic, normative, and extrinsic. J. Sport Psych. 1:170–175, 1979.

91. Snyder, E.E., and E. Spreitzer: Social Aspects of Sport, 2nd ed. Englewood Cliffs, N.J.: Prentice-Hall, 1983.

92. Spreitzer, E., and E.E. Snyder: The psychosocial functions of sport as perceived by the general population. Int. Rev. Sport Sociol. 10(3):87–93, 1975.

93. Spreitzer, E., and E.E. Snyder: Socialization into sport: an exploratory path analysis. Res. Quart. 47:238–245, 1976.

94. Springer, F.: The experience of senior colleges that have discontinued football. In An Inquiry into the Need for and Feasibility of a National Study of Intercollegiate Athletics (Appendix I). Edited by G. Hanford. American Council on Education, Wash., D.C., 1974.

95. Stephens, T.: Secular trends in adult physical activity: exercise boom or bust. Res. Quart. *58*:94–105, 1987.

96. Stevenson, C.L.: Socialization effects of participation in sport: a critical review of the research. Res. Quart. *46*:287–299, 1975.

97. Stevenson, C.L., and J.E. Nixon: A conceptual scheme of the social function of sport. In Sport Sociology: Contemporary Themes. 2nd ed. Edited by A. Yiannakis et al. Dubuque, Iowa: Kendall/Hunt, 1979, pp. 16–22.

98. Sugden, J., and A. Yiannakis: Politics and the Olympics. Newsletter of the N. Am. Soc. for Sociol. of Sport. *2(1)*, 1980.

99. Thomas, C.L.: Factors important to women participants in vigorous athletics. In Sports Medicine and Physiology. Edited by R.H. Strauss. Philadelphia: Saunders, 1979, pp. 304–319.

100. Ullrich, E.: System-environment relationships in American universities: a theoretical model and exploratory study. Ph.D. dissertation, The Florida State University, 1971.

101. Ulrich, C.: The Social Matrix of Physical Education. Englewood Cliffs, N.J.: Prentice-Hall, 1968.

102. Webb, H.: Professionalization of attitudes toward play among adolescents. In Aspects of Contemporary Sport Sociology. Edited by G.S. Kenyon. Chicago: The Athletic Institute, 1969, pp. 161–178.

103. Williams, J.F.: The Principles of Physical Education. Philadelphia: Saunders, 1927.

104. Yetman, N., and D.S. Eitzen: Black Americans in sports: unequal opportunity for equal ability. Civil Rights Digest. *5*:20–34, 1972.

105. Zaharieva, E.: Olympic participation by women: effects on pregnancy and childbirth. JAMA. *221*:992–995, 1972.

BIBLIOGRAPHY

1. Coakley, J.J.: Sport in Society: Issues and Controversies. 4th ed. St. Louis: Times Mirror/Mosby, 1990.

2. Eitzen, D.S., and G.H. Sage: Sociology of North American Sport. 3rd ed. Dubuque, Iowa: Wm. C. Brown, 1986.

3. Leonard, W.M.: A Sociological Perspective of sport. 2nd ed. Minneapolis, Minn.: Burgess, 1984.

4. Loy, J.W., B.D. McPherson, and G.S. Kenyon: Sport and Social Systems: A Guide to the Analysis, Problems, and Literature. Reading, Mass.: Addison-Wesley, 1978.

5. Redekop, P.: Sociology of Sport: An Annotated Bibliography. New York: Garland, 1988.

6. Robertson, I.: Sociology. 2nd ed. New York: Worth, 1981.

7. Snyder, E.E., and E.A. Spreitzer: Social Aspects of Sport. 2nd ed. Englewood Cliffs, N.J.: Prentice-Hall, 1983.

6

PHYSICAL ACTIVITY, GROWTH, AND DEVELOPMENT

INTRODUCTION

Following birth, children grow and develop according to similar patterns until maturity (adulthood). This growth and development process includes physical, cognitive, social-psychologic, and motor aspects, all of which are interrelated. That is, the child grows and develops as a whole person interacting with the physical and social environment. The scope of this chapter will be limited to (1) physical growth and motor performance, and (2) the effects of exercise on physical structural and functional growth. For a thorough discussion of the interactive effects of physical activity and cognitive, as well as social-psychologic development in children, the interested reader is referred to the text by Zaichkowsky and colleagues.[54]

To some, the word growth means simply getting bigger. Actually, growth has several meanings, two of which are important for our purposes. In its simplest context, growth refers to an increase over time in physical size of the whole body or any of its parts. The latter includes body segments, but also alterations in the internal organs (e.g., heart size) and in tissue components (e.g., fat cell size and number, and blood hemoglobin concentration). However, the term growth is also used to indicate the process by which the body attains a mature (adult) state, which certainly does not involve increase in size of all body parts, tissues and organs over a particular span of time. This point is effectively illustrated in Figure 6–1, in which the general growth curves, as a function of final adult size (100%), for lymphoid, neural, general, and genital classifications, each proceed at a markedly different rate. In addition, it is necessary to distinguish between growth and three related terms: (1) development, (2) maturation, and (3) readiness.

Development refers to an increase with age in capacities, skill and complexity of function. Thus, the child develops neuromuscular control and motor skills, as well as psychologic attributes, including sensory and reasoning skills, attitudes, and personality. *Maturation* refers to the development of body size, structure, functions, and capacities via an inherent genetic program. That is, these characteristics follow the same general sequence in all children, but they progress at different rates. One is more mature at a given chronologic age to the extent that skeletal development, sexual maturity, or some other marker is farther advanced than average. *Readiness* is a form of maturation which refers to the particular time when the young child reaches a state when neurologic and muscular capacities have evolved to the point that particular motor skills can be learned when one is motivated and taught properly.

Typically, growth in terms of change over time, merely describes the outcomes of underlying biologic processes as affected by assorted environmental influences. However, this information is of great practical use if one is appropriately cognizant of individual variability. Unfortunately, this individual variability in various aspects of structural growth and function, as well as physical performance, can be due to combinations of hereditarian and envi-

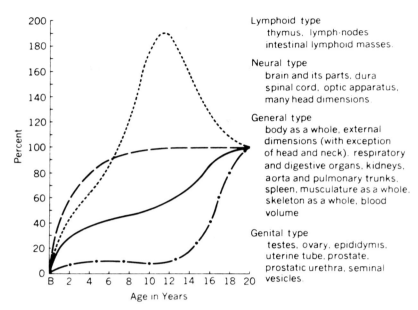

FIG. 6–1. The major types of postnatal growth of the various parts and organs of the body. The several curves are drawn to a common scale by computing their values at successive ages in terms of their total postnatal increments (to 20 years). (From Scammon, R.E.: The measurement of the body in childhood. In The Measurement of Man. J.A. Harris et al. Minneapolis: Univ. of Minnesota Press, 1930, p. 193.)

ronmental factors of varying importance. The latter point underlines the fundamental weakness of the cross-sectional method, in which children of various ages are measured at a given time. While this enables one to describe quickly how children of a certain age differ in one or more growth parameters, it does not permit effective analysis of the broad range of differences among children in their physical growth and performance, as well as their individual responses to particular environmental influences. The longitudinal method, in which measurements are taken on selected subjects over a period of time, can address these deficiencies, but is not without problems. In addition to the time needed and expense involved, substantial family mobility makes it difficult to study complete groups of children over prolonged periods. Further, even in relatively short-term longitudinal growth studies, it is essential to utilize a control group—particularly during rapid periods of growth. This point is well illustrated in Figure 6–2. In this study of the effects of 5 months' vigorous training

of 14 to 15-year-old females, there were almost as many subjects who gained body weight as those who lost. However, the mean body weight increase for adolescent girls this age over 5 months is 3½ pounds, about 1 pound of which would be body fat. The second panel of Figure 6–2, however, indicates that all subjects lost body fat, on average 5 pounds. Thus, while the "control" group was gaining 3½ pounds of body weight, including 1¼ pounds of fat, over the 5-month period, the exercise training group did not gain any weight and lost an average of 5 pounds of fat.

STAGES OF PHYSICAL GROWTH AND DEVELOPMENT

The most rapid stage of growth is prenatal, which is beyond the scope of this chapter. Postnatal stages of growth include: (1) infancy, the first year; (2) early childhood, ages 1 to 5 years; (3) late childhood, 5 to 11 years; (4) adolescence, ages 11 to 18 years; and (5) adulthood (matur-

Units in pounds

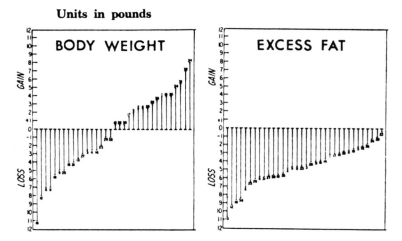

FIG. 6–2. Differential analyses of pre- and post-study measurements of body weight and excess fat in 34 adolescent girls undergoing 5 months of physical training. (Modified from Jokl, E.: Nutrition, Exercise and Body Composition. Springfield: Charles C Thomas, 1964, p. 80.)

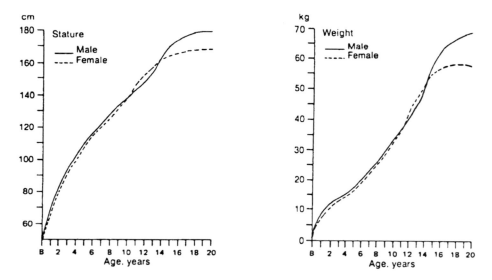

FIG. 6–3. Stature- and weight-attained curves (distance curves) for boys and girls. (From Malina, R.M.: Growth and Development: The First Twenty Years. Minneapolis, Minn.: Burgess, 1975, p. 19.)

ity). As can be seen in Figure 6–3, growth in body height and weight is similar for boys and girls through late childhood (10½ to 11 years), when girls enter puberty and the adolescent growth spurt about 2 years earlier than boys. There is a period of rapid growth from birth to about 3 years of age, which is somewhat greater for height than body weight. The rate of growth in both height and weight is relatively constant from 3 to 10 years.

Adolescence, the transitional stage between late childhood and adulthood, is marked by rapid growth, including body weight gains that peak at about 12 years in girls and age 14 in boys (see Fig. 6–4). Girls, on average, are typically slightly taller and heavier than boys from ages 11 to 13. This growth spurt is triggered by a programmed endocrine response and, in addition to maturation of secondary sex characteristics, results in the occurrence of substantial body size, proportion and composition differences between the sexes. By age 14 years, girls have reached 98½% of adult height, while boys, on average, are only at 91½%, and will continue to grow until 18 years of age. While girls continue to gain body weight until age 17, as is evident in

Figure 6–5, a higher proportion is due to an increased fat percentage of body weight. There is little gender difference in percent fat during childhood (i.e., up to about 11 years), and lean body mass and total body potassium are nearly the same for boys and girls until age 13, when the girls' values level off and boys continue to increase for several more years. Boys grow proportionally in shoulder and hip width, but as shown in Figure 6–6, girls' shoulder to hip width ratio falls steadily during adolescence.

GENETIC AND ENVIRONMENTAL EFFECTS ON GROWTH AND DEVELOPMENT

One's growth and developmental potential, as well as its pattern, is preset by heredity, but both can be notably affected by numerous environmental factors. Thus, each child inherits a genetic predisposition to attain a certain height and body weight, a certain number of muscle fibers, and numerous other structural characteristics that affect functional capacities and physical performance throughout life. Further, the

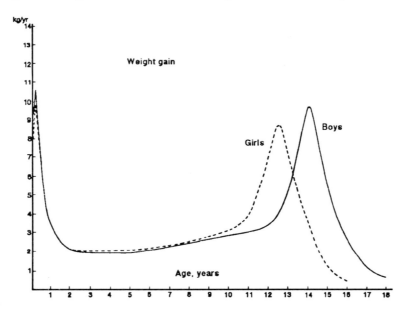

FIG. 6–4. Velocity curves for weight in boys (—) and girls (---). (From Tanner, J.M., R.H. Whitehouse, and M. Takaishi: Standards from birth to maturity for height, weight, height velocity, and weight velocity: British children, 1965, Part I. Arch. Disease Childh. 41:454–471, 1966.)

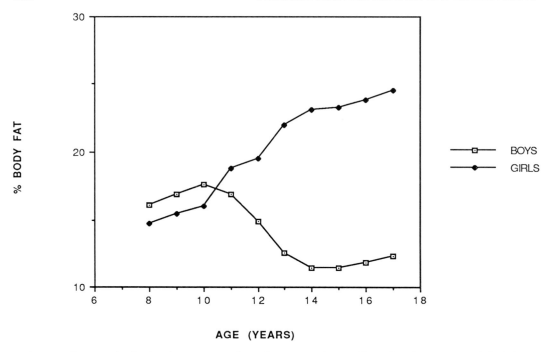

FIG. 6–5. Percent body fat during growth and aging in boys (▫) and girls (♦). (Modified from Cheek, D.B.: Human Growth: Body Composition, Cell Growth, Energy, and Intelligence. Philadelphia: Lea & Febiger, 1968, p. 700.)

rate at which we are able to develop the expression of this structural and functional potential, called maturation, is largely genetically determined. Several environmental factors have been shown to affect bodily growth. Particularly important are nutrition, disease, socioeconomic status, and physical activity.

It is well known that being either short or tall, thin or heavy, runs in families, but this is only suggestive evidence of here-

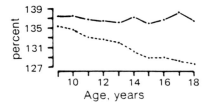

FIG. 6–6. Change in shoulder and hip width ratio during adolescence (Shoulder/Hip ×100). (From Malina, R.M.: Growth and Development: The First Twenty Years. Minneapolis, Minn.: Burgess, 1975, p. 22.)

ditarian influence, as individual familial factors, including eating and activity habits are intermingled. One approach to determining the relative influence of heredity and environment on body weight, is to compare the correlation between the weights of parents and their adopted children and their natural children, r = 0.15 and 0.50, respectively, in one study.[53] While this suggests that heredity is of importance in determining one's body weight, an r of 0.50 is not impressive for predictive purposes. However, it must be understood that parents transmit their heritage relative to structural growth potential, not just their own height, body weight, etc.

A more powerful technique for addressing the relative impact of heredity and environment over a normally encountered range of the latter, is to compare the variability in a group of identical (monozygotic, MZ) twins to that of a group of fraternal (dizygotic, DZ) twins of the same sex. The latter are no more likely to be genetically alike than other natural siblings of the same sex, while MZ twins have identical genotypes arising from the same fertilized egg. Thus, variability in their physical attributes will be due solely to environment, while that of DZ twin pairs will be due both to environmental and genetic factors. In one study using this design,[26] body weights of MZ (15 pair) and DZ (10 pair) twins from the same socioeconomic class, ages 7 to 13 years, were compared. The r between MZ twins was 0.96, while that between DZ twin pairs was 0.68.

The effects of environmental factors, such as nutrition, disease, and socioeconomic status are most readily illustrated in conditions of deprivation relative to that experienced by the vast majority of children in the United States. Severe nutritional restriction experienced currently by many children in third-world countries, particularly in terms of protein calories, results in significant decrements in height and weight, as well as muscle mass and bone density, compared to children of high socioeconomic status.[31] Short-term disease does not alter growth, but chronic nutritional deficiency appears to accentuate disease states that may compound the effect on growth.[31] In either case, if the effect is not too prolonged, the body's inherent compulsion to fulfill its innate growth potential prevails, even to the extent of a "catch-up" phase to normal body size. Decrements in growth have been demonstrated in numerous countries, including the United States, according to significantly divergent socioeconomic status. At first, this seems totally due to nutritional deficiency, but researchers contend that there are other important aspects, including greater number of children in poorer families, difference in sleep and rest patterns, and greater incidence of disease in children of poorer families.[49]

A related phenomenon of apparently predominant environmental impact on growth is the well-known secular trend of increased height and body weight. In Western European countries and the United States, children are considerably taller and heavier than 100 years ago. Figure 6–7 shows that the increase in height

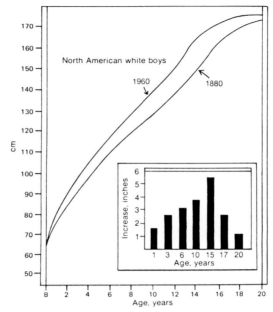

FIG. 6–7. Schematic curves for mean height for 1880 and 1960. Insert shows differences between the curves at selected ages. (From Meredith, H.V.: Change in the stature and body weight of North American boys during the last 80 years. In Advances in Child Development and Behavior. Edited by L.P. Lipsitt and C.C. Spiker. New York: Academic Press, 1963, pp. 69–114.)

of North American boys between 1880 and 1960 is greatest at age 15 years, with much less difference at ages 17 and 20. This same trend occurs for body weight, and is due to the fact that children over this time period have reached maturation at an earlier age. For example, in the 1800s it was not uncommon for males to continue growing in height until the early 20s, whereas now most American males reach maximum stature by age 18. American female's age at menarche (first menses) in 1880 was 14.6 years, while today the average is about 12.5 years. Causes of the secular trend in growth undoubtedly are tied primarily to improved socioeconomic conditions, better nutrition and less illness, as it was not evident in Western Europe from 1750 to 1830,[20] nor in third world countries today. Further, the trend has leveled off in Sweden during the past 25 years and, more recently, in the United States.[49] Thus, it appears that when most of a country's children are well nourished, enjoy better health care and living conditions, they reach their full growth potential.

Asmussen[4] astutely observed that in spite of an increase in height and weight of Olympic athletes from 1932 to 1960, body proportions remained constant. Thus, present-day taller athletes appear geometrically similar to their predecessors, but with at least proportionally larger muscles and greater body weight. Shephard[46] emphasizes that this would contribute to improved world records in running, jumping, and especially in throwing events. More important factors, however, include improvements in training, technique, equipment and facilities, as well as increased world population and much more universal "searching" of this population for individuals with the best athletic potential.

MATURATIONAL READINESS AND MOTOR SKILL DEVELOPMENT IN INFANCY AND EARLY CHILDHOOD

One indication that intrinsic factors are prominent in shaping human motor development is the orderly sequence of events in postural and locomotor development of infants. Rarick[42] cites the gradual and well-regulated progression of those primary motor abilities which precede creeping, crawling, standing, and walking. There is a cephalocaudal sequence of motor development proceeding from head and neck, to the upper trunk and arms, and then to the lower trunk and leg. Studies of motor development of the child's first 2 years indicate that enforced early practice does not benefit performance of reflex movements or rudimentary skills such as turning over, crawling, or walking. While early practice of more complex tasks results in improved early performance, a child who practices when "naturally" ready, catches-up rather rapidly and thus, learns more efficiently.[54] Studies of MZ twin pairs and DZ twin pairs exposed to the same range of normal environment during their first 2 years, reveal that MZ

correlations in motor development are consistently higher than those for DZ twins, again indicating that genetics plays the primary role.[9]

From 2 to 5 years of age, children develop proficiency in locomotor skills, usually in the progression of running, jumping, hopping, galloping, and skipping. In addition, they develop basic climbing skills, balancing ability, and initiate learning of throwing and catching skills. Rarick[42] contends that maturation of central nervous system integration plays the most prominent role in developing running, jumping, and throwing skills, rather than learning to synthesize discrete movement patterns. There is little difference between boys and girls in body size or composition at this age. Thus, some cultural impact on motor skill development is evidenced, in that by 5 years, boys perform galloping and can run, jump, and throw better, while girls tend to hop and skip better.[44] It seems likely that this difference would disappear if young boys and girls were uniformly afforded more early opportunity for appropriately directed movement expression (Fig. 6–8).

GROWTH, DEVELOPMENT, AND MOTOR PERFORMANCE IN LATE CHILDHOOD

From ages 5 to 11 years, there is little gender difference in body size or composition. Nonetheless, there are consistent gender differences in motor performances, with girls achieving better performance on flexibility (sit and reach) and on tasks requiring fine motor coordination. Boys consistently outperform girls of the same age in the standing long jump, (Fig. 6–9) running speed, and especially in throwing for distance.[19] These gender differences may seem readily attributable to practice effects, but hand grip strength (not usually practiced by boys or girls) is also consistently greater (approximately 10%) for boys during this period. Andres and colleagues[3] have presented interesting evidence suggesting a much more subtle effect, that of a culturally induced sex-inappropriateness. They found that there was no sig-

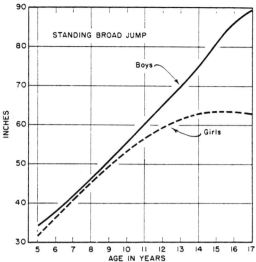

FIG. 6–9. Standing broad jump distance as a function of age. (From Espenschade, A.: Motor development. In Science and Medicine of Exercise and Sports. Edited by W.R. Johnson. New York: Harper, 1960, p. 433.)

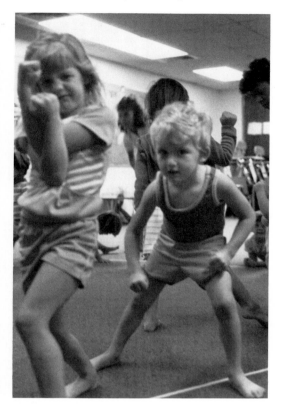

FIG. 6–8. A rich opportunity for appropriately directed movement expression is essential for the development of fundamental motor skills in early childhood for both boys and girls. (Photograph courtesy of Susan W. Stinson, Department of Dance, University of North Carolina at Greensboro.)

nificant difference in grip strength between 56 boys and 40 girls, ages 4 to 6 years, yet when questioned, 72% of the children thought that boys were actually stronger. Only 15% of the girls and 2% of the boys felt girls were stronger. The authors speculated that young girls may very early avoid participation in activities which they perceive to develop strength or other physical attributes more appropriate to males. This notion is of particular importance, in that physical performance tests demand both attentiveness to the task as well as motivation.

Klissouras[26] studied MZ and DZ twins, ages 7 to 13 years, from the same socioeconomic class, with both groups of twins

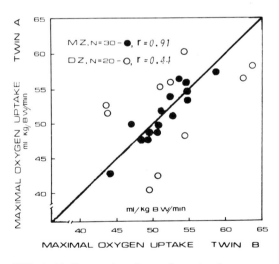

FIG. 6–10. Intrapair values of maximal oxygen uptake for MZ and DZ twins. Shaded area represents magnitude of the error of measurement. (From Klissouras, V.: Heritability of adaptive variation. J. Appl. Physiol. 31:338–344, 1971.)

engaged in the same range and amount of school and recreational physical activity. As shown in Figure 6–10, the variability in maximal oxygen uptake amongst MZ twin pairs was much less (r = 0.91) than among the DZ twin pairs (r = 0.44). Similarly divergent correlations were observed for maximum heart rate and maximal blood lactate following a treadmill run to exhaustion. Klissouras[28] also observed similarly divergent correlations in 1,000 meter run time (MZ twin pair r = 0.98; DZ twin pair r = 0.69). He concluded that maximum aerobic and anaerobic capacities, as well as middle-distance running performance, were primarily genetically determined in normally active children.

GROWTH, DEVELOPMENT, AND PHYSICAL PERFORMANCE DURING ADOLESCENCE

During adolescence, gender differences in physical performance are substantially increased over those existent in earlier years. In most cases, this is due primarily to differential physical growth and development changes, although there is evidence for a substantial cultural bias in certain cases. The girls' growth spurt during adolescence precedes by 2 years that of boys, beginning about 10½ years and ending about age 14½. Further, the female sex hormone, estrogen, tends to increase body fat at the expense of greater increase in lean tissue. Boys continue to grow in height, weight, and muscle mass through age 18. The principal male sex hormone, testosterone, increases from 10 to 20 times that in pre-pubertal years from ages 13 to 17. This induces large increases in muscle mass and is associated with significant reductions in percent body fat.[11] Lung and heart size grow proportional to lean body mass and hence, more so in boys than girls. There is little gender difference in hemoglobin concentration before adolescence, but a 20% increase occurs in boys during adolescence, with no change in girls.[52]

Girls' performance in the standing long jump (Fig. 6–9) plateaus at age 14, and even decreases slightly over the next 3 years. Boys' performance increases

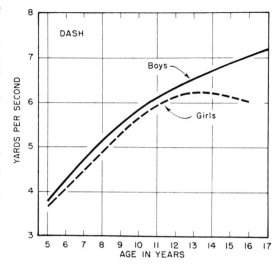

FIG. 6–11. Dash speed as a function of age. (From Espenschade, A.: Motor development. In Science and Medicine of Exercise and Sports. Edited by W.R. Johnson. New York: Harper, 1960, p. 432.)

throughout adolescence. A similar pattern is illustrated in sprinting speed in Figure 6–11. Divergent gender differences in adolescent body size and composition changes would appear to account in large part for the increasing disparity in standing long jump and sprint performance. Boys are increasing muscle mass to body weight ratio throughout this period, while girls actually have somewhat less muscle mass relative to body weight at age 17 than at age 13. The females' middle-distance running performance would also be adversely affected even more because of the male's increased hemoglobin concentration. However, there appear to be no clear gender differences in muscle fiber type[15] or in maximal strength and power output per unit of cross-sectional muscle area.[23]

The previously identified cultural bias relative to female performance in strength,[3] also seems evident upon careful analysis of school children gender differences in sprint speed (Fig. 6–11). At age 17, females sprint speed is 5.9 yards per second vs 7.2 for boys, a ratio of 0.82. The current world record for 100 meters (where we can assume that the female and male record holders were equally well endowed and privi-

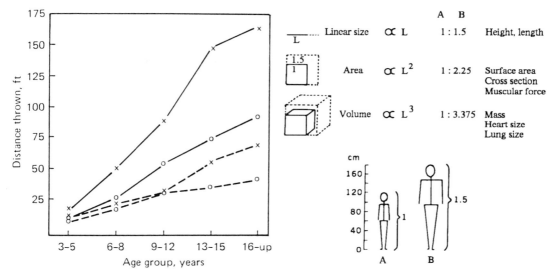

FIG. 6–12. Softball throw for distance in boys (x) and girls (o) using the dominant (—) and nondominant (---) arms. (From Wilmore, J.: Athletic Training and Physical Fitness. Boston: Allyn & Bacon, 1977, p. 186.)

FIG. 6–13. Schematic illustration of the influence of dimensions on some static and dynamic functions in geometrically similar individuals. A and B represent two persons with body height 120 and 180 cm respectively. ($\propto$ = proportional to.) (From Astrand, P.-O., and K. Rodahl: Textbook of Work Physiology. 3rd ed., New York: McGraw-Hill, 1986, p. 393.)

leged in training experience) is 9.83 and 10.76 seconds for males and females, respectively. This ratio is 0.91, with the difference between it and the 0.82 ratio for the normally active school children representing the gender "cultural gap" for sprinting in 17-year-old school children.

In gender comparisons of normally active adolescents and young adults, throwing and upper body strength appear particularly affected in association with the significantly smaller shoulder width in females relative to body weight.[31] Young adult females' arm extensor and flexor strength per unit body weight is about $\frac{1}{2}$ that of males. Undoubtedly, this contributes significantly to the substantial gender difference in the dominant arm softball throw for distance depicted in Figure 6–12. Boys progressively widen their throwing superiority throughout adolescence. However, the two dashed lines, denoting throwing performance of boys and girls using the nondominant arm (presumably reflecting no practice by either sex), show no difference until age 12, when the boys

gradually achieve better performance. At age 17, the nondominant arm gender difference is about 25 feet, while that for the dominant arm is about 75 feet. In this comparison, then, only about $\frac{1}{3}$ of the dominant arm gender difference is due to "non-practice" differences observed in nondominant arm throw performance.

To understand the expected magnitude of growth in various structures and function in children, it is helpful to examine the concept of scaling, or body dimension analysis. This relationship is illustrated in its simplest form, relative to changes in body dimensions of length (L), area (L^2), and volume (L^3) in Figure 6–13. In order for body dimension analysis to predict accurately changes in area, volume, and related biologic quantities, including body mass, the body must remain nearly constant in proportions and in density. Fortunately, this is the case during late childhood (5 years to puberty). During adolescence, body composition changes in both sexes, with males gaining a somewhat greater proportion of lean weight to total body weight and females a greater proportion of body weight as fat. The advantage of dimensional analysis is that it enables one to parcel out the amount of growth "due to" increased stature and dimensionally associated areas, volumes and related biologic quantities from what is actually observed. The difference between what is predicted and what is observed is then properly attributed to changes in body composition, or in the case of performances closely related to structural and functional growth, to refinement of neuromuscular coordination, maturation of the cardiorespiratory system, etc. For example, if an 18-year-old boy is 6 feet tall, as opposed to his height of 4 feet at age 7, the proportional increase is 1:1.5. At age 7, his grip strength was 35 lbs. and, since muscular force is proportional to cross-sectional area, we would expect an increase proportional to L^2 (i.e., 2.25 times), or 35 × 2.25 = 79 lbs. However, the average 18-year-old boy's grip strength is about 125 lbs. The difference between the observed (125 lbs.) and predicted (79 lbs.) values has been attributed primarily to changes in body composition and refinement of neuromuscular function during adolescence.[5]

EFFECTS OF MATURATION ON GROWTH, DEVELOPMENT, AND PHYSICAL PERFORMANCE

In previous sections of this chapter, growth, development, and physical performance in children have been described and analyzed in terms of group averages for boys and girls as a function of chronologic age. It was also mentioned that growth to adulthood entails two primary genetic components: (1) one that influences the individual's final adult size, and (2) another that influences the rate or speed at which that size is being attained, i.e., the maturation rate.[50] Thus, while the sequence of maturation to adult size is nearly uniform, children achieve various stages (whether identified by skeletal age, age at menarche, or some other marker) at different chronologic ages.

Because of the intense growth spurt dur-

ing adolescence, individual maturation rate—often referred to as biologic age—exerts profound effects on body size and composition, as well as physical performance. Evidence of similar biologic age in females—menarche—occurs usually at about 12, but can vary from 10½ to 13 years. Boys also evidence by skeletal age or other markers similar variability, entering puberty from age 12 to 15 years. As shown in Figure 6–14, height at the mid-point (12 years) of female adolescence varies from about 57½ inches (146 cm) to 62 inches (158 cm), respectively, in early and late maturing individuals. Body weight in early and late maturing girls varies even more than expected by dimensional analysis. Thus, early maturing girls tend to be not only taller, but heavier (and fatter) through adolescence.

In a ninth grade class of 14-year-old boys, it would not be unusual to find one or two individuals who would deviate by 4 inches in height and more than 25 lbs. from the average-sized boy of 65 inches and 120 lbs. Early maturing boys are taller than average, but are usually proportionally heavier with broader hips, shorter legs, and greater trunk length and muscularity. These differences in body height and weight—for both boys and girls—exert substantial influence on individual functional capacities and physical performance achievement during early adolescent years. A comparison of a pair of early and late maturing 12-year-old boys to a similar contrasted pair of girls is given in Table 6–1. Boy B is substantially taller and heavier, and has better physical performance scores than boy A (late maturer), especially in grip strength and the softball throw for distance. The early maturing girl (D) is also substantially taller and heavier than her late maturing counterpart (C). She is also stronger and has a substantially longer softball throw. However, the early maturing girl (D) has no advantage in the dash and jump, probably because she has a greater percent body fat than her late maturing counterpart.

While early maturing girls are bigger and stronger than late maturing girls during the early and middle years of maturation (8 to 14 years), late maturing girls tend to remain

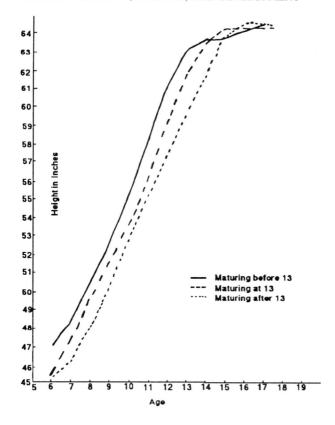

FIG. 6–14. Growth in height of early, average, and late maturing girls from 6 to 18 years. (From Richey, H.G.: The blood pressure in boys and girls before and after puberty: its relation to growth and maturity. Amer. J. Dis. Children. 42:1281–1330, 1931.)

Table 6–1. Height, Weight, and Physical Performance Comparison of Early and Late Maturing 12-Year-Old Boys and Girls*

	Boys		Girls	
Parameter	A	B	C	D
Skeletal age (yrs)	9.9	14.3	10.9	13.6
Height (in.)	54.3	61.1	57.3	63.5
Weight (lbs.)	77	102	82.5	147
Grip strength (lbs.)	43	61	45	55
35-yd. dash (sec.)	5.6	5.2	6.1	6.1
Standing long jump (in.)	60	65	53	52
Softball throw (ft.)	89	114	46	80

*Modified from Malina, R.M.: The nature of physical growth and development. In Singer, R.N., et al.: Physical Education: An Interdisciplinary Approach. New York: Macmillan, 1972, pp. 273–274.

more slender than their early maturing counterparts between 15 to 18 years, which gives them an advantage in numerous physical performances as their muscle mass increases without as much body fat as early maturing girls. This probably encourages prolonged participation in sport and further skill development.[47] Malina and colleagues[32] have shown that age at menarche is substantially delayed in U.S. national intercollegiate track and field competitors (average of 13.6 years for all events) compared to 12.2 years of age for nonathletes.

The comparison of early and late maturers' average grip strength, shown in Figure 6–15, clearly illustrates a gender difference. Early maturing boys tend to maintain body size and performance advantages over their late maturing counterparts through 17 years of age.[24] In fact, as shown in Figure 6–16, when boys who had the best strength scores at 11½ years of age (average about 75th percentile for four tests) were compared to the "weak" group (average of 15th percentile at age 11½ years) over a 6-year longitudinal study, the strong boys got stronger and the weak boys did poorer at age 17½ years (solid lines). Most of the strong boys were muscular and well above average height and weight, and thus early maturers at age 11½. It seems likely that the wider disparity in strength at age 17½ years was due in large part to the continued vigorous activity through adolescence in the strong group, together with the weak group's tendency to avoid vigorous activity in which they experienced little success.[24]

In view of the latter comparison, it would seem logical to expect that male athletic success could be rather easily predicted from a well-selected physical performance battery administered in early adolescence. However, this comparison of extremes in strength had absolutely no individual overlap. When individuals between the 50th and 75th percentile at age 11½ years were followed, a substantial number improved at a greater rate over the ensuing 6 years and became stronger than some of the members of the strong group.[24] In another growth study of male interscholastic athletic team participants,[13] it was found that only 25% had been rated as outstanding athletes in late elementary and junior high school years, and an additional 30% during junior high school only. Thus, 45% of the high school athletes had "arrived" from a less than outstanding observational prognosis during elementary and/or junior high school.

THE EFFECT OF PHYSICAL ACTIVITY ON GROWTH AND DEVELOPMENT

Much of the knowledge of the effects of physical activity on growth of human body structure (i.e., bone, muscle, and fat), as well as physiologic function, has been obtained on adults. This review, however, will focus on the effect of physical activity on the growth and development of chil-

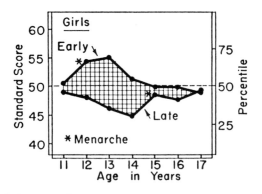
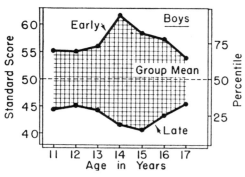

FIG. 6–15. Growth curve scores (right grip) for early and late maturing girls and boys expressed in percentiles. (From Jones, H.E.: Motor Performance and Growth. Berkeley: Univ. of California Press, 1949, pp. 59 and 64.)

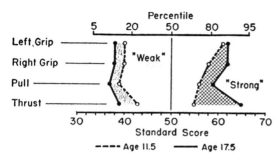

FIG. 6–16. Percentile profiles of contrasting groups (strength measurements). Key: (---) 11.5 and (—) 17.5 years. (From Jones, H.E.: Motor Performance and Growth. Berkeley: Univ. of California Press, 1949, p. 152.)

dren and adolescents. Particular attention will be given to the range of activity, including: (1) immobilization, (2) normal, habitual activity, (3) additional or special physical education programs, and (4) intensive training programs in competitive sports. However, it must be emphasized that physical activity is only one of several environmental factors influencing the genetic predisposition for each child's growth and thus, clear identification of optimum levels for particular goals is elusive. Finally, there is little research available that addresses the question of what happens in children and adolescents following intense activity; i.e., is there a "permanent" impact, as opposed to the transient effects routinely demonstrated in adults?

Bones are not solid unchanging structures; rather, they are a dynamic tissue with continuous cell exchange. In addition to adequate calcium and vitamin D in the diet, physical activity appears essential to maintain appropriate levels of calcium in the bone tissue throughout life.[29] There is no evidence of even intense physical activity affecting long bone growth or stature in humans.[10] However, there is evidence that bone width and density can be increased via prolonged, sustained activity.[7] None of these studies have used control groups, so it is possible that selectivity of individuals most likely to succeed in the athletic population studied accounted for differences observed. The observations of Buskirk and co-workers[12] on tennis players' dominant hand and forearm bones showed them to

be notably larger than on the nondominant limb (i.e., each subject served as his own control).

An exceptional example of how bones can grow in response to unusual weight bearing stress was reported by Houston.[22] A boy born without the larger tibia bone in his lower right leg, had the smaller fibula surgically moved to assume the tibia's normal locale at 2 years of age. After 18 months the fibula, which was doing the ordinary work of the tibia, had increased in size approximating that of the tibia in the contralateral limb. No studies have addressed the persistency effect, so that even if intense exercise does cause changes in bone width and density of well-nourished children, it may be of minimal impact unless at least threshold maintenance activity is adhered to through one's adult years.

Skeletal muscle adaptations to exercise training have been reviewed in detail earlier (Chapter 3). Apparently, no studies have been done on the effects of physical activity levels of youth and adolescents on muscle structure and function. In adults, lean tissue alterations with physical activity level are usually accompanied by reciprocal changes in body fat, often without appreciable changes in body weight.[2,37] The magnitude of change in body composition (leanness/fatness) effected by physical training depends on both its intensity and duration. However, this is much more difficult to quantify in growing children, as there are changes in body weight and composition due to the growth process, per se.

BODY COMPOSITION

EFFECTS OF ADDITIONAL PHYSICAL EDUCATION. There is some evidence that well designed supplemental physical education programs can decrease body fat (usually with a near proportional increase in lean tissue) in otherwise normally active school children. Coonan and co-workers[14] reported a study of 500 10-year-old boys and girls who were divided into three groups: (1) control, which received the regular physical education program of 3½ hours of motor skills work per week; (2) an experimental group that received 1¼ hours per day of fitness training; and (3) a second experimental group that participated for 1¼ hours per day in motor skill activities. At the end of the 14-week experiment, children in the fitness training group showed a significant reduction in subcutaneous fat at four skinfold sites. Neither the children who received equivalent extra time in motor skills activities, nor the control group, experienced any change in subcutaneous fat.

Thus, it appears that the type of extra physical activity, rather than just more time in the usual motor skill centered physical education program, is crucial to effecting changes in body fat. For example, Dutch 12- and 13-year-old boys, who had daily 1 hour sessions of the same program normally taken 3 times per week, did not differ in body fat from the control group.[25] Similarly, 1 hour per day extra physical education in a Canadian study[48] did not alter body fat in children ages 6 to 12 years from that of the control group. Parizkova[39] studied a group of boys over 4 years, beginning at age 11 years, who were then exposed to different amounts of physical education, sports participation, and physical training. The least active group participated in regular physical education 2½ hours per week, while the most active group trained 6 hours per week. At age 15, the least active group showed a non-significant decrease in body fat from 17.1 to 16.5%, while the physically trained group showed a decrease from 16.1 to 9.9% of body weight.

EFFECTS OF ATHLETIC TRAINING. The effect of physical training for athletic competition in several sports on body composition during adolescence has been studied in boys and girls by Parizkova.[40] A 5-year study of girls, from ages 12 to 17 years, showed no significant difference in height and body weight between the gymnastics and control groups. Body fat was the same in both groups at age 12 (17% of body weight), but by age 17 years, the gymnasts had about 30% less fat (and proportionally more lean tissue) than the control group.

However, prolonged intense training during adolescence does not preclude some expression of the female's hormon-

ally induced increase in percent body fat. Parizkova[40] studied boys and girls over 3 years of swim training from ages 11 to 14 years. There was no significant gender difference in height and body weight throughout the study, nor in body fat or lean body mass during the first 2 years. However, during the last year, the girls actually gained fat equivalent to 3% of body weight, while the boys experienced a greater lean body mass gain.

PHYSICAL ACTIVITY AND THE OBESE CHILD. Increased childhood obesity has been linked to lower levels of habitual physical activity.[41] In fact, there is considerable evidence that obese children actually eat less calories than their normal weight counterparts, but are less active and, when active, are less vigorous in their participation.[35] This has led to considerable effort in developing summer camp "rehabilitative" programs for obese children with a strong exercise component. Successful programs usually incorporate: (1) a well-balanced diet, with moderate restriction of calories, (2) a large increase in physical activity, but with gradual increase in intensity, and with a variety of games, sports, and fitness activities, (3) a strong education and counseling component, and (4) a follow-up component (i.e., is what has been learned being effectively applied upon return to the home?).[38] As shown in Figure 6–17, the body density (greater body density equals lower fat) changes of 11- and 12-year-old boys and girls during 8 weeks of summer camp (1959) are substantial, but about half of the effect is lost before the next year's camp (1960), which brings the obese children closer to the normal weight children's body density.

There is increasing interest in the use of physical activity programs, initiated early in life, as a preventive of obesity development. Obesity develops both from an increase in fat cell size and number, each increasing rapidly during infancy and again, less rapidly during adolescence.[21] Experiments in growing animals, from ages approximating the range of human infancy through adolescence, show that heavy exercise early in life substantially reduced fat cell size and number compared

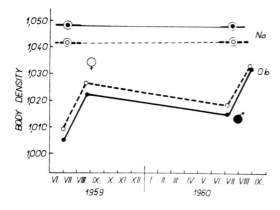

FIG. 6–17. Body density changes in obese and normal children during two years (11–12 years). (From Parizkova, J.: Physical activity and body composition. In Human Body Composition: Approaches and Application. Edited by J. Brozek. Oxford: Pergamon, 1965, p. 168.)

to the nonexercising controls.[36] Further, when the exercise training group assumed normal activity during adult years, they maintained a persistently reduced fat cell number from that of the controls, although their average fat cell sizes became similar. Since fat cell number in humans does not appear to increase in the adult years,[21] and it is difficult for most individuals to maintain substantially reduced fat cell size,[8] the importance of restricting fat cell development early in life is readily apparent.

PHYSIOLOGIC FUNCTION AND MOTOR PERFORMANCE

Enhanced growth in physiologic function, such as improved aerobic and anaerobic capacities, and in motor performance, has been routinely observed upon utilization of supplemental physical education programs in which no impact on normal height or body weight change was seen. For example, Canadian children who participated in 1 hour per day additional physical education beyond the usual 40 minutes per week, over a 6-year period from ages 6 to 12, did not differ significantly in height, weight or subcutaneous fat from those children who did not receive the supplemental program. There was also little difference in the more basic performances, such as the standing long jump and 50 yard dash. However, substantial differences in muscular endurance, strength, and cardiorespiratory endurance were observed.[47]

Ekblom[17] noted that if intense physical training was undertaken by previously nontrained young adults, they reached a plateau in 6 to 18 months that represented an upper limit well below Olympic performers, even when they continued maximum training for 5 years. He then decided to train six 11-year-old boys very hard for 3 years to examine the question of when in life this upper limit is set. The boys increased steadily in body weight, lung size, heart volume, and maximal aerobic capacity, but had only 20% greater values than a control group of boys followed over the same 3-year span. If this were a critical period of aerobic capacity development to raise the upper limit characteristic of adult years, one would expect an increase of 50 to 100% over the control group, rather than the observed 20% value. Indeed, Weber and colleagues[51] observed that 10 weeks of intense aerobic training of MZ twins, ages 10, 13, and 16 years, yielded somewhat greater effects at ages 10 and 16 years. In fact, the normally active MZ twin controls, age 13, increased their aerobic capacity almost as much as their twin counterparts who trained. The authors concluded that the popular notion that more might be gained by introducing the training stimulus at the time when the body height and weight growth is strongest, was not supported by their results.

No comparable studies of whether strength training can yield greater results if imposed at a particular time of adolescent growth have been reported. Normally active boys follow a well-defined pattern of peak growth in which that for height occurs 6 months prior to that for body weight, with peak muscle growth about half way between.[50] Peak muscular strength increase occurs several months after. This is not surprising, since strength has a central neural component, as well as a muscular hypertrophy component.[16]

Children, especially adolescents, generally achieve greater changes in both strength and endurance following several months training than do their normally active young adult counterparts. Bailey and colleagues[7] suggest that this is likely due to an enhancing effect of the inherent growth process, per se. Nonetheless, these changes appear transient without continued vigorous physical activity participation, as shown by Klissouras.[27] A pair of MZ twins who had lived together and were both highly active between ages 8 to 15 years were studied. At age 15, one twin became interested in cars, assumed a relatively sedentary lifestyle and at the time of study 3 years later, was a traveling salesman. His maximum oxygen uptake (aerobic capacity) was 36 ml/min/kg of body weight. His twin brother remained active throughout this period, training for high school sports team participation. His aerobic capacity was 49 ml/min/kg, which is about that for the average nontrained young adult male. Assuming the trained twin had not increased his maximum aerobic capacity appreciably with 3 additional years training in late adolescence, the previously active twin had lost about 30% of his aerobic capacity. The results of this study also substantiate the overriding impact of a genetic ceiling on maximum aerobic capacity, in that several years of intense training left the trained twin only at an average value for normally active young adult males and far below that required for an Olympic caliber endurance athlete.

ATHLETIC PARTICIPATION EFFECTS ON CHILDREN'S PHYSICAL GROWTH AND DEVELOPMENT

There has been a continued increase in sports competition for youth, involving more intense physical training regimens. There are now organized programs for children of elementary and junior high school ages (6 to 14 years of age), including competition in baseball, football, soccer, swimming, gymnastics, and track. Programs for girls have increased at an even more rapid rate. Medical concern regarding the effects of this early training and competition has focused on the physical growth process, cardiorespiratory system, and orthopedic problems attendant to bone and joint stress. This concern is well founded, in that children are not merely scaled down adults. For example, they do not possess a fully-developed skeletal system, or proportionally-developed cardiorespiratory and thermoregulatory function. Further, they proceed through the physical growth and development process at widely varied maturational rates for any given chronologic age. The latter is of particular importance in age-group team sport competition where individuals may vary several years in maturation and biologic age, as well as body size. Given the closer correlation between body size and physical performance, it seems more appropriate to organize teams according to the child's size rather than chronologic age.[33]

From previous discussion of rather limited research, it appears that athletic training and competition does not, in itself, affect the child's growth in height and body weight. However, the young athlete is usually leaner (i.e., has a lesser percentage of body weight as fat) than his nontrained counterpart. Further, the trained young athlete has substantially enhanced physiologic function and physical performance capacity. However, there have been few follow-up studies of children engaged in intense training and competition over a number of years. A classic study by Ericksson and co-workers[18] consisted of a 10-year follow-up on 30 top competitive girl swimmers, first studied between ages 12 to 16 years following several years of training. When first studied, some girls were swimming 4 to 4½ hours per day, covering as much as 12 kilometers. At that time, they had significantly larger lung size, heart volume, and total hemoglobin, as well as a 45% greater maximal aerobic capacity than their normally active age-matched controls. During the 10 years following the initial study, all the girls had ceased training for at least several years and few participated in regular vigorous physical activity. Instead, they were occupied with professional and/or domestic duties of a predominantly sedentary nature, such that their maximal aerobic capacity had been reduced by more than 25%. However, their lung size and heart volume were relatively unchanged. The authors concluded that there were no harmful effects evident from the previous years' intense training by these women, and that they retained structural advantages for superior endurance performance should they initiate vigorous activity again.

As discussed earlier, girls who succeed in certain sports, including track and field, gymnastics, and figure skating, experience menarche significantly later (1½ to 3 years) than do their nonathletic counterparts. It is not known, however, whether delayed menarche is due to prolonged early sport training or is just a characteristic of those who succeed in these sports. For example, delayed menarche (and attendant sexual maturation) is associated with less percentage of body fat, which could contribute to enhanced performance in many female athletic endeavors. Also of concern has been the temporary cessation or irregularity of menses, once initiated, that is prevalent amongst individuals of the same athletic groups.[45] Marker[34] has reported that athletes with late menarche experienced no ill effects with respect to their reproductive function, based on data obtained subsequently at childbirth. Further, there was no relationship between age at menarche and that at first parturition among athletes from numerous sports.

Orthopedic problems, particularly prevalent in many competitive sports are a special consideration for the growing child and adolescent. They are susceptible to the same musculoskeletal injuries as adults, such as contusions, sprains, and strains, as well as long bone and stress fractures. In addition, children are susceptible to three major types of musculoskeletal injuries due to incomplete growth: (1) those to the growth plate; (2) injuries to the epiphysis (the end of the long bone); and (3) avulsions, or the pulling away of major musculotendinous insertions from the bone. It is particularly important to understand that these injuries are often incurred over some period of time (microtrauma), rather than from single severe contact (macrotrauma), such as in a long bone fracture.

Macrotraumatic injury to the growth plate and epiphyses of long bones is an important concern, which usually is initially well treated with appropriate medical care. However, Larson[30] cautions that the skeletal element should be followed subsequently to ensure no restriction in future activity. In addition to acute separation (macrotrauma), recurrent overstress of a musculotendinous unit can result in chronic irritation and pulling away of the apophysis from the bone (microtrauma). This malady occurs rather frequently with increased intensive training in gymnastics, soccer, and swimming.

Much greater occurrence of a related orthopedic problem, "little league elbow," existed until the mid-1960s, when a medical report showed conclusively via x ray that young pitchers were experiencing epiphyseal injuries.[1] Barring of throwing the curve ball and limiting the number of innings pitched per week has virtually eliminated this problem. A new concern is the use of heavy weights in training associated with youth sports competition, including reports of fracture of the radial epiphysis growth plate in adolescents.[43]

SUMMARY

1. The child's growth and development includes an interrelated expression of physical, cognitive, social-psychologic, and motor aspects. In this chapter, only physical growth and motor performance, and the effects of exercise on physical structural and functional growth, were examined.

2. In its simplest context, growth refers to an increase over time in physical size of the whole body or any of its parts. Growth is also used to indicate the process by which the child's body attains the mature, adult state.

3. Development refers to an increase with age in capacities, skill and complexity of function. Maturation refers to the development of body size, structure, functions and capacities via an inherent genetic program.

4. Growth in body height and weight are similar in boys and girls through late childhood (10½ to 11 years), when girls enter puberty and the adolescent growth spurt about 2 years earlier than boys. The boys' adolescent growth rate is greater

than that for girls, and is characterized by changes in body composition, such that more of the boys' body weight gain during adolescence is lean tissue. The proportion of lean tissue in girls decreases somewhat during adolescence.

5. Studies comparing identical twins and fraternal twins of the same sex, living in normally encountered environmental conditions, show a preeminent effect of heredity on body growth and motor performance.

6. Severe nutritional restriction experienced currently by many children in third-world countries, particularly in terms of protein calories, results in significant reductions in height and weight, as well as muscle mass and bone density, compared to children of high socioeconomic status.

7. While all young children exhibit an inherent orderly sequence of events in postural and locomotor development, the time that each occurs varies considerably. A gender cultural impact occurs by age 5, when boys outperform girls in running, jumping, and throwing, while girls hop and skip better.

8. There is no gender difference in body size or composition from ages 5 to 11 years. Boys, however, continue to outperform girls of the same age in jumping, running, and especially throwing. Girls have better performance in flexibility and on tasks requiring fine motor coordination.

9. During adolescence, girls' running, jumping, and throwing performances plateau, which is associated with an earlier plateau of height and body weight than for boys, and an increase in the proportion of fat weight to body weight.

10. Boys' running, jumping, and throwing performances increase through age 18 years, which is associated with continued growth in height and body weight and an increase in the proportion of lean weight to body weight.

11. While the sequence of maturation to adult size is nearly uniform, children achieve various stages (whether identified by skeletal age, age at menarche, or some other marker) at different chronologic ages.

12. Early maturing children are taller and heavier than other children during early adolescence. This larger body size is associated with enhanced physical performance in boys, but is not so pronounced in early maturing girls who increase in body fat during adolescence.

13. Late maturing girls remain more slender than their early maturing counterparts, which facilitates performance in gymnastics and certain track and field events during adolescence.

14. While early maturing boys maintain body size and performance superiority over the latest maturing boys throughout adolescence, some intermediate maturing boys grow at a more rapid rate, eventually surpassing some of the early maturing boys in late adolescence.

15. Vigorous physical activity does not affect long bone growth, but does increase bone diameter and density.

16. Vigorous physical activity during childhood and adolescence has no effect on height and relatively little impact on body weight, as increased lean mass is often effectively balanced by reduced body fat.

17. Increased physical activity levels in obese children have been found to be an effective adjunct to a well-balanced diet, with moderate restriction of calories, in achieving a more optimal body weight.

18. There is no evidence that enhancing the training stimulus during the early adolescent growth spurt results in greater body structural and functional growth.

19. Children are not merely scaled down adults, as their skeletal system is not fully developed, nor do they have proportionally developed cardiorespiratory and thermoregulatory function.

20. Heavy exercise training in young children, which results in a greater rate of tissue breakdown than repair over time, can lead to orthopedic injury of the bone and the musculotendinous insertion to the bone.

REFERENCES

1. Adams, J.E.: Injury to the throwing arm: a study of traumatic changes in the elbow joints of boy baseball players. Calif. Med. *102*:127–132, 1965.
2. Adams, W.C., M.M. McHenry, and E.M. Bernauer: Long-term physiologic adaptations to ex-

ercise with special reference to performance and cardiorespiratory function in health and disease. Am. J. Cardiol. *33*:765–775, 1974.

3. Andres, F.F., C.R. Rees, S.A. Weiner, and D.J. Weiss: Actual and perceived strength differences. JOPERD. *52(5)*:20–21, 1981.

4. Asmussen, E.: Growth and athletic performance. FIEP. *34*:22, 1964.

5. Asmussen, E.: Growth in muscular strength and power. In Physical Activity: Human Growth and Development. Edited by G.L. Rarick. New York: Academic Press, 1973, pp. 60–79.

6. Astrand, P.-O., and K. Rodahl: Textbook of Work Physiology: Physiological Bases of Exercise. 3rd ed. New York: McGraw-Hill, 1986.

7. Bailey, D.A., R.M. Malina, and R.L. Rasmussen: The influence of exercise, physical activity, and athletic performance on the dynamics of human growth. In Human Growth (Vol. 2). Edited by F. Falkner and J.M. Tanner. New York: Plenum Press, 1978, pp. 475–505.

8. Bjorntorp, P.: Interrelation of physical activity and nutrition on obesity. In Diet and Exercise: Synergism in Health Maintenance. Edited by P.L. White and T. Mondeika. Chicago: Amer. Med. Assoc., 1982, pp. 91–98.

9. Bouchard, C.: Genetics and motor behavior. In Psychology of Motor Behavior and Sport. Vol. II. Edited by D.M. Landers and R.W. Christina. Champaign, Ill.: Human Kinetics, 1977, pp. 257–273.

10. Broekhoff, J.: The effect of physical activity on physical growth and development. In Effects of Physical Activity on Children. Amer. Acad. of P.E. Papers, No. 19. Edited by G.A. Stull and H.M. Eckert. Champaign, Ill.: Human Kinetics, 1986, pp. 75–87.

11. Brooks, G.A., and T.D. Fahey: Exercise Physiology: Human Bioenergetics and Its Applications. New York: Macmillan, 1985.

12. Buskirk, E.R., K.L. Anderson, and J. Brozek: Unilateral activity and bone and muscle development in the forearm. Res. Quart. *27*:127–131, 1956.

13. Clarke, H.H.: Proceed. of 8th Am. Med. Assoc. Nat. Conf. on Medical Aspects of Sports. Chicago: Amer. Med. Assoc., 1967, pp. 49–57.

14. Coonan, W.T., et al.: Daily physical education: a review of current Australian research projects. In Movement and Sport Education: Proc. of the VII Commonwealth and Int'l. Conf. on Sport, Physical Education, Recreation, and Dance. Edited by M.L. Howell and J.E. Saunders. Queensland, Australia: Univ. of Queensland, Dept. of Human Movmt. Studies, Vol. 6, 1982, pp. 239–245.

15. Costill, D.L., et al.: Skeletal muscle enzymes and fiber composition in male and female track athletes. J. Appl. Physiol. *40*:149–154, 1976.

16. de Vries, H.A.: Physiology of Exercise For Phys-

ical Education and Athletes. 4th ed. Dubuque, Iowa: Wm. C. Brown, 1986.

17. Ekblom, B.: Physical training of normal boys in adolescence. Acta Paediatr. Scand. *(Suppl. 217)*:60–62, 1971.

18. Eriksson, B.O., et al.: A physiological analysis of former girl swimmers. Acta Paediatr. Scand. *(Suppl. 217)*:68–72, 1971.

19. Espenschade, A.: Motor development. In Science and Medicine of Exercise and Sports. Edited by W.R. Johnson. New York: Harper & Bros., 1960, pp. 419–439.

20. Harrison, G.A., et al.: Human Growth. An Introduction to Human Evolution, Variation and Growth. Oxford: Clarendon Press, 1964.

21. Hirsch, J., and J. Knittle: Cellularity of obese and non-obese human adipose tissue. Fed. Proceed. *29*:1516–1521, 1970.

22. Houston, C.S.: The radiologist's opportunity to teach bone dynamics. J. Canad. Assoc. Radiol. *29*:232–238, 1978.

23. Ikai, M., and T. Fukunaga: Calculation of muscle strength per unit cross-sectional area of human muscle by means of ultrasonic measurements. Arbeitsphysiol. *26*:26–32, 1968.

24. Jones, H.E.: Motor Performance and Growth. Berkeley: University of California Press, 1949.

25. Kemper, H.C.G., et al.: Invloed van Extra Lichamelijke Opvoeding. Amsterdam: Posthuma & Snabel, 1974.

26. Klissouras, V.: Heritability of adaptive variation. J. Appl. Physiol. *31*:338–344, 1971.

27. Klissouras, V.: Genetic limit of functional adaptability. Arbeitsphysiol. *30*:85–94, 1972.

28. Klissouras, V.: Prediction of potential performance with special reference to heredity. J. Sports Med. *13*:100–107, 1973.

29. Krolner, B., B. Toft, S.P. Nielsen, and E. Tondevold: Physical exercise as a prophylaxis against involutional bone loss: a controlled trial. Clin. Sci. *64*:541–546, 1983.

30. Larson, R.L.: Physical activity and the growth and development of bone and joint structures. In Physical Activity: Human Growth and Development. Edited by G.L. Rarick. New York: Academic Press, 1973, pp. 32–59.

31. Malina, R.M.: Growth and Development: The First Twenty Years. Minneapolis, Minn.: Burgess, 1975.

32. Malina, R.M., A.B. Harper, H.H. Avent, and D.E. Campbell: Age at menarche in athletes and non-athletes. Med. Sci. Sports. *5*:11–13, 1973.

33. Malina, R.M., and G.L. Rarick: Growth, physique and motor performance. In Physical Activity: Human Growth and Development. Edited by G.L. Rarick. New York: Academic Press, 1973, pp. 125–153.

34. Marker, K.: Influence of athletic training on the maturity process. In The Female Athlete. Edited

by J. Borms, M. Hebbelinck, and A. Venerando. Basel, Switzerland: Karger, 1981, pp. 117–126.

35. Mayer, J.: Overweight. Causes, Cost, and Control. Englewood Cliffs, N.J.: Prentice-Hall, 1968.

36. Oscai, L.B., et al.: Exercise or food restriction: effect on adipose tissue cellularity. Am. J. Physiol. 227:901–904, 1974.

37. Parizkova, J.: Impact of age, diet, and exercise on man's body composition. Ann. N.Y. Acad. Sci. 110:661–674, 1963.

38. Parizkova, J.: Physical activity and body composition. In Human Body Composition: Approaches and Applications. Edited by J. Brozek. Oxford: Pergamon, 1965, pp. 161–176.

39. Parizkova, J.: Longitudinal study of the development of body composition and body build in boys of various physical activity. Human Biol. 40:212–225, 1968.

40. Parizkova, J.: Body composition and exercise during growth and development. In Physical Activity: Human Growth and Development. Edited by G.L. Rarick. New York: Academic Press, 1973, pp. 97–124.

41. Pate, R.R.: A new definition of youth fitness. Physician Sportsmed. 11(4):77–83, 1983.

42. Rarick, G.L.: The emergence of the study of human motor development. In Perspectives of the Academic Discipline of Physical Education. Edited by G.A. Brooks. Champaign, Ill.: Human Kinetics, 1981, pp. 163–189.

43. Ryan J.R.: Fracture of the distal radial epiphysis in adolescent weight lifters. Am. J. Sports Med. 4:26–28, 1976.

44. Seefeldt, V., and J. Haubenstricker: Patterns, phases, or stages: an analytical model for the study of developmental movement. In The Development of Movement Control and Coordination. Edited by J.A.S. Kelso and J.E. Clark. New York: Wiley, 1982, pp. 309–318.

45. Shangold, M.M.: Sports and menstrual function. Physician Sportsmed. 8(8):66–72, 1980.

46. Shephard, R.J.: The Fit Athlete. London: Oxford University Press, 1978.

47. Shephard, R.J.: Physical Activity and Growth. Chicago: Year Book Medical, 1982.

48. Shephard, R.J., et al.: Un programme complementaire d'education physique. Etude prelimi-

naire de l'experience pratiquee dans le district de Trois Rivieres. In Facteurs limitant l'endurance humaine. Les techniques d'amelioration de la performance. Edited by J.R. LaCour. France: Universite de St. Etienne, 1977, pp. 43–54.

49. Sinclair, D.: Human Growth After Birth. 4th ed. New York: Oxford University Press, 1985.

50. Tanner, J.M.: Growth at Adolescence. 2nd ed. Oxford: Blackwell, 1962.

51. Weber, G., W. Kartodihardjo, and V. Klissouras: Growth and physical training with reference to heredity. J. Appl. Physiol. 40:211–215, 1976.

52. Wintrobe, M.M., et al.: Clinical Hematology. 8th ed., Philadelphia: Lea & Febiger, 1981.

53. Withers, R.F.J.: Problems in the genetics of human obesity. Eugenics Rev. 56(2):81–90, 1964.

54. Zaichkowsky, L.D., L.B. Zaichkowsky, and T.J. Martinek: Growth and Development: The Child and Physical Activity. St. Louis: Mosby, 1980.

BIBLIOGRAPHY

1. Bailey, D.A., R.M. Malina, and R.L. Rasmussen: The influence of exercise, physical activity, and athletic performance on the dynamics of human growth. In Human Growth (Vol. 2). Edited by F. Falkner and J.M. Tanner. New York: Plenum Press, 1978, pp. 475–505.

2. Gallahue, D.L.: Understanding Motor Development: Infants, Children, Adolescents. 2nd ed., Indianapolis: Benchmark, 1989.

3. Jones, H.E.: Motor Performance and Growth. Berkeley: University of California Press, 1949.

4. Malina, R.M.: Growth and Development: The First Twenty Years. Minneapolis, Minn.: Burgess, 1975.

5. Rarick, G.L. (editor): Physical Activity: Human Growth and Development. New York: Academic Press, 1973.

6. Shephard, R.J.: Physical Activity and Growth. Chicago: Year Book Medical, 1982.

7. Sinclair, D.: Human Growth After Birth. 4th ed. New York: Oxford University Press, 1985.

8. Zaichkowsky, L.D., L.B. Zaichkowsky, and T.J. Martinek: Growth and Development: The Child and Physical Activity. St. Louis: Mosby, 1980.

EXERCISE AND AGING

INTRODUCTION

Aging and a relatively fixed life span are characteristic of all living things. They do, however, differ across species, and this appears to be largely a function of a genetically based cellular aging clock. That is, when embryonic cells from different animal species are grown in test tubes, their ability to continue growth and division is proportional to their maximum life span.[25] However, even in a similar environment, there are large individual differences within a species in aging and length of life. This also appears to have a strong genetic component, in that death due to natural causes differs only by an average of 3 years in MZ (identical) twin pairs, but by 8 years in DZ twin pairs.[62]

The expression of one's age in terms of functional capacities is affected not only by cellular deficiencies characteristic of advancing years, but also by one's physical activity level. The development of chronic disease also increases notably in the elderly and adversely affects functional capacity, as well as health and well-being. However, there is increasing evidence that one's lifestyle, including their physical activity level, has a significant effect on the development of numerous chronic disease states. While there is no evidence of prolonging the human life span beyond its approximate 125 years, there is increasing evidence that positive lifestyle behaviors, including regular exercise, can reduce the mortality rate of certain chronic diseases.[50] The role of exercise in enhancing the functional capacity, health, and well-being of the expanding proportion of elderly individuals in our population is becoming increasingly well defined. However, though there is strong evidence of a positive impact on enhancing the quality of life, if not at least some increase in length of life, how this occurs and by what means, are yet to be identified definitively. Further, since older individuals have reduced functional reserve and may have advanced chronic disease, there appears to be an increased risk of too much activity at a given time, which needs to be better identified and attended to in prescribing the appropriate type, amount, and intensity of physical activity for the elderly.[23,64,73]

PHYSIOLOGIC AGING

Physiologic aging is defined as one's functional state at any given age. It represents a composite effect of genetic influence on the chronologic age of an individual and of the environment, particularly one's physical activity level. Typically, the normally active individual's functional capacities increase with age until about 20 years of age, and remain essentially constant until age 30. Thereafter, as shown in Figure 1–3, the average sedentary person evidences decreases in all basic functional capacities, though at varied rates. For example, nerve conduction velocity decreases 10% by age 70 from the value observed at age 30 years,[63] while maximal aerobic capacity ($\dot{V}O_{2max}$) declines by more than 40%.[5]

The larger decline in $\dot{V}O_{2max}$ is, in part,

213

Table 7–1. Decline in Maximal Cardiorespiratory Parameters with Age*

Parameters	Age (yr)	
	30	70
$\dot{V}O_2$ max (l/min)	3.28	1.95
Maximal heart rate (beats/min)	190	150
Maximal stroke volume (ml)	115	95
Maximal (a–v) O_2 difference (ml/liter)	150	137

*Data from Astrand, P.-O., and K. Rodahl: Textbook of Work Physiology: Physiological Bases of Exercise. 3rd ed, New York: McGraw-Hill, 1986, p. 409.

due to the fact that it represents an integrated multiple organ system response to maximal exercise. Thus, as seen in Table 7–1, $\dot{V}O_{2max}$ decreases 40% from age 30 to 70 years, while maximal heart rate decreases by about 20%, maximal stroke volume by 17% and oxygen extraction (a-v O_2 difference) by about 10%. The decline in maximal heart rate from 190 to 150 beats per minute from age 30 to 70 (which occurs even in individuals who exercise regularly), is clear evidence that aging results in a gradual loss of the body's capacity for effective response to environmental challenge.[62] However, as can be seen in Figure 7–1, there is wide disparity in a normally

active population in a multiple organ system response to maximal exercise. While $\dot{V}O_{2max}$ varies consistently through age 60, there is greater variation in the 7th decade due, in part, to greater disparity in daily physical activity levels. Thus, it is difficult to differentiate how much of the decline with age is due to aging, per se, as opposed to disuse atrophy and/or disease.

Whatever the relative effect of the inherent aging process and chronic disease state of an individual, numerous physiologic functions deteriorate with age in the normally active adult. In this section, those functions that influence the elderly person's ability to perform basic physical ac-

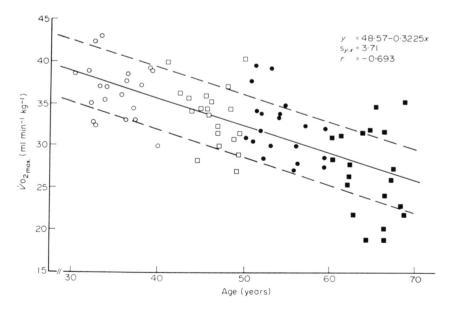

FIG. 7–1. Individual and group mean relationship of maximal oxygen uptake and age in sedentary middle-aged males. (From Adams, W.C. et al.: Multistage treadmill walking performance and associated cardiorespiratory responses of middle-aged men. Clin. Sci. 42:355–370, 1972.)

tivities necessary in a normal lifestyle with a reasonable margin of reserve, are reviewed.

SKELETAL SYSTEM

Peak bone mass is attained at about 30 years of age, being about 40% higher in males than in females, and approximately 15% greater in blacks than Caucasians.[72] As shown in Figure 7–2, there is a rapid increase in bone mineral loss (relative to age 30 years), beginning about age 50. However, the rate of bone mineral loss of females is nearly double that of males, ages 50 to 80 years, and is associated with comparably elevated incidence of bone fracture due to reduced bone density and tensile strength.[15,66] This condition of decreased bone mass, with increased susceptibility to fracture, is called osteoporosis. It is caused by persistent calcium imbalance, which may be due to decreased calcium intake in the diet, altered endocrine function relative to absorption and retention, skeletal blood flow, and inactivity. Osteoporosis is now a major health problem among the steadily expanding number of elderly persons in Western countries.[29] Individuals most susceptible to osteoporosis and increased rate of fracture are white women, particularly those who experience early menopause.

Joints which form the articular surface between adjoining bones entail joint capsules with synovial fluid, ligaments, and tendons that all show deterioration with aging. This condition, referred to as osteoarthritis contributes to joint stiffness, which reduces flexibility, i.e., the range of motion.[1]

NEUROMUSCULAR SYSTEM

Sensory function important to effective physical performance, including hearing and vision losses in normal persons, is compromised with advancing age. Accordingly, there is some reduction in reaction time, but the major reduction in motor task performance is due to an increased central processing time.[67]

Age related skeletal muscle mass decline

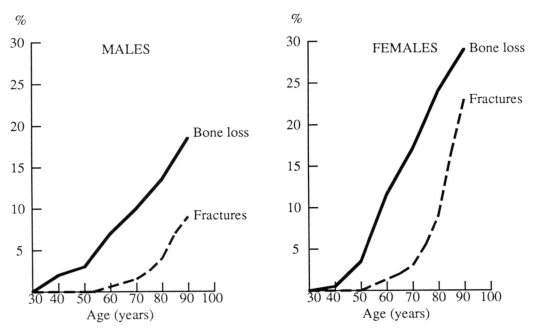

FIG. 7–2. Relationship between bone loss and cumulative probability of bone fracture. (Modified from Garn, S.M.: Adult bone loss, fracture epidemiology and nutritional implications. Nutrition. 27:107–115, 1973.)

in adults is well documented.[13] About 1/3 of the muscle fibers existent at age 20 are lost by age 70,[43] which contributes significantly to the muscle mass decrease,[20] as does reduced size of existent muscle fibers, primarily limited to type II fibers.[20,32,42] It seems that there is variation in particular muscle groups, which may be related to the relative level of normal activity in sedentary older individuals.[21] Further, this selective response is associated with muscle enzymatic activity changes that have important implications in terms of reduced muscular power and strength.[13] Thus, advancing age is accompanied by a loss of strength and, to a lesser extent, a reduced speed of movement. Hand grip strength declines about 25% from age 30 to 70 years (Fig. 1–3), though isometric strength of other muscle groups declines at different rates.[4] Muscular endurance, expressed as the ability to continue a specific task, decreases but the relative work capacity measured as 50% of one's maximum strength is unaffected by age.[42]

CARDIORESPIRATORY SYSTEM

Age related decrease in maximum aerobic endurance performance is due primarily to decreased $\dot{V}O_{2max}$. Until recently, most studies of $\dot{V}O_{2max}$ decrease with age had utilized the cross-sectional method. Figure 7–3 shows a cross-sectional comparison of sedentary females' $\dot{V}O_{2max}$ decrease with age, in combination with a 6-year longitudinal follow-up that yielded closely comparable results.

Reduced maximum cardiac output, which occurs due to numerous structural changes in the heart and blood vessels with age, accounts for most of the decreased $\dot{V}O_{2max}$. The heart muscle loses contractile strength and stiffens with age, which delays filling time and reduces stroke volume.[8] The arteries lose elasticity with age, become narrower, thus increasing resistance to blood flow. As shown in Figure 7–4, this results in increased systolic blood pressure at any given submaximal workload in older individuals (50 to 70 years) compared to their younger (30 to 40 years of age) normally active counterparts. Further, the older group's systolic blood pressure at the highest submaximal workload was slightly greater than 90% of their maximal value, while that for the younger group was 80%. This means that the heart is working harder at the same submaximal workload in older individuals. Venous valves deteriorate with age, and this contributes to reduced venous return, increased ventricular filling time, and to reduced maximal stroke volume.[8]

Muscle mass is reduced with age, as are mitochondrial volume and associated enzymes. The latter contributes to reduced oxygen extraction with age, but there appears to be little change in maximal muscle blood flow per unit of muscle mass.[3,57] Oxygen pick-up at the lung is reduced with age at about the same rate as maximal cardiac output, so there is little change in the ventilation perfusion ratio.[8] In addition to an increase in alveoli size and resultant loss of respiratory efficiency with age, decreased elasticity of the lungs, and weakened respiratory muscles, can result in an increased oxygen cost for breathing a given amount of air.

BODY COMPOSITION

Body weight for the adult man and woman of average height (70 and 65 inches, respectively), increases at a rate of about 1/2 pound per year during middle-age.[44] However, as mentioned earlier in this section, there is a significant loss in both bone mineral and muscle mass after age 30 to 40 years in sedentary people. With this decrease in lean body weight, fat weight increases more than that indicated by increased body weight. Thus, average body weight that is fat increases in males from about 15% at age 25, to 28% at age 65. The average female's body fat increases from about 25 to 39% of body weight during this 40-year period.[11] Little data on body composition changes have been obtained by the longitudinal method. In one study of sedentary middle-aged men over 12 years (from 32 to 44 years), a gain of 14 lbs. body weight and more than equivalent amount of body fat gain was observed.[9]

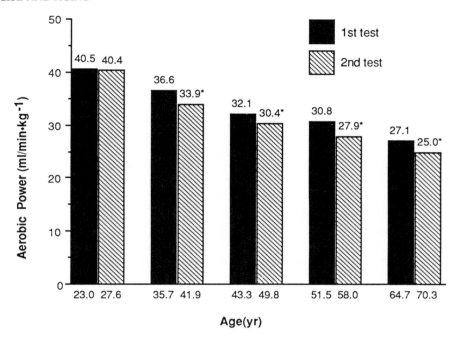

FIG. 7–3. Loss of aerobic power ($\dot{V}O_{2max}$) with age in females. Subjects were tested twice approximately 6 years apart. All groups significantly decreased in aerobic power at the second testing (*), with the exception of the youngest group (23.0 to 27.6 years). (Modified from Plowman, S.A., B.L. Drinkwater, and S.M. Horvath: Age and aerobic power in women: a longitudinal study. J. Gerontol. *34*:512–520, 1979.)

This resulted in increased body fat from 16 to 22%.

Reasons for this creeping fat gain during middle-age are not entirely clear. One factor, as shown in Figure 7–5, appears to be that basal metabolic rate (BMR) declines about 2% per decade after 20 years of age. The consistently lower values for females per unit of body weight are apparently due to a greater proportion of total weight as fat, which is less metabolically active.[31] Steadily decreased BMR with age, together with reduced physical activity level, is not equivalently matched by decreased caloric intake, though Keys and colleagues have presented data that individual daily caloric intake is actually less than it was a generation ago.[30]

EXERCISE AND PHYSIOLOGIC AGING

As previously stated, the adult's functional capacities decline with age due both to genetic and environmental factors. The most profound environmental influence is one's physical activity level, which extends from weeks to several months of inactivity typified by bedrest and space flight (with zero gravity effects on human movement), to years of continued high level competition in some individuals into the 6th decade and beyond. In essence, then, there now exists a continuum of physical activity levels (and their physiologic consequence) not previously available for analysis.

BEDREST DECONDITIONING EFFECTS

Surprisingly to those who perceive that years of sedentary activity produces the lowest functional capacity in humans, there is abundant evidence that several weeks of bedrest (or space flight) incurs substantial impairment in previously normally active individuals. There is also increasing awareness that prolonged bedrest

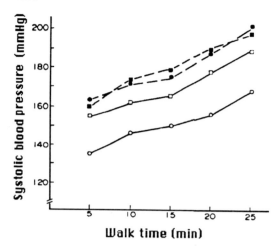

FIG. 7–4. Group mean systolic blood pressure response to increasing submaximal workloads (as indicated by oxygen uptake) for normally active males in the 4th, ○; 5th, □; 6th, ● and 7th,■ decade. (Modified from Adams, W.C. et al.: Multistage treadmill walking performance and associated cardiorespiratory responses of middle-aged men. Clin. Sci. 42:355–370, 1972.)

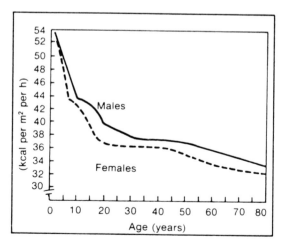

FIG. 7–5. Basal metabolic rate as a function of age and sex. (Adapted from Altman, P.L., and D.S. Dittmer. Metabolism. Bethesda, MD: Federation of American Societies for Experimental Biology, 1968, p. 345, as depicted in McArdle, W.D., F.I. Katch, and V.L. Katch. Exercise Physiology. 2nd ed., Philadelphia: Lea & Febiger, 1986, p. 132.)

can adversely affect the clinical condition of hospitalized patients.[35] Physiologic effects observed in these conditions, which appear to be due primarily to enforced inactivity, include bone and muscle atrophy, loss of flexibility, and cardiorespiratory deterioration. Even 2 to 4 weeks of bedrest induces substantial muscle atrophy, accompanied by significant loss in muscular strength and endurance.[18] Bone demineralization, reflected in increased calcium loss, occurs primarily in the weight-bearing bones, with the loss of contracting muscle force on bones due to reduced activity in bedrest being of lesser importance.[58] Prolonged weightlessness experienced by astronauts can result in as much as 1% bone mineral loss per week.[71] Connective tissue in ligaments, fascial sheaths of the muscles, and tendons become dense and shortened with prolonged disuse, thus substantially limiting normal range of motion.[38]

The cardiorespiratory system deteriorates progressively during bedrest, with $\dot{V}O_{2max}$ decreasing as much as 25% within 3 weeks.[59] While the recumbent position appears primarily responsible for decreased plasma volume, blood pressure regulation and venous return, other aspects of cardiorespiratory function impairment can be largely attributed to the reduced activity level.[10] These include reduced heart volume, maximal stroke volume, and muscle blood flow, as well as marked reductions in oxidative enzyme activity of the muscles.[61]

PROLONGED CHAIR REST
DECONDITIONING EFFECTS

An interesting study of young adult males strapped lightly in a chair for 16 hours per day while performing routine cockpit control tasks and reading, revealed significant deconditioning effects within 10 days.[39] Although 8 hours each day was spent in bedrest, the other 16 hours of continuous chair rest provided gravitational effects and increased hydrostatic pressure below the diaphragm. Nonetheless, decreased blood volume, reduced blood pressure regulation and exercise tolerance were observed, which were attributed primarily to the restricted body movement over the 10-day period. Lamb[38] contends that only slightly less extreme hypokinesis is present in the lifestyle of many office workers who sit at their desks 8 hours a day and then drive to their homes to sit for several more hours before retiring to bed.

HABITUAL ACTIVITY LEVELS IN THE MIDDLE-AGED AND ELDERLY

Most American adults' jobs do not entail sufficient physical demands to preserve the peak functional capacities characteristic of young adults in their 20s. Hence, it is primarily through vigorous leisure-time activity that middle-aged and elderly adults can incur a sufficient stimulus to produce a training effect.[24] While the proportion of adults engaging in vigorous leisure-time activity increased from 1978 to 1985,[69] as shown in Figure 1–4, there is a steady decline from 40% at age 25 to 20% at age 70, and less than 10% at age 80. Further, nearly 50% of adults over 65 reported only sedentary leisure-time activity (such as playing cards) in the 1985 survey.[69]

Since the body adapts to the physical demands it routinely experiences, it is clear that most older adults do not get sufficient physical activity in amount or intensity to prevent progressive deconditioning with advancing age. As many of the effects of hypokinesis are qualitatively similar to those of aging, the overall effect on exercise capacity, cardiorespiratory function, disuse atrophy and loss of cells, is greater than if either were operational alone.[7] This is a particularly important problem in the elderly, as continued disuse leads to debilitation and a further desire to remain inactive and eventually to spend more time in bed.[8]

LOSS OF FUNCTIONAL RESERVE WITH AGE

Young[74] has astutely emphasized that the progressive decrease in cardiorespiratory capacity and muscular strength with age and disuse results in a critically compromised ability of the elderly to perform what would seem to be routine activities. For example, he estimates that a woman of 20 years may use only 50% of her maximum voluntary strength of the quadriceps muscles in rising slowly from an armless chair, while this effort exceeds 85% of an 80-year-old woman's quadriceps strength. Similarly, a pleasantly rapid walk at 4 miles per hour on level pavement necessitates an energy expenditure equivalent to about 1.2 liters per minute of oxygen for the average size man (72 kg). This energy demand remains essentially constant through one's lifetime, and represents only 33% of the average young adult male's $\dot{V}O_{2max}$. However, it constitutes about 50% of the average male's $\dot{V}O_{2max}$ at age 55, and over 85% at 85 years of age.

TRAINABILITY AND AGE

When previously sedentary older adults undertake progressively intensified exercise training programs, they experience notable physiologic changes, though not necessarily by the same means or to the same degree as young adults. The magnitude of change in strength and $\dot{V}O_{2max}$ is less in older adults undertaking training at the same percent of maximum as young adults. However, their percent change in strength[2,22,46] and $\dot{V}O_{2max}$[12,22,60] are similar. In a recent study[22] of healthy males and females in their 70s, no significant gender difference was observed in the effects of 26 weeks of endurance training or Nautilus resistance training on $\dot{V}O_{2max}$ and strength improvements, respectively.

Since the older person is, on average, more deconditioned than the young adult upon initiating training, one might expect a greater percent improvement in individuals with lower initial values, as has been observed in young adults.[59] Perhaps the primary answer to this apparent somewhat reduced trainability with advancing age lies in the muscle cells, in that older individuals appear to increase strength primarily via improvements in neural function, with much less muscle hypertrophy than in young adults.[46] Similarly, older adults evidence little, if any change in muscle oxygen extraction during maximal work following endurance training. This apparent decrease in trainability in the elderly may be due to an aging related impairment in the muscle cell's capability for protein synthesis and chemical regulation.[44]

EFFECTS OF EXERCISE TRAINING ON PHYSIOLOGIC AGING

In general, the effect of a properly prescribed exercise training program in the elderly is to reverse body structure and functional deconditioning effects induced by hypokinesis. On the other hand, there is little evidence that exercise training alters the aging process itself.[26]

In cross-sectional studies, athletes have routinely been found to have greater bone mineral mass than do sedentary individuals of the same sex.[65] This does not establish a cause and effect relationship, since greater bone mineral content may be a selective requisite for athletic success. However, Montoye and colleagues[45] found that senior tennis players, mean age of 64 years with 40 years of playing experience, had a 13% greater bone mineral mass in the humerus and an 8% greater bone mineral mass in the dominant arm compared to their nondominant arm. This difference was about double that for nonathletes of similar age.[27] The effect of exercise training on bone mineral mass and the development of osteoporosis in previously sedentary older females will be analyzed in a later section.

Flexibility, or range of motion in various joints of the body, increases significantly in the elderly following 6 to 12 weeks of stretching (Fig. 7–6), general calisthenics, and/or rhythmic activities. In one study using a control group,[48] 40 women ranging in age from 65 to 88 years were randomly assigned to the control or experimental group. Following initial measurements of flexibility in six major joints in both groups, the experimental group participated in a specially designed exercise and dance program for 1 hour, 3 times per week, for 12 weeks. They increased flexibility at all six joints, ranging from 8% at the shoulder joint to 48% at the ankle joint, while the control group showed decreases of 2 to 5%

in all joints. It appears that this improved flexibility in previously sedentary elderly individuals is primarily due to stretching of muscle, tendons, and joint connective tissue.[8]

There is no evidence of increased fiber number in older subjects undergoing strength training.[19] However, the area of fast-twitch type II fibers is increased with heavy resistance training in older men.[2] Further, low resistance, high repetition strength training has been shown to elicit some increase in size of type I fibers in older individuals (ages 55 to 65 years), as well as greater size increases in type II fibers.[41] Strength training may not induce an increase in total muscle cross-sectional area in elderly persons, as the increased proportion of intramuscular fat and connective tissue in sedentary individuals may be proportionally decreased with training.[41]

Muscle strength has been observed to decrease very little with age up to 60 years in muscle groups that are frequently used. For example, Petrofsky and Lind[51] found no difference in hand grip strength between ages 22 and 62 years in a group of machine workers involved in daily arm exercise. Strength training in previously sedentary older individuals appears to produce about the same percentage increase in strength as that incurred by their young adult counterparts.[47] Aniansson and Gustafsson[2] observed increased quadriceps muscle strength in men over age 70 following training that was of similar percentage change as that seen in a young adult training group. Larsson[41] found no difference between knee extensor strength changes following training in men ages 20 to 39 years compared to men ages 55 to 65 years.

While Aniansson and Gustafsson[2] observed significant increases in both strength and type II fiber area following strength training of elderly men, Moritani and deVries[47] observed little change in estimated muscle cross-sectional area following training in their older subjects (67 to 72 years of age). However, maximal muscle activation level (reflective of the amount of motor unit discharge and recruitment), as measured by electromyography, increased in near direct proportion to strength. Thus, these elderly subjects appeared to increase

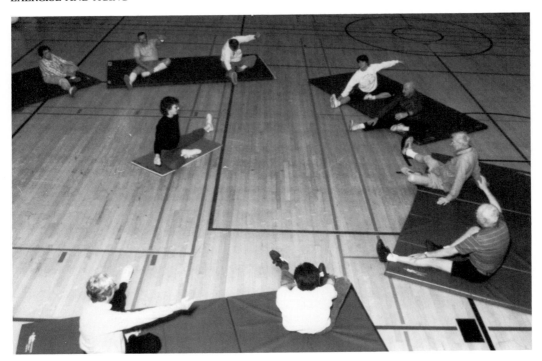

FIG. 7–6. A major cause of declining flexibility in older adults is lack of movement in joints on a daily basis. Training programs incorporating stretching of muscle, tendon and joint connective tissue on a regular basis preserve this important aspect of fitness in older persons.

strength following training primarily by changes in central nervous system function related to motor unit recruitment and activation, and very little by muscle hypertrophy. Larsson[41] suggests that loss of strength with age is not affected primarily by mean muscle fiber area, but by some combination of decreased fiber number, impaired neuromuscular contractile coupling, and decreased activation of high threshold motor units.

A cross-sectional study[68] suggests that training may have important effects on retarding decreased central nervous system function with age via improved processing of relatively simple visual auditory stimuli and the initiation of simple and complex movements in response to the stimuli. Both simple and complex reaction times, as well as movement time, were significantly less in older racket sport participants and runners than in sedentary controls of similar age and a young adult sedentary control group. Subsequently, Spirduso[67]

has suggested that physical condition influences the impaired age-movement initiation relationship, either directly through a manipulation of the neurotransmitter dopamine, or by manipulating some other system that interacts with catecholamines.

There is a significant increase in $\dot{V}O_{2max}$ in previously sedentary older persons following endurance training. It is accompanied by improved ventilatory capacity, but with no change in pulmonary gas exchange.[49] Increased maximal oxygen transport is effected solely by increased maximal stroke volume, as maximal heart rate and hemoglobin concentration do not change with training in the elderly.[60,70] Muscle oxygen extraction, as reflected by a-v O_2 difference, does not appear to change with training in older people. However, an increased oxygen uptake in the muscles following training in the elderly is achieved by increased muscle blood flow and oxidative enzyme activity.[70] Since there is also increased venous return, endurance training of the elderly improves $\dot{V}O_{2max}$ primarily via enhanced cardiovascular function.[56]

Much interest has arisen from the media recognized research reports that highly trained endurance athletes in their 60s and 70s have a higher $\dot{V}O_{2max}$ than do sedentary young adult males.[6,53] This had led to speculation that intensive endurance training continued into old age might actually delay the aging process. Close inspection of the lines depicted in Figure 7–7 seems to refute this notion. The lower line indicates the decline in $\dot{V}O_{2max}$ with age in sedentary males. The top line shows consistently higher values, but a parallel decline for champion master's track runners and walkers, ages 40 to 75 years, who had continued training. Both of these lines were plotted from cross-sectional data of individuals differing in age. Of particular interest is the more rapid decline in $\dot{V}O_{2max}$ for a group of champion middle-distance

runners, all of whom had become sedentary 20 or more years before retest at a mean age of 57 years (shown as open squares at mean ages of 24 and 57). The top line in Figure 7–7 suggests that the trained master's athletes merely maintain their higher $\dot{V}O_{2max}$ into old age if they continue to train, but do not forestall the effects of the aging process. However, a 10-year longitudinal follow-up study reported by Pollock et al.[55] showed that 11 of these athletes who continued to train intensively, including regular competition (from age 50 to 60 years), experienced only a 3% decline in $\dot{V}O_{2max}$ compared to the approximate 8% decline evidenced in the top line of Figure 7–7.

RISKS OF EXERCISE IN THE ELDERLY

Evidence of the benefits of exercise training in reducing the effects of a sedentary

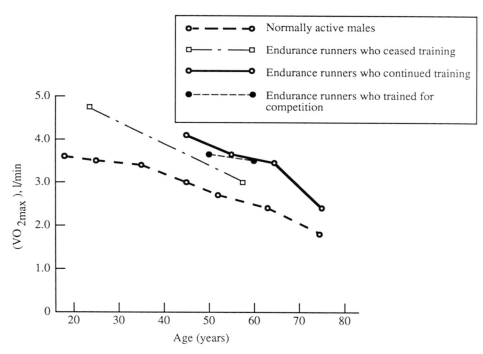

FIG. 7–7. Group mean change in aerobic power ($\dot{V}O_{2max}$) with age in male middle-distance runners (trained and nontrained) and normally active males. (Modified from Noble, B.J.: Physiology of Exercise and Sport. St. Louis: Times Mirror/Mosby, 1986, p. 477; Pollock, M.L. et al.: Physiological characteristics of champion American track athletes 40 to 75 years of age. J. Gerontol. 29:645–649, 1974; Pollock, M.L. et al.: Effect of age and training on aerobic capacity and body composition of master athletes. J. Appl. Physiol. 62:725–731, 1987; and Robinson, S. et al.: Physiological aging of champion runners. J. Appl. Physiol. 41:46–51, 1976.)

lifestyle on physiologic aging has been emphasized in the preceding discussion, but with little mention of possible adverse effects. The latter occur most frequently from poorly-designed exercise programs, though the potential for injury or death, exists even in well-designed programs.[23] Most injuries from health-oriented exercise are due to overuse, rather than to trauma-type injuries experienced more often in sports participation.[16] Older persons will not only be prone to exercise-induced overuse injury following a prolonged period of sedentary activity, but also to enhanced risk of adverse acute responses to exercise because of their more advanced level of chronic disease, including hypertension, diabetes, and coronary heart disease. The latter will be examined in detail in a subsequent chapter.

MUSCULOSKELETAL INJURIES

Kraus and Conroy[36] reviewed available evidence on the mortality and morbidity from injuries in sports and recreation, and found a striking discrepancy of epidemiologic data relevant to establishing participation risks in organized competitive sports and that for physical recreation. Koplan et al.[34] observed that data establishing risks associated with participation in aerobic activities that people choose to enhance health and fitness were particularly lacking. However, there were limited data that establish important distinctions concerning the potential for exercise mode (i.e., walking, jogging/running, rhythmic calisthenics—generally in the form of aerobic dancing, cycling, and swimming) and amount (frequency, intensity, and duration) in inducing musculoskeletal injuries.

Koplan et al.[33] studied the injury rates in 2,500 male and female runners for 1 year. They found that 35% developed orthopedic injuries sufficient to reduce weekly training mileage. However, risk of injury was associated with increasing mileage, with 65% of those who ran more than 50 miles per week experiencing an injury sometime during the year. This observation is consistent with Garrick's report of 2/3s occurrence of overuse injuries (com-

pared to acute injuries) in runners seen at a large sports medicine facility serving primarily recreational athletes.[16] Pollock et al.[54] conducted an experimental study of the effects of overuse in terms of training frequency and duration in previously sedentary men, 20 to 35 years of age. Training intensity was between 85 to 90% of maximum HR, with the men attempting to complete a 20-week jogging program. In one part of the study, three groups trained for 30 minutes per day, for either 1, 3, or 5 days per week. Injury (sufficient to prevent training for 1 week) incidence for the three groups was 0, 12, and 39%, respectively. In another group that trained at the same intensity for 45 minutes, 3 days per week, injury incidence was 54%. In a subsequent analysis of these data, Pollock[52] concluded that training programs for beginning joggers at 85 to 90% of maximum HR for 45 minutes, 5 days per week, cause too many injuries to be recommended for health/fitness enhancement.

Koplan et al.[34] speculate that those whose training mode is walking, would be susceptible to similar weight-bearing injury hazards as those for jogging, but there are no data for direct comparison. However, it seems highly probable that the musculoskeletal strain incurred from more restricted excursions of the body's center of gravity during walking would result in reduced incidence of injury. This is of particular importance to older persons, as well as to the significantly overweight, who can achieve an effective training HR (usually above 75% of age-adjusted HRmax) while walking at a brisk pace (i.e., about 4 mph).

Those who engage in rhythmic calisthenics done to music, i.e., aerobic dancing, also appear to experience significant overuse injury incidence similar to that of joggers.[16] However, Koplan et al.[34] contend that though aerobic dancing is a popular form of exercise (especially among females) there is no systematic collection of data on injuries associated with the number and age of participants, and the time of participation.

Non-weight bearing exercise, particularly bicycling and swimming, have been recommended as an effective means of reducing musculoskeletal injury.[14] Bicycling, however, results in accidents causing significant incidence of acute injury. In a random survey of bicycle accidents and injuries in a college population, ranging in age from 17 to 66 years,[37] 13% reported involvement in an accident within the past year. Sixty-two percent of those involved in an accident sustained an injury, with 1/3 significant enough to require medical attention (though only 8% of the accidents were police-reported). The authors concluded that, if these trends are accurate for other populations, studies based on hospital or police records fail to give an accurate assessment of bicycle related accidents and injuries.

Though there is a significant mortality from swimming each year, Koplan et al.[34] conclude that it is unlikely that most of the persons who died were swimming for exercise. These authors contend that there are only isolated data identifying swimming-induced morbidity in competitive athletes, including musculoskeletal injury of the shoulder, and no data on the prevalence, incidence, or natural history of these or other adverse events in noncompetitive, health/fitness oriented swimmers. Lap swimming, water-jogging, and water aerobics/calisthenics appear particularly appropriate for older persons who are more likely to be overweight, as well as obese adults who are more susceptible to orthopedic problems when engaged in weight-bearing activities.[14,17]

REDUCTION OF MUSCULOSKELETAL INJURY CAUSED BY EXERCISE TRAINING. In addition to medical screening and providing exercise prescription appropriate for reducing potential hazards of exercise for patients with various chronic disease conditions, it is vital to individualize exercise training to one's age and fitness level in order to reduce the incidence of musculoskeletal injury. The elderly experience a greater risk of degenerative arthritis, as well as osteoporosis that leads to increased incidence of bone fracture.[29] Larson and Bruce[40] contend that the ideal exercise program for an aging society has yet to be identified, and remains a difficult task in a population that varies more physiologically with advancing age. They maintain that exercise should

be dynamic, varied and fun, easily accessible, and without adverse sequelae if it is to become habitual. Further, they contend, "No pain, no gain does not apply to a strategy of lifelong regular exercise. Brisk, regular walking is a popular, accessible form of exercise that may be sufficient to induce a training effect, especially in the elderly."[40:784] Indeed, Kannel[28] asserts that a vigorous walking program may be more prudent for middle-aged flabby, deconditioned persons in order to minimize the considerable musculoskeletal side effects experienced in strenuous exercise. Further, exercise training for the older adult should proceed by gradual progression from an initial light to moderate intensity.[23]

SUMMARY

1. Aging, in terms of one's physiologic capacities, is effected not only by cellular deficiencies characteristic of advancing years, but also by one's habitual physical activity level; this combination defines physiologic aging.

2. Decrements in physiologic response with age occur at a greater rate for integrative parameters than for their attendant components.

3. The middle-aged and elderly population experience losses in skeletal, neuromuscular, and cardiorespiratory capacity, as well as changes in body composition (i.e., loss in bone and muscle, and a gain in fat).

4. As many of the effects of hypokinesis are qualitatively similar to those of aging, the overall effect on exercise capacity, cardiorespiratory function, disuse atrophy and loss of cells is greater than if either were operational alone.

5. With physiologic aging, functional reserve is decreased in the middle-aged and elderly, such that performance of the same task as that done when a young adult constitutes a greater percentage of maximum capacity.

6. Since most U.S. adults' jobs do not entail vigorous activity levels, it is primarily through vigorous leisure-time activity that the middle-aged and elderly can incur

sufficient stimulus to produce a training effect.

7. In general, the effects of a properly prescribed exercise training program in the elderly is to reverse body structure and functional deconditioning effects induced by hypokinesis. On the other hand, there is little evidence that exercise training alters the aging process itself.

8. When previously sedentary older adults undertake progressively intensified exercise training, they experience notable physiologic changes, though not necessarily by all of the same means, or to the same degree, as do young adults.

9. Appropriately prescribed exercise training can produce significant functional improvements in the middle-aged and elderly adults' muscular strength and endurance, flexibility, movement efficiency, and cardiorespiratory capacity.

10. Adverse effects of exercise training in older adults, especially musculoskeletal injuries, occur primarily from overuse, and have a higher incidence than in young adults, unless activity levels are initiated at a low intensity and increased slowly.

REFERENCES

1. Adrain, M.J.: Flexibility in the aging adult. In Exercise and Aging: The Scientific Basis. Edited by E.L. Smith and R.C. Serfass. Hillside, N.J.: Enslow Publ., 1981, pp. 45–57.
2. Aniansson, A., and E. Gustafsson: Physical training in old men with special reference to quadriceps muscle strength and morphology. Clin Physiol. 1:87–98, 1981.
3. Asmussen, E.: Aging and exercise. In Environmental Physiology: Aging, Heat and Altitude. Edited by S.M. Horvath and M.K. Yousef. New York: Elsevier/North-Holland, 1981, pp. 419–428.
4. Asmussen, E., and K. Heeboll-Nielsen: Isometric muscle strength in relation to age in men and women. Ergonomics. 5:167–169, 1962.
5. Astrand, P.-O., and K. Rodahl: Textbook of Work Physiology: Physiological Bases of Exercise. 3rd ed., New York: McGraw-Hill, 1986.
6. Barnard, R.J., G.K. Grimditch, and J.H. Wilmore: Physiological characteristics of sprint and endurance Masters runners. Med. Sci. Sports Exer. 11:161–171, 1979.
7. Bortz, W.M.: Disuse and aging. JAMA. 248:1203–1208, 1982.
8. Brooks, G.A., and T.D. Fahey: Exercise Physiology: Human Bioenergetics and Its Applications. New York: Macmillan, 1985.
9. Chien, S., et al.: Longitudinal measurements of blood volume and essential body mass in human subjects. J. Appl. Physiol. 39:818–824, 1975.
10. Convertino, V.A.: Exercise responses after inactivity. In Inactivity: Physiological Effects. Edited by H. Sandler and J. Vernikos-Danellis. New York: Academic Press, 1986, pp. 149–187.
11. Durnin, J.V.G.A., and J. Womersley: Body fat assessed from total body density and its estimation from skinfold thickness: measurements on 481 men and women aged from 16 to 72 years. Br. J. Nutr. 32:77–97, 1974.
12. Ekblom, B., et al.: Effect of training on circulatory response to exercise. J. Appl. Physiol. 24:518–528, 1968.
13. Fitts, R.H.: Aging and skeletal muscle. In Exercise and Aging: The Scientific Basis. Edited by E.L. Smith and R.C. Serfass. Hillside, N.J.: Enslow Publ., 1981, pp. 31–44.
14. Foss, M.L., and D.A. Strehle: Exercise testing and training for the obese. In Nutrition and Exercise in Obesity Management. Edited by J. Storlie and H.A. Jordan. New York: Spectrum, 1984, pp. 93–121.
15. Garn, S.M.: Bone loss and aging. In The Physiology and Pathology of Aging. Edited by R. Goldman and M. Rockstein. New York: Academic Press, 1975, pp. 39–57.
16. Garrick, J.G.: Characterization of the patient population in a sports medicine facility. Physician Sportsmed. 13(10):73–76, 1985.
17. Goodman, C., and M. Kenrick: Physical fitness in relation to obesity. Obesity Bariat. Med. 4:12–15, 1975.
18. Greenleaf, J.E., and S. Kozlowski: Physiological consequences of reduced physical activity during bedrest. In Exercise and Sport Sciences Reviews. Vol. 10. Edited by R.L. Terjung. Philadelphia: Franklin Institute, 1982, pp. 84–119.
19. Grimby, G.: Physical activity and muscle training in the elderly. Acta Med. Scand. Suppl. 711:233–237, 1986.
20. Grimby, G., and B. Saltin: The aging muscle. Clin. Physiol. 3:209–218, 1983.
21. Grimby, G., B. Danneskiold-Samsoe, K. Hvid, and B. Saltin: Morphology and enzymatic capacity in arm and leg muscles in 78–82-year-old men and women. Acta Physiol. Scand. 115:124–134, 1982.
22. Hagberg, J.M., et al.: Cardiovascular responses of 70- to 79-yr-old men and women to exercise training. J. Appl. Physiol. 66:2589–2594, 1989.
23. Haskell, W.L.: Physical activity and health: need to define the required stimulus. Am. J. Cardiol. 55:4D–9D, 1985.
24. Haskell, W.L., H.J. Montoye, and D. Orenstein: Physical activity and exercise to achieve health-

related physical fitness components. Public Health Rep. *100*:202–212, 1985.

25. Hayflick, L.: The cell biology of human aging. N. Engl. J. Med. *195*:1302–1308, 1976.

26. Holloszy, J.O.: Exercise, health, and aging: a need for more information. Med. Sci. Sports Exer. *15*:1–5, 1983.

27. Huddleston, A.L., D. Rockwell, D.N. Kulund, and R.B. Harrison: Bone mass in lifetime tennis athletes. JAMA. *255*:1107–1109, 1980.

28. Kannel, W.B.: Exercise and sudden death. JAMA. *248*:3143–3144, 1982.

29. Kelsey, J.L.: Epidemiology of osteoporosis and associated fractures. *In* Bone and Mineral Research/5. Edited by W.A. Peck. New York: Elsevier Science Publ., 1987, pp. 409–444.

30. Keys, A.: Body composition and its change with age and diet. *In* Weight Control: A Collection of Papers Presented at the Weight Control Colloquium. Edited by E.S. Eppright, P. Swanson, and C.A. Iverson. Ames, Iowa: Iowa State College Press, 1955, pp. 18–28.

31. Keys, A., H.L. Taylor, and F. Grande: Basal metabolism and age of adult men. Metabolism. *22*:579–587, 1973.

32. Kiessling, K.H., et al.: Enzyme activities and morphometry in skeletal muscle of middle-aged men after training. Scand. J. Clin. Lab. Invest. *33*:63–69, 1974.

33. Koplan, J.P., et al.: An epidemiological study of the benefits and risks of running. JAMA. *248*:3118–3121, 1982.

34. Koplan, J.P., D.S. Siscovick, and G.M. Goldbaum: The risks of exercise: a public health view of injuries and hazards. Public Health Rep. *100*:189–195, 1985.

35. Kottke, F.: The effects of limitation of activity upon the human body. JAMA. *196*:117–122, 1966.

36. Kraus, J.F., and C. Conroy: Mortality and morbidity from injuries in sports and recreation. Ann. Rev. Publ. Health. *5*:163–192, 1984.

37. Kruse, D.L., and A.A. McBeath: Bicycle accidents and injuries. Am. J. Sports Med. *8*:342–344, 1980.

38. Lamb, D.R.: Physiology of Exercise: Responses & Adaptations. (2nd ed.) New York: Macmillan, 1984.

39. Lamb, L.E., P.M. Stevens, and R.L. Johnson: Hypokinesia secondary to chair rest from 4 to 10 days. Aerospace Medicine. *36*:755–763, 1965.

40. Larson, E.B., and R.A. Bruce: Exercise and aging. Ann. Intern. Med. *105*:783–785, 1986.

41. Larsson, L.: Physical training effects on muscle morphology in sedentary males at different ages. Med. Sci. Sports Exer. *14*:203–206, 1982.

42. Larsson, L., and J. Karlsson: Isometric and dynamic endurance as a function of age and skeletal muscle characteristics. Acta Physiol. Scand. *104*:128–136, 1978.

43. Lexell, J., K. Henriksson-Larsson, B. Winblad,

and M. Sjostrom: Distribution of different fibre types in human skeletal muscle. 3. Effects of aging on vastus lateralis studied in whole muscle cross-sections. Muscle Nerve. *6*:588–595, 1983.

44. McArdle, W.D., F.I. Katch, and V.L. Katch: Exercise Physiology: Energy, Nutrition, and Human Performance. 3rd ed., Philadelphia: Lea & Febiger, 1991.

45. Montoye, H.J., E.L. Smith, D.F. Fardon, and E.T. Howley: Bone mineral in senior tennis players. Scand. J. Sports Sci. *2*:26–32, 1980.

46. Moritani, T., and H.A. deVries: Neural factors versus hypertrophy in the time course of muscle strength gain. Am. J. Phys. Med. *58*:115–130, 1979.

47. Moritani, T., and H.A. deVries: Potential for gross muscle hypertrophy in older men. J. Gerontol. *35*:672–682, 1980.

48. Munns, K.: Effects of exercise on the range of joint motion in elderly subjects. *In* Exercise and Aging: The Scientific Basis. Edited by E.L. Smith and R.C. Serfass. Hillside, N.J.: Enslow Publ., 1981, pp. 167–178.

49. Niinimaa, V., and R.J. Shephard: Training and oxygen conductance in the elderly. II. The cardiovascular system. J. Gerontol. *33*:362–367, 1978.

50. Paffenbarger, R.S., R.T. Hyde, A.L. Wing, and C.H. Steinmetz: A natural history of athleticism and cardiovascular health. JAMA. *252*:491–495, 1984.

51. Petrofsky, J., and A.R. Lind: Aging, isometric strength and endurance, and cardiovascular responses to static effort. J. Appl. Physiol. *38*:91–95, 1975.

52. Pollock, M.L.: How much exercise is enough? Physican Sportsmed. *6*(6):50–64, 1978.

53. Pollock, M.L., H.S. Miller, and J. Wilmore: Physiological characteristics of champion American track athletes 40 to 75 years of age. J. Gerontol. *29*:645–649, 1974.

54. Pollock, M.L., et al.: Effects of frequency and duration of training on attrition and incidence of injury. Med. Sci. Sports. *9*:31–36, 1977.

55. Pollock, M.L., et al.: Effect of age and training on aerobic capacity and body composition of master athletes. J. Appl. Physiol. *62*:725–731, 1987.

56. Reddan, W.G.: Respiratory system and aging. *In* Exercise and Aging: The Scientific Basis. Edited by E.L. Smith and R.C. Serfass. Hillside, N.J.: Enslow Publ., 1981, pp. 89–107.

57. Richardson, D., and R. Schewchuk: Comparison of calf muscle blood flow responses to rhythmic exercise between mean age 25- and 74-year-old men. Proc. Soc. Exp. Biol. Med. *164*:550–555, 1980.

58. Rodahl, K., et al.: Physiological changes during prolonged bed rest. *In* Nutrition and Physical Activity. Edited by G. Blix. Stockholm: Almqvist & Wiksell, 1967, p. 107.

59. Saltin, B., et al.: Response to submaximal and maximal exercise after bed rest and training. Circulation. *38*(Suppl. 7):1968.

60. Saltin, B., L.H. Hartley, A. Kilbom, and I. Astrand: Physical training in sedentary middle-aged and older men. II. Oxygen uptake, heart rate and blood lactate concentration at submaximal and maximal exercise. Scand. J. Clin. Lab. Invest. 24:323–334, 1969.

61. Saltin, B., and L.B. Rowell: Functional adaptations to physical activity and inactivity. Fed. Proceed. *39*:1506–1513, 1980.

62. Shephard, R.J.: Physical Activity and Aging. Chicago: Year Book Medical, 1978.

63. Shock, N.: The physiology of aging. Sci. Amer. *206*(1):100–110, 1962.

64. Siscovick, D.S., et al.: Physical activity and primary cardiac arrest. JAMA. *248*:3113–3117, 1982.

65. Smith, E.L.: Bone changes in the exercising older adult. *In* Exercise and Aging: The Scientific Basis. Edited by E.L. Smith and R.C. Serfass. Hillside, N.J.: Enslow Publ., 1981, pp. 179–186.

66. Smith, E.L., C.T. Sempos, and R.W. Purvis: Bone mass and strength decline with age. *In* Exercise and Aging: The Scientific Basis. Edited by E.L. Smith and R.C. Serfass. Hillside, N.J.: Enslow Publ., 1981, pp. 59–87.

67. Spirduso, W.W.: Reaction and movement time as a function of age and physical activity level. J. Gerontol. *30*:435–440, 1975.

68. Spirduso, W.W., and P. Clifford: Replication of age and physical activity effects on reaction and movement time. J. Gerontol. *33*:26–30, 1978.

69. Stephens, T.: Secular trends in adult physical activity: exercise boom or bust. Research Quart. Exer. Sport. *58*:94–105, 1987.

70. Suominen, H., et al.: Effects of 8 weeks' endurance training on skeletal muscle metabolism in 56–70-year-old sedentary men. Eur. J. Appl. Physiol. *7*:173–180, 1977.

71. Tilton, F.E., J.J.C. Degioanni, and V.S. Schneider: Long-term follow-up of Skylab bone demineralization. Aviat. Space Environ. Med. *51*:1209–1213, 1980.

72. Trotter, M., and B.B. Hizon: Sequential changes in weight, density, and percentage ash weight from an early fetal period through old age. Anat. Rec. *179*:1–18, 1974.

73. Vuori, I., M. Makarainen, and A. Jaaskelainen: Sudden death and physical activity. Cardiol. *63*:287–304, 1978.

74. Young, A.: Exercise physiology in geriatric practice. Acta Med. Scand. Suppl. *711*:227–232, 1986.

BIBLIOGRAPHY

1. Astrand, P.-O., and G. Grimby (editors): Physical Activity in Health and Disease. Acta Med. Scand. Suppl. *711*:1–244, 1986.

2. Ostrow, A.C.: Physical Activity and the Older Adult. Princeton, N.J.: Princeton Book Co., 1984.

3. Shephard, R.J.: Physical Activity and Aging. Chicago: Year Book Medical, 1978.

4. Shock, N.: The physiology of aging. Sci. Amer. *206*(1):100–110, 1962.

5. Smith, E.L., and R.C. Serfass (editors): Exercise and Aging: The Scientific Basis. Hillsdale, N.J.: Enslow, 1981.

8

THE MODERN CONCEPT OF HEALTH

INTRODUCTION

It is becoming increasingly well understood that health implies more than freedom from disease or observable physical defect. The former prevalent definition that one was either sick or healthy was useful when the predominant public health problem was illness (morbidity) and death (mortality) due to infectious disease. That the development of modern sanitation, public health methods and antibiotic drugs has nearly eradicated most of these diseases is evident in the contrast of mortality rates in the U.S. in 1900 as opposed to that in 1981 shown in Table 8–1. In 1900, four major infectious disease categories (pneumonia and influenza, tuberculosis, diarrhea and enteritis, and nephritis) accounted for 628 deaths per 100,000 live population. The death rate attributed to the three major chronic diseases (heart disease, CNS vascular lesions, and cancer) totaled 308 per 100,000 live population. In 1983, however, the major causes of death were primarily attributable to chronic disease, with only pneumonia and influenza, amongst infectious diseases, remaining on the top ten list. Heart disease, cancer, and CNS vascular lesions now account for over two-thirds of the deaths in the U.S. each year. Other chronic diseases now on the top eight list include chronic obstructive pulmonary disease, diabetes, and cirrhosis of the liver.

As shown in Table 8–2, life expectancy at birth increased from 49.2 years in 1900 to 69.7 in 1960. This was due primarily to the control of infectious diseases which had previously caused high infant and early childhood mortality. The relatively smaller increases at age 50 and 70 years from 1900 to 1960 reflects the reduced impact of infectious disease mortality in older adults. However, with this improvement in public health, more of our population reached adult middle-age where they became increasingly susceptible to death via chronic, degenerative disease. Indeed, since the mid-1920s, our major public health problem has stemmed from progressive cardiovascular disease and cancer which evolve over years, usually without observable symptoms. There is accumulating evidence though, that these diseases are not merely inevitable with advancing years, but rather are substantially dependent upon one's lifestyle.[9] This contention will be examined in a later section.

While mortality rates provide one important indicator of public health problems, people live from day to day experiencing both acutely evident ill health of various magnitudes (as in transitory respiratory infection or injury from accident which may be minor or have significant long-term effects), together with the increasing predisposition to chronic disease states, some of which do not lead to early death (e.g., arthritis). An analysis of days of bed disability reveals that disease conditions, such as upper respiratory infections, arthritis, mental disorders, and fractures/dislocations are extremely important relative to heart disease and cancer.[69] This presents the medical profession with a complex challenge in attending effectively to the public's health care needs.

Table 8–1. Mortality Rates Per 100,000 Live Population from the 8 Leading Causes of Death in 1900 and 1981*

	1900			1981	
Rank	Cause	Rate	Rank	Cause	Rate
1	Pneumonia and influenza	202.2	1	Diseases of the heart	328.7
2	Tuberculosis	194.4	2	Cancer	184.0
3	Diarrhea and Enteritis	142.7	3	Vascular lesions affecting central nervous system	71.3
4	Diseases of the heart	137.4	4	Accidental deaths (all kinds)	43.9
5	Vascular lesions affecting central nervous system	106.9	5	Chronic obstructive pulmonary disease	25.7
6	Nephritis	88.6	6	Pneumonia and influenza	23.4
7	Accidental deaths (all kinds)	72.0	7	Diabetes mellitus	15.1
8	Cancer	64.0	8	Cirrhosis of the liver	12.0

*From the National Office of Vital Statistics, United States Public Health Service, 1983.

TOWARD A MODERN DEFINITION OF HEALTH

The World Health Organization (WHO) defined health in 1960 as "A state of complete physical, mental and social well-being, and not merely the absence of disease or infirmity."[70] This definition is more inclusive of the basic dimensions of human health, which obviously include more than the physical aspect. However, it remains deficient, in that it fails to recognize that health (a state of well-being) can coexist with chronic disease development. Further, one can have a relatively minor pain or illness, or a permanent physical handicap, and yet not evidence any manifestation of chronic disease.

Terris[62] contends that the WHO definition of health is not realistic, as it indicates an either/or dichotomy. He astutely notes that health (a state of well-being) can coexist with disease, such as the slow progression of atherosclerosis (leading to coronary heart disease) or cancer without evidence of symptoms that one is ill. Figure 8–1 depicts a health-illness continuum in which, from left to right, one becomes progressively less well and only at the midpoint, progressively more ill. Also shown in the bottom two panels are the effects on the reciprocal qualities of body function and disease. This analysis correctly identifies the usual occurrence of response, i.e., feeling well or ill, relative to function as chronic disease progresses. It does not, however, seem applicable to mental and social well-being aspects of health. To this end, Hoyman[25] has proposed a health concept, with several levels of health and illness. At the top of Hoyman's scale is *optimal health*, which entails a nearly complete state of physical, mental, and social well-being. The effects of modern life upon man are too complex to expect near perfect function in all dimensions of health, but this

Table 8–2. Average Life Expectancy Comparisons for 1900, 1960, and 1981*

Age	Average Life Expectancy 1900 (years)	Average Life Expectancy 1960 (years)	Average Life Expectancy 1981 (years)	Increase 1960 vs 1900 (years)	Increase 1981 vs 1960 (years)
At birth	49.2	69.7	74.2	20.5	4.5
At age 10 yrs	51.1	62.1	65.3	11.0	3.2
At age 50 yrs	21.2	25.2	28.1	4.0	2.9
At age 70 yrs	9.3	11.3	13.5	2.0	2.2

*Modified from National Office of Vital Statistics, United States Public Health Service, 1983.

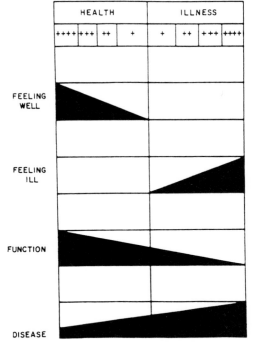

FIG. 8–1. Illustration of the health-illness continuum: relation to function and disease. (From Terris, M.: Approaches to an epidemiology of health. Am. J. Pub. Health. 65:1037–1045, 1975.)

weight and blood pressure, does not smoke, and exercises regularly significantly reduces the risk of heart attack. In addition to recognizing that an underlying chronic disease may be advancing rapidly in an otherwise apparently healthy person, the modern concept of health also connotes that it is not a static, permanent condition, but rather a quality of life that is in a continually dynamic state. Further, the modern definition of health includes a mental dimension which can have demonstrable physical effects (e.g., stress-induced elevation in blood pressure and indigestion), even before diagnosed mental illness is manifested. Thus, health is a complex integrative and dynamic quality of human life that currently defies precise assessment.

BASIC DIMENSIONS OF HEALTH

Those who are in accord with the modern concept of health, contend that it encompasses an integrated balance of mental, physical, social, and spiritual components. Edlin and Golanty[21] have identified this perspective as the holistic view of health, and further state:

Such a view recognizes the interrelatedness of the physical, psychological, emotional, social, spiritual, and environmental factors that contribute to the overall quality of a person's life. No part of the mind, body, or environment is truly separate and independent.[21:6]

This statement is of particular significance, in that it integrates man's health—multidimensional—in the environment. The interaction remains largely a mystery, but it is instructive to examine the components. In this section, the fundamental dimensions of health identified by Hoyman in Figure 8–2, viz., physical fitness, mental health, and spiritual faith, will be discussed. In the following section, the basic determinants of health, including heredity and the environment, will be examined.

PHYSICAL FITNESS

Many consider that physical fitness relates only to one's ability to perform daily

level is useful as an ultimate goal to which individuals can aspire, though only rarely achieve. Other levels are essentially in accord with Terris' model, in that function (well-being) and disease are seen as a continuum.

It is obvious, then, that health and disease are not just complete opposites; there are degrees of each. While most people would agree that a sick person could become more ill, there are many who fail to realize that a well person can become healthier. The latter notion is of increasing importance, as it represents a vital defense against the development of the most prevalent chronic diseases—coronary heart disease and cancer—which reach advanced stages before symptoms are evident. One who follows appropriate health precepts—e.g., no smoking and a high fiber diet, reduce their risk of lung and colon cancer, respectively. Similarly, one who eats a low-animal fat diet, maintains normal body

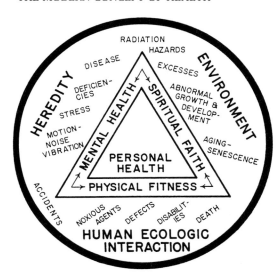

FIG. 8–2. The personal health triangle: physical fitness, mental health, and spiritual faith. In this conceptualization, health is determined by heredity, environment, and human ecologic interaction. (From Hoyman, H.S.: Our modern concept of health. J. School Health. 32(7):253–264, 1962.)

tasks with efficiency (skill), without undue fatigue, and with ample reserve to enjoy vigorous leisure-time activities and to meet unforeseen emergencies. For most adults, however, their primary work—whether in the home or elsewhere—is largely devoid of demanding physical effort. Thus, they become "adapted" to a relative state of physical disuse which, when one engages in occasional vigorous leisure-time activity, results in undue fatigue and perhaps physical injury. A margin of reserve for unforeseen emergencies is obviously absent, though the individual does retain the level of fitness necessary to perform routine sedentary tasks. Clearly, this individual is not physically fit to enjoy abundant, fruitful living, and the quality of life is effectively compromised. Further, there is an increasingly impressive body of knowledge which effectively documents that prolonged sedentary activity (i.e., hypokinetics) has a deleterious effect on one's health and well-being. In view of this important expanded role for physical fitness in alleviating the effects of hypokinetics upon numerous

chronic diseases in the adult population, a revision of the previously accepted definition is needed. Pate has proposed that the following statement be added to the definition given at the beginning of this section to make it complete: ". . . and demonstration of physical activity traits and capacities that are consistent with minimal risk of developing hypokinetic diseases."[50:82]

Cureton[14] has identified three components of physical fitness: (1) physique, (2) organic efficiency, and (3) motor fitness. One's physique, a primarily inherited component, essentially represents the relationship of height to weight. If the latter is much greater than average for height due to excess fat, then physical performance will be hindered; however, if excess weight for height is due to greater than average muscle mass, many types of physical performance will be facilitated. The influence of physique, particularly in terms of excess weight (and body fat) on one's health will be discussed later in this chapter.

Organic efficiency refers to the quality of function in fundamental organ systems that facilitate physical fitness, including particularly the muscular, nervous, cardiovascular, respiratory, and endocrine systems. The capacity of each is dependent in varied degrees upon hereditarian predisposition, as well as one's physical activity level (some more so than others). Since physical performance depends on an effective integrated response of all these organ systems, a weakness in one causes reduced organic efficiency and physical fitness. Cardiorespiratory endurance and the aerobic exercise that develops it have been linked with reduced risk of coronary heart disease.[13,37] Hence, optimal function of the cardiorespiratory system has significant health related implications.

As shown in Figure 8–3, motor fitness is dependent upon certain aspects of other physical fitness components, viz., body composition (physique) and cardiorespiratory endurance (organic efficiency). It is also composed of seven other elements that collectively are well related to athletic performance potential.[50] This relationship is perhaps more apparent when each is defined, as follows:

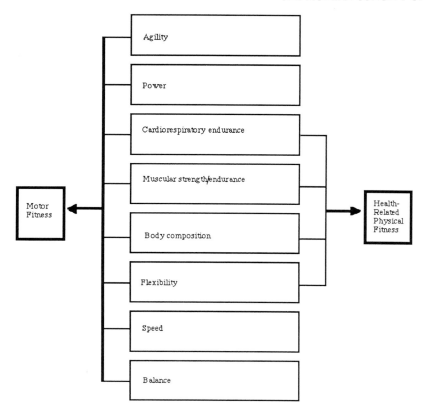

FIG. 8–3. Components of motor fitness and health-related physical fitness. (From Pate, R.R.: A new definition of youth fitness. Physician Sportsmed. *11(4)*:77–83, 1983.)

1. *Agility.* Ability to change direction of the entire body in space with speed and accuracy.
2. *Power.* The rate at which one can do work; exemplified by activities that demand the production of explosive force, such as jumps or throwing events in track and field.
3. *Muscular strength.* Represents the maximum amount of force developed in a single muscular contraction.
4. *Muscular endurance.* The capacity of muscle groups to sustain performance; relates to the ability to apply submaximal force repeatedly, or to sustain an isometric muscular contraction for a prolonged period.
5. *Flexibility.* Emphasizes the ability to move the body parts through their full range of motion. It is largely dependent on the suppleness of the muscle, ligament and tendon complex of a joint.
6. *Speed.* The ability to perform body movement(s) rapidly.

7. *Balance.* The ability to maintain equilibrium via the interrelationship of internal and external forces while stationary (static) or moving (dynamic).

Also indicated in Figure 8–3 is that muscular strength and endurance, as well as flexibility, have been identified as elements of health related fitness. This is due to the substantial clinical evidence that low back pain—a relatively common malady that causes much disability[4]—is associated with weakness of the abdominal muscles and lack of flexibility in the lower back and hamstring musculature.[29] Kraus[32] has developed an appropriate lower back/hamstring stretching and abdominal muscle strengthening program that has been shown to ameliorate many low back pain cases. It has been successfully adapted for use in YMCA adult fitness programs as a preventive measure.

MENTAL HEALTH

Just as the modern definition of health means more than freedom from illness, so mental health refers to more than absence of clinically manifested emotional disturbance. Thus, there are levels of mental health which, however, are not possible to identify precisely. For example, some who suffer from severe emotional disturbance may exhibit continuous mild-mannered and otherwise apparent symptom-free behavior before displaying an abrupt pathologic behavior.[27] Others may demonstrate perceived abnormal behavior on frequent occasion, but never evidence clear symptoms of emotional disturbance, or seek or obtain psychologic assistance. Nonetheless, there is increasing agreement amongst mental health workers as to the traits that characterize individuals with good mental health.[27]

Jahoda[28] analyzed the characteristics of mentally healthy people and those with emotional disturbance, finding that they differed in six fundamental characteristics. Each is identified with supporting summary below.

1. SELF-CONCEPT. A good self-concept, or self-image, appears fundamental to good mental health. It depends on one's ability to cope with environmental input, which is influenced by reality perception and appropriate reaction regarding personal identity factors such as self-insight, self-pity, and self-acceptance. People with a good self-concept feel comfortable about themselves, making the most of their abilities. They recognize their flaws and abilities, but are not overly concerned about them. They spend little time being worried, fearful, anxious, or jealous.[35]

2. REALITY PERCEPTION. Feeling good about oneself in any environment could be due to an unrealistic perception or to capable temporary coping strategies, rather than to correct assessment and response. Realistic people understand the difference between what is and what should be. Further, they correctly perceive what they can change, while unrealistic individuals often become "hung-up" on what should be. Insel and Roth[27] contend that realistic people accept evidence that contradicts what they believe or want to believe and,

if it seems important, modify their beliefs accordingly.

3. INTEGRATION. A mature, mentally healthy person possesses a unifying outlook on life which permits shaping one's life with wisdom and perspective. Such persons are usually able to cope constructively with numerous routinely adverse problems which might otherwise result in anxiety, frustration, guilt, resentment, and/or hostility. They can also cope with adversity without developing a "big me and little you complex." In addition to emotional balance, people with effective integrative understanding of themselves and their environment usually evidence a deeper understanding of life.

4. AUTONOMY. Persons who enjoy good mental health are able to function well without making undue demands on others. Further, they are sensitive to how they feel and their natural impulses, and trust them to guide their actions. They do not feel compelled to act because they fear disapproval or rejection. Rather, they are capable of creative adjustment as well as appropriate conformity to cultural expectations. Such persons can accept or reject alternatives and make plans and decisions to carry them out. While they have a well-developed inner life, they effectively alternate periods of solitude and reflection with creative activities and social life that enables them to share life with others with compassion.

5. ENVIRONMENTAL MASTERY. The ability to take life as it comes and master it is another important aspect of mental health. This involves two related central themes—one success, the other creative adjustment. Adequacy in work, family life, recreation, citizenship, and human relationships; efficiency in meeting situational requirements and in problem-solving; and, the ability to create and contribute within the limits of one's capacities are all interrelated factors in environmental mastery.[25]

6. SELF-ACTUALIZATION. This aspect of good mental health arises from the work of Maslow regarding satisfaction of needs and motivation of human behavior, discussed in Chapter 4. This level of need is addressed only after other, more basic, needs have been effectively satisfied. Self-actualization involves creative, free expression according to one's compulsion without direct need for evaluation by others. Those who evidence self-actualiza-

tion are oriented toward the future and an expectation of growth in experience for the anticipated value in personal terms.

From the above discussion, it should be apparent that good mental health does not mean complete freedom from anxiety and dissatisfaction. Such a state is only rarely achieved for short periods of time by perhaps a few people (thus constituting a state of optimal mental health). Further, many people may experience acute and/or chronic deficiencies in achieving good mental health in one or more parameters. Any persistent problem can also contribute to the occurrence of psychosomatic disease in which body (somatic) changes occur in part because of mental-emotional concerns. A good example is resting blood pressure which increases notably with acute perceived stress but, more importantly, can remain elevated over prolonged periods due to persistent emotionally charged situations.[72]

SPIRITUAL FAITH

Hoyman[25] contends that man's spiritual nature and human aspirations compel him to seek a feeling of belongingness in the universe, rather than viewing oneself as an alien in an indifferent and meaningless world. Hoyman elaborates on the meaning and the importance of considering spiritual faith as a basic dimension of health.

Human life is essentially a quest for personal identity and fulfillment, social sensitivity, ethical insight and moral responsibility, and spiritual meaning. "Spiritual faith" is intended to signify that man is searching for some deeper, more unifying, meaning to his life than mere existence or survival. A truly healthy person seeks to transform and transcend himself and to justify his life through spiritual aspiration and faith that link up the brute facts of his existence with ideal ends . . . for us to ignore the spiritual dimension of man in conceptualizing his health would be to deal with man de-humanized, for moral and spiritual values are central to human personality and mental health.[25:260]

Edlin and Golanty[21] contend that spirituality is an important integrated element with mind and body in the attainment of health. This holistic view:

acknowledges that an objective, scientific explanation of the workings of the physical body contributes to a greater understanding of the mechanisms of disease and hence illness prevention and the attainment of health. But it also recognizes that many people have inner experiences that are subjective, mystical, and for some religious, and that these experiences may affect health as well. By recognizing that the spiritual aspects of being can be important to health, the holistic philosophy is in accord with such centuries-old traditional philosophies as the Hinduism of India, Taoism of China, and Buddhism of Tibet, Japan, and other Asian countries.[21:19–20]

DETERMINANTS OF HEALTH

Hoyman's modern concept of health depicted in integrative form previously (Fig. 8–2), identifies three fundamental determinants of health: (1) heredity, (2) environment, and (3) human ecologic interaction. While it is convenient to attribute disease occurrence to a single cause, this is not usually the case, in that almost all depend on an integration of the three determinants of health. For example, even some genetic defects can be due to fetus chromosomal mutation arising from environmental substances, such as chemicals, x rays, and atomic radiation.[21] Nonetheless, it is instructive to examine evidence of the effects of heredity and environment on disease incidence, as well as their interaction and that of human ecologic interaction in man's efforts to live a healthier life.

HEREDITY

About 5% of all humans are born with hereditary defects that result in anatomic or physiologic abnormalities. In addition, predisposition to the occurrence of many other diseases, including some types of mental disorders, are due in part to one's genetic makeup. In fact, all diseases are partly a result of heredity, in the sense that one who is genetically "weaker" in a critical respect is more susceptible to the environmental influences concerned in the etiology of the particular disease in question.

Hereditary factors are dominant in such basic physical features as one's height, body type, eye color, and facial features. Of these basic physical features, one's body type is of particular importance in affecting health potential. The idea that body type is related to general health and disease susceptibility is of ancient origin. For example, Hippocrates (460 to 370 B.C.) defined two fundamental body types, a long, thin type and a short, thick type. Even at that time, the former was considered particularly subject to tuberculosis, while the latter had a predisposition toward diseases of the vascular system.[12]

In the late 1940s, Sheldon and colleagues[58] developed a detailed body typing procedure, called the somatotype. Their method consists of evaluating the relative predominance of the three embryonic body layers (endoderm, mesoderm and ectoderm) evidenced in one's physique on an equal increment scale from 1 through 7. The endodermic layer develops into the viscera, i.e., intestines, stomach, liver, and fat tissue; the mesoderm into muscle, connective tissue, and bone; and the ectoderm into skin and nervous tissue. It is essential to realize that everyone has varying degrees of all three primary components manifested in their somatotype. For instance, a physique with an adjudged somatotype of 3 4 4 indicates a slightly lower than average amount of endomorphy (3), and an average degree of mesomorphy (4) and ectomorphy (4). This individual is properly categorized as a medial type since his physique exhibits no component predominantly. An individual characterized by a linear appearance with a high height to body weight ratio, would have a predominant ectomorphic rating, i.e., 1 2 6. Conversely, a predominant endomorph (i.e., 7 2 2) would exhibit a rotund appearance and a low height to body weight ratio. A predominant mesomorph (i.e., 2 7 1) would have a lower than average height to body weight ratio, but would evidence a trimmer and much more muscular appearance than the endomorph.

In addition to providing evidence that one's somatotype is primarily attributable to heredity, Sheldon and colleagues have demonstrated a substantial difference in weight gain with age. As depicted in Figure 8–4, predominant endomorphs gain weight at a far more rapid rate during early middle-age than does the individual with a medial somatotype. The predominant mesomorph (2 7 1), however, gains weight only at a slightly greater rate than the medial type. McCloy and Young[44] contend that this is likely due to endomorphs possessing a larger amount of digestive organs per unit of body height than do ectomorphs and medial types. Endomorphs, therefore would be expected to have comparatively more area from which to absorb food than do ectomorphs and medial types, and hence would tend to put on more weight through middle age.

More recent evidence also suggests that obesity has a predominant hereditarial factor. Mayer[41] found that less than 10% of children of normal weight parents were obese, while when both parents were obese, prevalence of obesity was 80%. Stunkard and colleagues[60] have reported a strong relation between the body mass index (body weight (kg)/height (m)²) of 540 adult adoptees (average age of 42 years) ranging from thin to obese, and their biologic parents, with no systematic relationship to that of their adoptive parents.

From the above discussion, it is apparent that certain body types, viz., endomorphs and meso-endomorphs are much more likely to become grossly overweight during middle-age, especially in sedentary life. Van Itallie[66] has urged greater emphasis on environmental intervention—particularly in terms of a moderate and defensive diet and relatively high physical activity levels—but more specifically targeted to obesity-prone individuals. He contends that these measures, though difficult for members of our sedentary and "food laden" society to accomplish, must become a constant effort if obesity-prone individuals are to reduce their risk of chronic illness and premature death.

ENVIRONMENT

Man's environment appears to be functioning increasingly as a double-edged

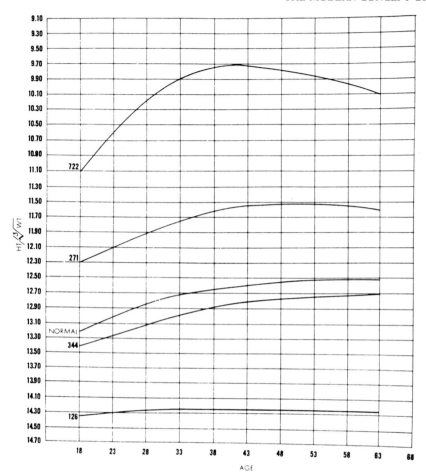

FIG. 8–4. Normal curve for height over the cube root of weight for American men by age, and for selected somatotypes: 1) Endomorph—722; 2) Mesomorph—271; 3) Most Common Somatotype—344; and 4) Ectomorph—126. (Adapted from Sheldon, W.H., et al.: Atlas of Men. New York: Harper and Bros., 1954, pp. 38, 126, 156, and 330.)

sword with respect to health and well-being. On the one hand, we are dependent on our biologic and physical environment for air, water, food, and shelter. Further, modern sanitation, public health methods, and antibiotic drugs have dramatically reduced morbidity and mortality from infectious diseases that were the most prevalent public health problem in the U.S. through the early 20th century. On the other hand, associated technologic progress has brought a new array of health problems that we are not yet coping with effectively. As more humans live a longer life, and in increasingly concentrated land masses typ-

ical of a highly technologically advanced society, they constitute an increased probability for adverse ecologic impact and thus, become a greater part of the growing environmental health problem.

For example, with increased concentration of the U.S. population in metropolitan areas (which now constitutes about 75% in 10% of the country's land mass), there are now only recently well-recognized problems of air, land, and water resource pollution. Trieff[63] has provided an effective integrative graphic of man's interrelationship with his environment showing adverse effects on health (Fig. 8–5). Man and the en-

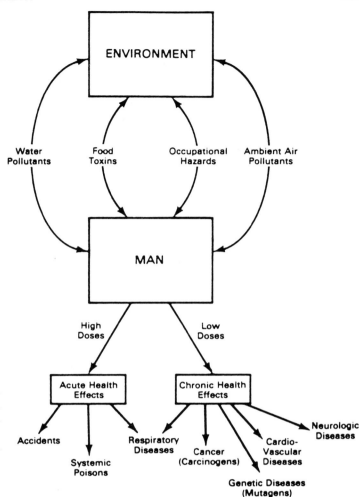

FIG. 8–5. The interrelationships between man and his environment, showing adverse effects on man's health. (From Trieff, N.M.: Environment and Health. Ann Arbor, Mich.: Ann Arbor Sci. Publ., 1980, p. 16.)

vironment are shown to interact regarding water pollution, food toxins, occupational hazards, and ambient air pollutants. That is, man's biologic and physical environment constitutes a challenge to health which can be diminished or enhanced by the sum of human action. High doses of toxic substances have acute health effects, while lower doses have the potential for the development of numerous serious chronic health effects. What is particularly perplexing about the latter, is that these effects can take years—even decades—to become clearly evidenced, and we are not yet well aware of their potential for significant chronic public health impact.

The sociocultural aspect is another important element of one's environment that significantly impacts health. The child's health is crucially dependent upon this aspect of the environment, which is interrelated with the biologic and physical environmental aspects.[20,25] While human socioculture appears universal in seeking to protect the life and health of its young, be it primitive or industrialized, it has harmful as well as beneficial effects on health. For example, we live in a society that has made rapid scientific and technologic development, part of which has produced virtual eradication of mortality due to infectious diseases and has recently aided in reducing the heart disease mortality rate 36% between 1968 and 1983.[51] However, scientific and technologic development and its wide diffusion in our culture has resulted in industrialization and urbanization, which have produced a more concentrated society and a near void in vigorous physical activity required of most humans since the early 1900s.

Industrialization and urbanization have also brought adverse health effects in our physical environment, including noise pollution and an alarming motor vehicular accident rate.[21] We live in a society with relatively free enterprise, in which a significant unevenness in distribution of wealth exists. Those near and below the poverty line have significantly poorer health, both in terms of increased morbidity and a higher mortality rate. Those of higher socioeconomic means enjoy better health care and lower morbidity and mortality rates. However, they are not immune to purchasing and using certain heavily advertised products that are injurious to good health. Thus, one's sociocultural environment, via interaction with biologic and physical aspects, presents both advantages and potential deterrents to human health.

HUMAN ECOLOGIC INTERACTION

Heredity supplies the basic organic structure, while one's environment provides substantial forces in shaping its function and direction. Man is unique, however, in that he has the capacity to profoundly affect his health potential and length of life. This is largely due to the fact that chronic disease development is caused by an interaction of numerous factors (i.e., multiple-causation theory), many of which are amenable to influence by one's personal decisions regarding health and health related behavior.

Hoyman further defines the concept of human ecologic interaction:

Man has great plasticity and flexibility of behavior, if not free will, and can learn by experience and make progress toward significant long range goals . . . as a self-conscious emergent from the interaction of his heredity and environment, he is capable of self-directed, unique behavior affecting his level of health.[25:262]

Hoyman, however, reminds us that human health is an ecologic resultant and thus, dependent on man's effective interaction with his environment. Though human ecology is not a new concept, its increased emphasis and resultant greater understanding presents important opportunities for individuals to understand more effectively how to achieve their health potential in the short-term, as well as how to influence long-term health advantages for humankind and other life forms.

While heredity is the primary influence on obesity in the normally encountered environment, appropriate intervention efforts yield important effects. There is also a steadily increasing body of knowledge concerning the effect of lifestyle on coronary heart disease, diabetes, and hypertension, which suggests a vital role for lifestyle intervention programs that include diet management, exercise, smoking cessation, and stress reduction. Fundamental though, is the realization that sound knowledge regarding health and health related behavior is not enough; the will to apply this knowledge is crucial to one's health enhancement.[35]

EVIDENCE THAT MAN IS FAILING TO ACHIEVE HIS HEALTH POTENTIAL

The most impressive evidence that we are failing to reach our health potential has been alluded to earlier in terms of the high mortality rate due to chronic, degenerative disease (Table 8–1). There is evidence that strongly suggests abundant room for improvement, though there has been a notable increase in adult life expectancy since 1960, primarily due to a reduction in deaths from coronary heart disease and stroke.[51] Young adults perceive that chronic illness is an "old-folks" syndrome, but they should appreciate that habits formed early in life can predispose one to early occurrence of chronic disease and reduced life expectancy.

LIFESTYLE DISEASES

Most of our principal public health concerns are properly identified not just as chronic, degenerative disease, but as life-style diseases.[21] In this section, the most prominent of these diseases, together with the principal predisposing conditions, will be discussed.

CARDIOVASCULAR DISEASE. Diseases of the heart and blood vessels (i.e., cardiovascular diseases) account for about 50% of the deaths each year in the United States, with over 20% occurring in individuals under age 65.[1] Heart attacks and strokes account for nearly 85% of deaths due to cardiovascular disease, which is of significance in that both heart attacks and strokes are due primarily to the progressive development of atherosclerosis.

Atherosclerosis is characterized by damage to the inner arterial walls (intima), and can occur at numerous locations in the body, including the aorta, coronary, carotid, and femoral arteries. The initiation and progression of atherosclerosis is not entirely clear. It appears that cholesterol and other fats are deposited on the intima, first evident as fatty streaks, then progressing to fibrous plaques which can eventually ulcerate and lead to additional scar tissue formation.[5] However mediated, the result is a progressive narrowing of the lumen (inner opening) of the main systemic arteries affected. Advanced atherosclerotic blockage in the coronary and carotid arteries is especially critical, in that both the heart and brain cannot continue their life-sustaining function beyond several minutes cessation of oxygen supply.

The heart does not receive its blood supply from within its chambers, but is nourished and has its waste products removed by its own circulatory system. Blood is supplied to the heart by the right and left coronary arteries and their many branches (Fig. 8–6). These branches divide and subdivide, until finally they become tiny arterioles which provide blood to the muscle fibers or cells of the heart. When the condition of the coronary arteries reaches the point where there is a restriction of the blood supply causing oxygen insufficiency, any unusual stress such as emotional excitement, exposure to cold temperature, or unusual physical activity may cause a type of heart attack called angina pectoris. The pain associated with this attack is generally short in duration and may be eased by terminating the stressful activity and resting quietly for a few moments.

If obstruction in the arteries continues, the possibility of a coronary thrombosis or occlusion increases. If an occlusion occurs, the blood supply to the heart muscle is obstructed and as a result, a part of the heart muscle dies and is replaced by scar tissue (myocardial infarction). The severity of the attack depends upon the size of the artery blocked and the amount of heart muscle it supplies. If it is near the top of the coronary artery, especially on the left side, death will likely occur. On the other hand, if the stoppage is in a tiny arteriole, the occlusion may go unnoticed and the heart usually recovers normal function. This occurrence is facilitated by a physiologic adaptive process referred to as collateral circulation. Bourne[7] contends that this process involves a linking up of nearby coronary arterial structure enabling blood flow to bypass the atherosclerotic obstruction.

What causes the atherosclerotic process that eventually induces the vast majority of heart attacks? Over a quarter century of intensive research has revealed no single cause, but rather that coronary heart disease is associated with numerous interrelated factors which increase one's risk. The American Heart Association has summarized the most important risk factors (Table 8–3). Major risk factors are categorized, in part, according to those which cannot be changed because one has no control over them. For example, males over 45 years have a mortality rate nearly double that of females. Even more significant is that adults with a family history of coronary heart disease have a 5 times greater risk than average if first-degree relatives have experienced a heart attack.[51] The role of genetic factors, however, is difficult to quantitate since environmentally influenced factors have a strong familial input. Major risk factors that can be changed include hyperlipidemia (high blood levels of cholesterol and triglycerides), hypertension, and cigarette smoking. Each are associated with more than double the average person's risk, and their combined effect may be more than additive.[51]

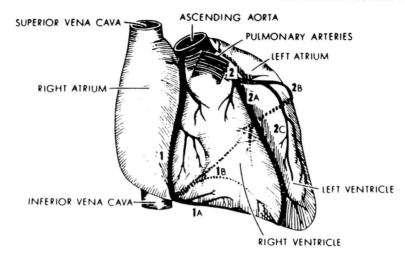

FIG. 8–6. Arteries of the heart. (From Adams, W.C. et al.: Foundations of Physical Activity. Champaign, Ill.: Stipes, 1968 (3rd edition), p. 126.)

1.	Right coronary artery	2.	Left coronary artery
1A.	Marginal branch	2A.	Anterior interventricular branch
1B.	Posterior interventricular branch	2B.	Circumflex branch
		2C.	Marginal branch

Recent research has suggested that the effects of hyperlipidemia on coronary heart disease may be much more complex than first thought. Both cholesterol and triglycerides are transported in the blood via a carrier called lipoproteins. It appears that low density lipoproteins are associated with transport and deposition of fat on the arterial wall, while high density lipoproteins appear associated with fat transport to the liver for excretion.[61] These observations are of particular interest, in that high levels of high density lipoprotein have been observed in adults who engage in aerobic training.[39]

Other risk factors for increased incidence of coronary heart disease identified in Table 8–3 are categorized as contributing factors. Each may exert an independent effect on coronary heart disease incidence, and/or have a direct effect on other risk factors. Since each have other important health implications, they will be discussed in a later section.

Hypertension. Less than 20,000 people die in the U.S. each year due to direct hypertensive disease. However, as alluded to above, hypertension is a primary risk factor which enhances heart attack and stroke mortality rates. Other primary risk factors

Table 8–3. Categorization of Coronary Heart Disease Risk Factors*

Major Risk Factors	*Other Contributing Risk Factors*
Factors That Can Be Changed	Obesity
Cigarette smoking	Physical inactivity
Hypertension	Stress
Blood cholesterol	Diabetes
Factors That Cannot Be Changed	
Heredity	
Age	
Sex	
Race	

*From 1990 Heart and Stroke Facts, American Heart Association, Dallas, Texas, pp. 18–20.

associated with enhanced occurrence of stroke include age, race, and sex.[1]

Classifications from normal through severe hypertension have been established by the 1984 Joint National Committee on Detection, Evaluation, and Treatment of High Blood Pressure.[52] Hypertension is usually identified by persistent diastolic blood pressure readings in excess of 90 mmHg. Using this criterion, approximately 60 million Americans are considered to have essential hypertension. As shown in Figure 8–7, the excess mortality rate rises rapidly at diastolic pressures in excess of 100 mmHg to more than double that for normals at 110 mmHg.

Blood pressure rises with age in American adults as it does in most other Western civilizations. While increased hypertension incidence with age is essentially non-existent in some primitive societies, it is evidenced in many developing African populations.[71] Reasons for the rise with age in the U.S., as well as its increased incidence in males, and in blacks at all ages compared to whites, are complex and currently under investigation.[10] A general consensus that hypertension reflects a strong genetic influence has developed from the collective observations of population studies and genetic analyses of relatives, young and adult

siblings, twins, and adopted children.[3] However, there is abundant evidence that one's lifestyle and environment are important determinants of high blood pressure, although the relative importance of each remains unclear.[71] Principal factors, other than genetics, that have been identified with the development of hypertension include: (1) obesity, (2) salt, (3) alcohol consumption, and (4) psychosocial tensions (stress).[10]

CANCER. The second leading cause of death in the United States is attributable to all forms of cancer, totaling in excess of 400,000 deaths per year. Figure 8–8 shows a continued increase in mortality rate due to all cancers from 1960 to 1978, which is in contrast to the substantially reduced mortality rates for coronary heart disease and stroke. However, there was a 10% drop in death rate in all cancers other than lung cancer, which more than doubled during this period. About 80% of all lung cancer deaths can be attributed to smoking.[11]

Cancer occurs in the human in numerous forms, but arises as a mutation of normal cell structure, and grows in an unregulated manner. The most common classification, carcinomas, originate from

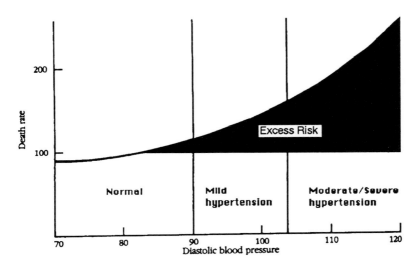

FIG. 8–7. Relationship of high diastolic blood pressure and risk of death. (From Edlin, G., and E. Golanty: Health and Wellness: A Holistic Approach. 2nd ed. Boston: Jones and Bartlett, 1985, p. 404.)

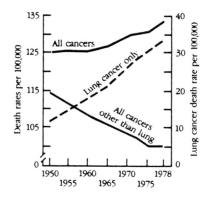

FIG. 8–8. Death rates per 100,000 population from all cancers, lung cancer, and all cancers other than lung cancer, 1950–1978. (From Health Consequences of Smoking: Cancer, Washington, D.C.: U.S. Department of Health and Human Services, 1982.)

epithelial tissue, grow rapidly, and can interfere with adjacent vital organ function at the site of the tumor or, via metastases (transfer through body circulation), can interfere with vital organ function at several sites.

Typically, cancer develops over many years before it is clinically evident. In addition to genetic predisposition, three principal categories of environmental agents, viz., radiation, selected viruses, and numerous chemicals, have been shown to induce cancer in experimental animals. Epidemiologic studies of humans confirm the important role of numerous environmental factors, including smoking, asbestos, ionizing radiation, and diet, on the increased incidence of cancer.[11]

DIABETES. Diabetes, most usually diabetes mellitus, is now ranked as the 7th leading cause of death in the United States. About 40,000 Americans die each year due to this disease, which afflicts over 10 million persons. Both morbidity and mortality rates for diabetes are increasing, largely because of increased incidence in adults.

Diabetes mellitus is a condition characterized by a deficiency or diminished effectiveness of the pancreatic hormone insulin in regulating blood glucose levels. There are two main clinical categories of diabetes: (1) Type I, which is characterized

by a lack of insulin production, and is generally manifested before age 40 (it requires regular injections of insulin for effective clinical management); and (2) Type II, which arises in the middle-aged or elderly, particularly in those who are obese, and is caused not by a lack of insulin production but by receptor site loss or insensitivity. Type II diabetes can usually be clinically managed by dietary means and/or by oral ingestion of a hypoglycemic drug.[15]

Type II diabetes tends to run in families, but the relative roles of heredity and environment are uncertain.[49] The mortality rate of diabetics is 8 times higher in the grossly obese (greater than 40% above standard weight) than in the normal weight diabetic.[19] Diabetes in adults is frequently accompanied by arteriosclerosis and is associated with abnormalities in large and small blood vessels, as well as capillaries. Diabetics have double the average mortality rate for heart attack and stroke.[1]

CHRONIC OBSTRUCTIVE PULMONARY DISEASE (COPD). COPD accounts for about 56,000 deaths annually in the United States. It is the fifth leading cause of death, and the mortality rate attributable to COPD is still increasing, largely due to the still high number of heavy smokers. Many adult patients with COPD can perform sedentary life functions, but physical activity capacity is severely compromised. With continued smoking, however, COPD progresses to the point where even breathing at rest becomes compromised.

There are three principal COPD conditions: (1) chronic bronchitis, (2) emphysema, and (3) asthma. Asthma can occur in combination with bronchitis and emphysema in adults, but also afflicts over 2 million children under the age of 17. Asthma is characterized by a sudden narrowing of the air passageways (spasm) in the bronchii and bronchioles, accompanied by secretion of thick mucus. The exact cause is unknown, but respiratory irritants such as dust, pollen, smoke, as well as cold and damp conditions, can precipitate an acute episode of expiratory wheeze and failure to achieve adequate ventilatory/perfusion ratio in the lung capillaries. Fortunately, asthma in individuals who have never smoked can be effectively managed with appropriate bronchodilator drug therapy.[6]

While asthma can also accompany chronic bronchitis and emphysema in adults who smoke, its effects are minimized by the progressive effect of the latter on pulmonary function. Bronchitis is characterized by chronic narrowing of the bronchii, and is exacerbated by extra mucus produced by respiratory irritants. The basic symptom is chronic cough, which is usually accompanied by increased sputum. This makes effective respiratory gas exchange more difficult due to the increased resistance to air flow through the pulmonary air passageways. Emphysema is a progressive disease often accompanying bronchitis that affects respiratory gas exchange at the alveoli. The loss in effective lung gas exchange structure causes "airtrapping," which results in increased difficulty in properly ventilating the blood circulating through the lung capillaries.

COPD appears to be largely environmentally induced. Heavy cigarette smoking is particularly implicated in chronic bronchitis and emphysema, although there is suggestive evidence that those living in areas of heavy environmental air pollution may be further compromised.[6]

EMOTIONAL DISORDERS AND MENTAL ILLNESS. The number of resident patients in state and county mental hospitals reached a peak of 560,000 in 1955 and has declined since by more than 50%. However, this was due primarily to advances in effective drug therapy management, which has led to a substantial increase in outpatients.[22] A careful analysis of patient illness observed in a general practice indicated that 12% was due to emotional disorders, but that a number of minor illness categories (i.e., gastrointestinal and skin) could be partially attributed to emotional distress.[17] Thus, our current public health concern entails not only diagnosed mental illness, but the increasing occurrence of psychosomatic disease.

Mental health extends from prolonged periods of primarily successful coping with one's environment and the fulfillment of personal needs, to the most severe mental illness of psychosis, in which there is prolonged gross impairment in one's psychologic functioning and ability to meet ordinary demands of life.[27] Being mentally healthy is a dynamic process involving effective adjustment to one's internal and external environment. Thus, all people face what seems to be an incredibly wide array of challenges in our exceedingly complex, rapidly changing society. Inability to meet these challenges—some recognized, others not—and to satisfy one's needs causes psychologic stress.

Some degree of stress is a natural part of life, and, in the case of physical performance improvement, is an essential component of the training process. However, as discussed in Chapter 3, well-designed training programs use graded amounts of stress, with regularly intervening periods of rest, i.e., "stress-reduction." Thus, stress consists of any demand placed on the organism by his biologic, physical, and social environment which disturbs homeostasis. Selye[56] has defined stress as a "nonspecific response of the body to any demand made upon it," and advanced the concept of a general adaptation syndrome. That is, any disturbing influence of sufficient magnitude will elicit a characteristic three-stage response to the stressor: (1) alarm, (2) resistance, and (3) exhaustion. Significant endocrine system response is intimately involved in the body's general reaction to the stressor. If of persistent psychologic origin, such as continued frustration and anger, or anxiety induced reaction, the body's ability to withstand stress extends only to a certain point and, once exceeded (exhaustive stage), results in tissue damage and health impairment.[56] Some examples of stress-induced psychosomatic illness include chronic indigestion and/or diarrhea, peptic ulcers, colitis, and migraine headaches.[59]

It is important to understand that since stress-related illness is mediated by the brain, the extent of the effects of stress are greatly dependent upon the individual's interpretation of particular events or situations. That is, the same situation, occurring on a repeated basis, can cause conflict, frustration, anxiety, and tension in one individual and elicit little effect on another person. This individual difference in perception and interpretation also accounts, in part, for the development of psychologic states, including severe depression and feelings of helplessness and intolerable despair, that characterize most individuals who commit suicide.[55] At least 200,000 people in the United States attempt suicide each year, with the annual death rate of nearly 30,000 now ranking suicide as the tenth leading cause of death.

ACCIDENTS. In the United States, accidents are now the single leading cause of death among individuals between the ages of 1 and 40 years.[64] Over 100,000 deaths each year are due to accidents, with half occurring from motor vehicular collision. That accidents have reached epidemic proportions is also affirmed by the estimated 10 million persons suffering injury each year, including 400,000 resulting in permanent, partial or total disability.[59]

The term accident suggests that it occurs due to unavoidable circumstances, such as an earthquake or tornado, or when one is a passenger in an airplane wreck. However, in many instances accidents are avoidable, though maybe not entirely due to the effort of all people involved. For example, the mortality rate due to accidents in the workplace has been reduced from 45 per 100,000 in 1937 to less than 15 per 100,000 in the 1980s.[48] In contrast, deaths from motor vehicular accidents increased through much of this period, though they have remained near 50,000 per year since the mid-1970s.

OBESITY. Public concern with being overweight—and, more importantly over-fat (i.e., obesity)—has increased dramatically since 1955. This is due primarily to the well-publicized observations of enhanced mortality in individuals above the average weight for young adults, ages 20 to 29 years, for a given height and sex group. However, there is no substantial difference in mortality until one's weight exceeds 20% above average, but then a rapid increase to more than double the mortality rate for individuals 50% above average weight.[8,57]

Overweight and Obesity. The most prevalent standard still used to assess one's desirable weight are the height-weight tables

Table 8–4.   Desirable Weights for Adult Men and Women (in indoor clothing)

| Height | | Men | | | Women | | |
Feet	Inches	Small Frame	Medium Frame	Large Frame	Small Frame	Medium Frame	Large Frame
4	10				102–111	109–121	118–131
4	11				103–113	111–123	120–134
5	0				104–115	113–126	122–137
5	1				106–118	115–129	125–140
5	2	128–134	131–141	138–150	108–121	118–132	128–143
5	3	130–136	133–143	140–153	111–124	121–135	131–147
5	4	132–138	135–145	142–156	114–127	124–138	134–151
5	5	134–140	137–148	144–160	117–130	127–141	137–155
5	6	136–142	139–151	146–164	120–133	130–144	140–159
5	7	138–145	142–154	149–168	123–136	133–147	143–163
5	8	140–148	145–157	152–172	126–139	136–150	146–167
5	9	142–151	148–160	155–176	129–142	139–153	149–170
5	10	144–154	151–163	158–180	132–145	142–156	152–173
5	11	146–157	154–166	161–184	135–148	145–159	155–176
6	0	149–160	157–170	164–188	138–151	148–162	158–179
6	1	152–164	160–174	168–192			
6	2	155–168	164–178	172–197			
6	3	158–172	167–182	176–202			
6	4	162–176	171–187	181–207			

Note: values include 5 lb of indoor clothing for men and 3 lb of indoor clothing for women, and 1-in heels for both. Data from the Metropolitan Life Insurance Company, 1983.

for men and women (Table 8–4). Clinically, overweight is usually taken to begin at 15% above desirable weight, while one who is 20% above desirable weight is considered to be obese. Using a similar height/weight relationship, the National Health and Nutrition Examination Survey[46] defined overweight as 20% above desirable weight. Using this standard, Van Itallie[66] reports an increasing prevalence from age 20 through 65 years in both males and females, which exceeds 30% for both sexes between ages 45 and 65 years.

There is little problem in identifying individuals who are grossly overweight and obese. However, an individual may be substantially overweight primarily on the basis of their bony structure and/or musculature, yet not be excessively fat (obese). Also, one may be of average, or near average weight and yet be obese. In one study of young adult men, 40% were found to be misidentified with respect to overweight as an indicator of obesity when a more direct method of assessing body fat was used.[67] With increasing public interest in the effects of obesity on one's health, more accurate, readily available indicators are now being used, including skinfold measurements of subcutaneous body fat. As approximately 50% of the total body fat is located immediately below the skin at numerous subcutaneous fat depots, measurement of skinfolds at several sites has been found to give a reasonably accurate estimation of total body fat. Measurement of just one site, over the tricep muscle (Fig. 8–9), has been found useful for screening purposes. Values given in Table 8–5 represent minimum levels for obesity in young adult men and women. These values fall within the 80th and 90th percentile of a sample of college males and females (Table 8–6), meaning that approximately ¼ of young adults are obese by these standards.

How Does One Become Obese? The underlying explanation for obesity is an intake of calories in excess of those expended by the body. Gordon cites Dr. Cyril MacBryde's summary of this condition:

A plethora of calories is the only explanation of obesity. The Law of the Conservation of Energy applies to the human body as surely as to any other machine which produces heat and

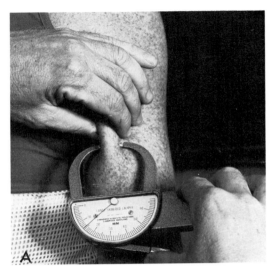

FIG. 8–9. Technique for obtaining the triceps skinfold thickness. (From McArdle, W.D., F.I. Katch, and V.L. Katch: Exercise Physiology: Energy, Nutrition, and Human Performance. 2nd ed. Philadelphia: Lea & Febiger, 1986, p. 497.)

performs work. When the intake of food, whether protein, fat or carbohydrate, exceeds in caloric value the expenditure as work and heat, the excess will be stored in the body tissues. Because of the relatively limited capacity of the body to store protein and carbohydrate, the greatest part of the excess is converted into and stored as fat. Thus, too much of any type of food is fattening.[24:162]

While the energy balance equation accounts for weight gain when caloric intake exceeds caloric expenditure, it does not tell us why certain individuals tend to obesity

Table 8–5. Obesity Standards in Young Adult Caucasian Americans*

Age (yrs)	Minimum Triceps Skin-Fold Thickness Indicating Obesity (millimeters)	
	Males	Females
18	15	27
19	15	27
20	16	28
21	17	28
22	18	28

*Modified from Seltzer, C.C. and J. Mayer: A simple criterion of obesity. Postgrad. Med. *38*:A101–A107, Aug., 1965.

Table 8–6.   Triceps Skinfold Thickness (in mm) for the 1st Through 9th Decile in College Males and Females*

| | Decile | | | | | | | | |
Sex	1st	2nd	3rd	4th	Mean	6th	7th	8th	9th
Males	7.1	9.1	10.6	11.8	13.0	14.2	15.4	16.9	18.9
Females	15.2	17.5	19.2	20.6	22.0	23.4	24.8	26.5	28.8

*Modified from Katch, F.I. and W.D. McArdle: Prediction of body density from anthropometric measurements in college-age men and women. Human Biol. 45:445–454, 1973.

more so than others. It is clear that obesity is not fully explained by the single adverse behavior of inappropriate eating in the setting of attractive foods.[47] Indeed research indicates that obesity is a heterogeneous disorder of multiple etiology. Factors of importance include fat cell number, excess caloric intake, decreased physical activity, metabolic and endocrine abnormalities, and behavioral predispositions.[47] Detailed analysis of each is beyond the scope of this chapter, though the role of physical activity on weight control will be discussed in Chapter 9.

Creeping Obesity. Creeping weight gain in men and women, which occurs from age 20 to 60 years, has been a consistent observation in the United States for 75 years.[2,45,46] This creeping weight gain amounts to about 15% between ages 20 and 60 years in males, with the average body weight for a 5 feet 11 inch tall male, increasing from 161 to 185 pounds. During the same interval, the average female, 5 feet 5 inches in height, increases from 134 to 154 pounds. Mayer[40] contends that this is not a natural biologic phenomenon of aging, but represents an inability of the body to diminish appetite proportional to reduced physical activity levels below a certain level. He further states:

I am convinced that inactivity is the most important factor explaining the frequency of "creeping" overweight in modern Western societies. Natural selection, operating for hundreds of thousands of years, made men physically active, resourceful creatures, well prepared to be hunters, fishermen or agriculturalists. The regulation of food intake was never designed to adapt to the highly mechanized sedentary conditions of modern life, any more than animals were made to be caged. Adaptation to these conditions without develop-

ment of obesity means that either the individual will have to step up his activity or that he will be mildly or acutely hungry all his life.[40:120]

Among individuals between the ages of 20 and 60 years, the number of daily calories required to maintain normal daily activities may decrease by 20%. This is due in part to a voluntary decrease in activity level, but also to a near 2% per decade drop in basal metabolic rate (which can be largely explained by decreased lean tissue that is metabolically more active than the fat tissue replacing it with advancing age).[30] Even if one assumes no loss in lean body weight with age, the creeping weight gain mentioned above has a striking effect on the percent body fat at age 60 for the average young adult male and female (Table 8–7). Thus, the prevalent creeping weight gain results in a percent body fat at age 60 which is at, or above, the level generally accepted as indicative of obesity.[42] In Figure 8–4, it was shown that creeping weight gain is not the same for all body types. Again, assuming that no lean tissue is lost with age, the average weight gains for four males, each 5 feet 11 inches in height, but of distinct somatotypes, is given in Table 8–8. It is clear that creeping weight gain in males is dramatically different for individuals of distinctly variant body types compared to the average male's values shown in Table 8–7. It seems probable that a similar variance exists for females, though there are no definitive data at present.

Dangers of Obesity. In the strictest sense, obesity is not a disease but an associative, perhaps partially causal, condition that significantly enhances the afflicted person with increased risk of morbidity and mortality, particularly in the cardiovascular, digestive, and endocrine systems. Obesity

Table 8–7. The Effect of Creeping Weight Gain From Age 20 to 60 Years on Percent Body Fat in the Average Male and Female Adult*

	Male				Female		
Body Weight (lbs)	Body Fat (%)	Lean Body Weight (lbs)	Age	Body Weight (lbs)	Body Fat (%)	Lean Body Weight (lbs)
161	15.0	136.8	20 yrs	134	24.0	101.8
185	26.1	136.8	60 yrs	154	33.9	101.8

*Assumes no change in lean body weight with age

Table 8–8. Average Body Weight and Body Fat Gain with Age in Adult Males of Varied Somatotypes*

Somatotype	Age, 20 Years			Age, 60 Years		
	Body Wt. (lbs)	Body Fat (%)	Lean Body Wt. (lbs)	Body Wt. (lbs)	Body Fat (%)	Lean Body Wt. (lbs)
Ectomorph (126)	122	7.5	112.9	125	9.7	112.9
Mesomorph (271)	200	15.0	170.0	231	26.4	170.0
Endomesomorph (651)	245	22.5	189.9	320	40.7	189.9
Endomorph (722)	253	30.0	177.1	321 +	44.8	177.1

*Assumes no change in lean body weight with age. +Body weight at age 45. Modified from Sheldon, W.H. et al: Atlas of Men. New York: Harper & Bros., 1954.

places undue strain on circulatory and renal function, and is associated with significantly increased incidence of cardiovascular disease, diabetes mellitus, gallbladder disease, renal disease, and musculoskeletal disorders—particularly in weight bearing joints.[65] Table 8–9 shows clearly the increased mortality rate (with 100 as the base value for normal weight men) from all causes, as well as for several leading causes of death. The relation appears to be exponential, in that increased mortality rate is more than double that of men 20% above average weight in men who are 40% above average weight. Earlier studies of insurance company policy owners had indicated a somewhat lower mortality rate for women who were overweight

Table 8–9. Increased Mortality Ratios in Adult Males as a Function of Being 20 and 40% Above Average Weight*

Cause of Death	Men 20% Above Average Weight		Men 40% Above Average Weight	
	Build Study 1979	American Cancer Society	Build Study 1979	American Cancer Society
Coronary heart disease	118	128	169	175
Cerebral "hemorrhage" (stroke)	110	116	164	191
Cancer	110	122	165	187
Diabetes	250	210	500	300
Digestive diseases	125	168	220	340
All causes	120	121	150	162

*From Van Itallie, T.B.: Obesity: adverse effects on health and longevity. Am. J. Clin. Nutr. 32:2723–2733, 1979.

Table 8–10.   Variations in Mortality Ratios by Weight in the American Cancer Society Study

Percentage of Average Weight	Mortality Ratios	
	Male	Female
80%	1.25	1.19
80%–89%	1.05	0.96
90%–109%	1.00	1.00
110%–119%	1.15	1.17
120%–129%	1.27	1.29
130%–139%	1.46	1.46
140% +	1.87	1.87

*Mortality ratios are expressed in relation to death rates of those 90 to 109% of average weight. From Lew, E.A. and L. Garfinkel: Variations in mortality by weight among 750,000 men and women. J. Chron. Dis. 32:563–576, 1979.

to the same degree as men. However, data from the American Cancer Society Study of the general population shown in Table 8–10 indicate a similar effect.

The association of obesity with coronary heart disease risk factors, including hypertension, elevated cholesterol, and diabetes, is most evident in the 20 to 44 years of age range.[66] Further important evidence of the deleterious effect of obesity on the incidence of coronary heart disease arises from the Framingham 26-year follow-up study which shows that obesity is an independent risk factor.[26] More recent studies suggest that the typically masculine deposition of fat in the abdominal area with advancing age, as opposed to the thighs and hips, is a better predictor of coronary artery disease risk than is the degree of obesity, per se.[34,36]

Thus, there is clear evidence of association between obesity and mortality, as well as morbidity predisposition. However, the etiologic relationship between obesity and diseases such as hypertension, coronary heart disease, and diabetes is complex, since they develop in individuals who have never been overweight. Moreover, some individuals who are obese never experience any detectable disease with which obesity is commonly associated.

MEANS TO AID MAN IN ACHIEVING HIS HEALTH POTENTIAL

There are many ways that effective improvement in the length and quality of human life can be made in the U.S. today. The following categories under which significant advances can be made are not necessarily organized in order of importance, but to facilitate a more coherent presentation.

REASSESS PREVALENT NOTIONS OF HEALTH CARE PROVISION

From previous discussion, it should be evident that our current major health problem is chronc degenerative disease. However, responsibility for addressing this concern remains primarily with the traditional health care delivery system—doctors, hospitals, insurance and pharmaceutical companies, and government. This system, according to Kristein and colleagues[33] is better organized to treat those who are sick, rather than helping people stay well. Further, costs to treat an ill person may be considerably above that necessary to keep the person well enough not to need hospitalization for an extended period. While government agencies are increasingly calling attention to the need for effective preventive medicine, only a minority of health insurance policies include coverage for preventive medical services. Few hospitals have organized significant service programs that effectively aid in alleviating the impact of chronic degenerative disease.[33]

The current health care delivery system, at least in terms of advancements in medical science and its application, has not only virtually eradicated infectious disease mortality but, more recently, has played a significant role in reducing coronary heart disease mortality. Further, there is strong reason to support medical research in facilitating discovery of answers to reduce the prevalence, and improve the effective treatment of chronic diseases. However, Insel and Roth[27] have argued strongly that the health care delivery system does not yet provide equitable service to the poor, in general, and minority groups in particular. This contention is substantiated, in part, by the overall mortality rates in the United States compared to many other technologically advanced countries with more equitably distributed health care service. For example, the infant mortality rate in this country is nearly double that in Sweden and ranks behind more than a dozen other countries. Life expectancy for blacks is still notably less than for Caucasians.[27]

Insel and Roth[27] emphasize, however, that no amount of innovations in medicine, medical technology, or in health care delivery can overcome the damage to health that people impose on themselves. Resistance to progressive degenerative disease requires preventive medicine, which entails a primary personal responsibility of each individual to adopt positive health related behavior and to minimize negative factors. Edlin and Golanty[21] also contend that a person's health is primarily the responsibility of the individual and that their primary goal should be prevention of disease via appropriate lifestyle modification.

BETTER EDUCATION OF THE PUBLIC RELATIVE TO PERSONAL HEALTH RESPONSIBILITY

Few Americans are aware of the necessity for personal responsibility to improve their health significantly. Most have been conditioned to believe that the health care delivery industry is responsible for maintaining health when, in fact, it is designed primarily for treating the ill. Instead, it needs to learn more about preventive medicine and health enhancement. In addition to concerns for adverse effects of the physical environment, such as air and water pollution, more concern needs to be given to adverse cultural environmental effects that favor adoption of negative health behaviors. The health care industry—particularly the medical profession, health insurance companies, and government—needs to collaborate in better educating the public, as well as in implementing new programs that encourage preventive med-

icine and individual responsibility in enhancing one's health status.

REDUCE ACCIDENTS

Significant reduction in industrial accident injuries and death rate during the past 40 years is direct evidence that improved health can be achieved by well-conceptualized preventive efforts. Sinacore and Sinacore[59] describe the use of epidemiology in safety research, which considers (1) the host (the person), (2) the agent (those things that inflict injury), and (3) the environment (e.g., highway design, weather, and visibility). Accordingly, efforts are made to reduce the hosts' susceptibility to accidents, render the agent less hazardous, and to modify the environment to make it more accident free. They contend that accident reduction has been achieved primarily via rearrangement of the environment and making agents less hazardous (e.g., utilization of shatterproof glass and padded fixtures in cars). Less success has been realized by accident prevention programs seeking to modify human behavior, yet Edlin and Golanty[21] stress that this area has the most potential of developing effective strategies for reducing accident proneness and drunk drivers (who now account for over one-half of the 50,000 highway fatalities each year).

INDIVIDUAL ADOPTION OF HEALTHY LIFESTYLES

This is the essence of Hoyman's fundamental determinant of health, human ecologic interaction, which represents man's unique capacity to interact with his genetic potential and environment to achieve his individual level of health. He can adopt largely favorable health habits, or succumb to a largely unhealthy lifestyle. The vital importance of this consideration is evidenced by the following quote from the 1979 U.S. Surgeon General's Report on Health Promotion and Disease Prevention:

Collectively, smoking, misuse of alcohol and other drugs, poor dietary habits, lack of regular exercise, and stress place enormous burdens on the health and well-being of many Americans today . . . Although helping people to understand the need for and to act to change detrimental lifestyles cannot be easy, the dramatic potential benefits clearly make the effort worthwhile.[16:138]

REDUCE SMOKING. Fielding[23] observed that cigarette smoking has been identified as the single most important source of preventable morbidity and premature mortality in each of the reports of the U.S. Surgeon General since 1964. The estimated annual excess mortality from cigarette smoking in the United States exceeds 380,000.[68] It is estimated that 170,000 deaths per year from coronary heart disease and 125,000 from cancer (80% of which are lung cancer deaths) are attributable to smoking. COPD accounts for another 62,000 smoking-related deaths.[23] Clearly, there is exceptional potential for improving the public's health by developing more effective means of preventing young people from initiating smoking, and by aiding current smokers to quit permanently.

Since 1973, a substantial downward trend in annual per capita (number of individuals 18 years and older) cigarette consumption has occurred; the 1983 figure of 3,494 down from 4,140 in 1974, was the lowest in 35 years.[23] Still, 35% of men and 29% of women smoked in 1983, though this was down from values of 52 and 34%, respectively, in 1965.

There are about 50 million people who currently smoke and 35 million ex-smokers.[31] Apparently, smoking cessation results in rather quick reduction in coronary heart disease risk, as the incidence of myocardial infarction in men under 55 years of age was similar to that of nonsmokers within 2 years.[54] On the other hand, lung cancer mortality rate in ex-smokers may not return to that of nonsmokers for 15 years, though it is only 40% that of current smokers after 5 years.[18] The mortality risk reduction for COPD in individuals who have already developed the onset of smoking-related respiratory symptoms upon smoking cessation, also may take 10 to 20 years to reach average mortality rates.[53]

STRESS REDUCTION. Edlin and Golanty[21] contend that stress reduction can be achieved by (1) eliminating the stressors in the environment, (2) controlling one's reaction to a given situation, or (3) reducing the magnitude of stress on the body by employing one or more effective techniques on a regular basis. Eliminating stressful situations depends upon one's ability to recognize them and limitations of control in changing the environment. Effective control of one's reaction to persistent stress is largely dependent on objective identification of problems, anticipation of their occurrence, and a "mind-set" that you can now handle it because you're properly prepared (i.e., it's no longer a significant stress).

The important consideration is that one not adopt a failure to cope strategy, including persistent negative thoughts, or reliance on alcohol or drugs for repeated temporary stress relief but which do not provide an effective solution. While stress reduction techniques do not identify the underlying problem, there is growing evidence of their effectiveness. These techniques, involving relaxation and/or cognitive strategies, were discussed in Chapter 4. Their effectiveness in the enhancement of health, however, has not been definitively documented.

ADOPT BETTER NUTRITIONAL HABITS. Efforts at adopting nutritional habits most consistent with preventive medicine have been compromised by two primary factors: (1) deeply ingrained dietary precepts which properly advocated high quality protein in animal and dairy products in prior times of noted deficiency, but which now often result in a diet far too high in fats commensurate with current health concerns; and (2) a "hurry-up" lifestyle with extensive media advertisement for a restricted array of foods that are usually high in simple sugars and/or fat content, and either ready to serve or quickly prepared. Nearly all Americans get enough food in terms of caloric content, but many suffer from malnutrition due to eating a restricted number of foods which often leads to deficiency of essential nutrients. Many also eat foods with high caloric content, especially fats and simple sugars, which contributes to overweight and obesity. Conversely, complex carbohydrate consumption, including dietary fiber content, has dropped.

These dietary habits are not consistent with preventive medicine, in that they are associated with increased incidence of obesity, hypercholesterolemia, and hypertension. Individuals who develop these conditions have increased risk of coronary heart disease, stroke, and diabetes. There is also evidence that the obese individual has a higher risk of cancer[11,38] as do individuals whose routine diet is high in animal products, especially fats, and low in complex carbohydrates.[11]

Given the high visibility of a restricted number of foods in media advertising and the conflicting nutritional information available, responsibility for gaining the most creditable information from one's physician, a dietician or nutritionist, rests largely with the individual. Further, acting on this information to eliminate unsound nutritional habits and replacing them with dietary choices consistent with preventive medicine and attainment of high levels of health remains ultimately the responsibility of each individual.

ADOPT MORE ACTIVE LIFESTYLES. The role of enhanced physical activity in alleviating chronic, degenerative disease amongst individuals living in our advanced technologic and sedentary (hypokinetic) society was examined in concept in Chapter 1. It was clearly evident that enough scientific evidence, together with public health agency recognition, had occurred to justify proper advocacy of enhanced activity levels for children and adults of all ages. Detailed information supporting this contention was developed for children in Chapter 6, and is discussed for adults in the following chapter.

INCREASE THE QUALITY OF LIFE. While most of the discussion in this section has focused on ways of reducing the mortality rate, this is only one marker of health. Its use is prompted primarily by the ready availability of mortality statistics and their wide acceptance as a fundamental criterion of public health status. McCloy[43] argued more than 40 years ago, however, that the length of life was not as important a criterion of health status as the richness and fullness of life. He contended that most adults lived poorly with regard to personal health habits, including lack of adequate exercise. The bottom line of Figure 8–10 depicts, in a qualitative sense, the all too frequently found curve of vitality. The top line represents the condition for which one should strive—and which could be achieved by many adults with appropriate attention to adopting lifestyles consistent with enhancing health status. McCloy contends that such people have high vitality not only in enhanced physical fitness, but also in mental outlook and attitude.[43]

SUMMARY

1. The development of modern sanitation, public health methods, and antibiotic drugs has nearly eradicated infectious diseases as a public health concern.

2. With virtual elimination of infectious diseases, chronic degenerative diseases, such as coronary heart disease, cancer, chronic obstructive pulmonary disease, diabetes, and cirrhosis of the liver have the highest mortality rate.

3. Health and disease are not just complete opposites; there are degrees of each. This means that not only can a person who is ill become well, but that a well person can become healthier.

4. Health encompasses an integrated balance of physical fitness, a mental component, and a spiritual dimension.

5. Physical fitness can be defined as the ability to (a) perform daily tasks efficiently, and without undue fatigue; (b) retain ample reserve to enjoy vigorous leisure time activities; and (c) demonstrate physical activity traits and capacities that are consistent with minimal risk of developing hypokinetic diseases.

6. Mental health extends on a continuum from prolonged periods of primarily successful coping with one's environment and the fulfillment of personal needs, to the most severe mental illness of psychosis, in which there is prolonged gross impairment of one's psychologic functioning

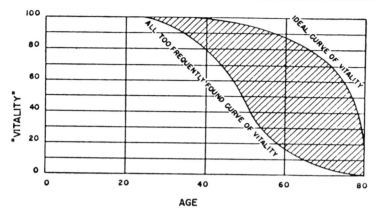

FIG. 8–10. Qualitative comparison of vitality levels with age for a physically active (top line) and sedentary population. (From McCloy, C.H.: Physical education for living. JOHPER. *16(1)*:18–20, and 48–51, 1945.)

and ability to meet even ordinary demands of life.

7. A healthy person generally seeks to transform and transcend himself, and to justify his life by searching for some deeper, more unifying, meaning to life than mere existence or survival.

8. Man's health is determined by an integrative expression of one's heredity, the environment, and human ecologic interaction.

9. About 5% of all humans are born with hereditary defects that result in anatomic or physiologic abnormalities. In addition, predisposition to the occurrence of many other diseases is due, in part, to one's genetic makeup.

10. Human health is both positively and negatively impacted by one's physical, biologic, and sociocultural environment. This means that technologic and scientific advances do not come without a "price."

11. Man has great plasticity and flexibility of behavior, if not free will, which enables each person to interact with his heredity and environment and effect self-directed, unique behavior affecting his level of health.

12. Most of today's principal public health concerns are properly identified not just as chronic, degenerative diseases, but as lifestyle diseases. They include cardiovascular disease, hypertension, cancer, diabetes, chronic obstructive pulmonary dis-

ease, emotional disorders and mental illness, accidents, and obesity.

13. Risk factors associated with increased incidence of coronary heart disease include heredity, age, sex, race, blood lipids, hypertension, and cigarette smoking. Other contributing factors include obesity, physical inactivity, stress, and diabetes.

14. Hypertension is a primary risk factor which enhances heart attack and stroke mortality rates. Principal predisposing factors for the development of hypertension include heredity, obesity, salt intake, alcohol consumption, and psychologic tension.

15. The mortality rate for lung cancer has tripled in the last 40 years at a time when the death rate due to all other forms of cancer has decreased.

16. Bronchitis and emphysema are chronic obstructive pulmonary diseases that arise primarily from prolonged heavy cigarette smoking.

17. Though the number of resident patients in mental hospitals has declined 50% in the last 30 years, this was due to advances in effective drug therapy management that permitted outpatient treatment. The total number of persons with diagnosed mental illness has actually increased, as have those with psychosomatic afflictions.

18. Accidents are the leading cause of death in the U.S. among individuals between the ages of 1 and 40 years. One-half

of the 100,000 accidental deaths each year occur as a result of motor vehicular collision.

19. Those who are grossly overweight for their sex and height are also overfat (obese). However, for most persons one's degree of obesity can best be determined by body composition assessment.

20. While heredity is the primary determinant of obesity, environmental factors, including caloric intake and physical activity level, also have a significant impact on one's body weight.

21. Obesity, in terms of an adult being 40% above average weight, is associated with a near doubling of mortality rate.

22. The nation's public health can be significantly enhanced by more uniform health care delivery across socioeconomic class and by increased attention to preventive medicine.

23. Increased efforts of effective communication to the public that one must assume a personal responsibility for health enhancement must be made if significant reduction in lifestyle disease effects is to be achieved.

24. Individual adoption of healthy lifestyles includes no cigarette smoking, stress reduction, adoption of better nutritional habits, increased physical activity, and a "mind-set" to enhance one's overall quality of life.

REFERENCES

1. American Heart Association. Heart Facts. Dallas: 1986.
2. Association of Life Insurance Medical Directors and Actuarial Society of America. Medico-Actuarial Mortality Investigation. Vol. 1. New York, 1912.
3. Bauer, J.: Genetics of essential hypertension. Acta Genet. Medic. Gemell. 17:577–583, 1968.
4. Belkin, S.C., and T.B. Quigley: Finding the cause of low back pain. Med. Times. 105(7):59–63, 1977.
5. Benditt, E.P.: The origin of atherosclerosis. Sci. Amer. 236(2):74–85, 1977.
6. Bouhuys, A.: The Physiology of Breathing. New York: Grune & Stratton, 1977.
7. Bourne, G.H.: Heart Disease. London: Wyman & Sons, 1955.
8. Bray, G.A.: Complications of obesity. Ann. Intern. Med. 103:1052–1062, 1985.
9. Breslow, L., and J.E. Enstrom: Persistence of health habits and their relationship to mortality. Prevent. Med. 9:469–483, 1980.
10. Castelli, W.P.J.: Risk factors. In Hypertension. Edited by P. Sleight and E.D. Freis. London: Butterworth Scientific, 1982, pp. 1–13.
11. Cimino, J.A., and H.B. Demopoulos: Determinants of cancer relevant to prevention, in the war on cancer. In Cancer and the Environment. Edited by H.B. Demopoulos and M.A. Mehlman. Park Forest South, Ill.: Pathotox, 1980, pp. 1–10.
12. Clarke, H.H.: Application of Measurement to Health and Physical Education. 4th ed. Englewood Cliffs, N.J.: Prentice-Hall, 1967.
13. Cooper, K.H., et al.: Physical fitness levels vs selected coronary risk factors: a cross-sectional study. JAMA. 236(2):166–169, 1976.
14. Cureton, T.K. Jr., et al.: Physical Fitness Appraisal and Guidance. St. Louis: Mosby, 1947.
15. Davidson, M.B.: Diabetes Mellitus: Diagnosis and Treatment. New York: Wiley, 1981.
16. Department of Health, Education and Welfare. Healthy People. The Surgeon General's Report on Health Promotion and Disease Prevention. Washington, D.C., U.S. Government Printing Office, 1979.
17. Dingle, J.H.: The ills of man. Sci. Amer. 229(3):77–84, 1973.
18. Doll, R., and A.B. Hill: Lung cancer and other causes of death in relation to smoking: a second report on the mortality of British doctors. Br. Med. J. 2:1071–1081, 1956.
19. Dublin, L.I., A.J. Lotka, and M. Spiegelman: Length of Life. New York: Ronald Press, 1949 (Revised edition).
20. Dubos, R.J.: Health and disease. JAMA. 174:505–507, 1960.
21. Edlin, G., and E. Golanty: Health & Wellness: A Holistic Approach. 2nd ed. Boston: Jones & Bartlett, 1985.
22. Eisenberg, L.: Psychiatric intervention. Sci. Amer. 229(3):117–127, 1973.
23. Fielding, J.E.: Smoking: health effects and control. N. Engl. J. Med. 313:491–498, 1985.
24. Gordon, E.S.: Metabolic and endocrine factors in weight control. In Weight Control. Edited by E.S. Epright, P. Swanson, and C.A. Iverson. Ames, Iowa: Iowa State College Press, 1955, pp. 160–165.
25. Hoyman, H.S.: Our modern concept of health. J. School Health. 32(7):253–264, 1962.
26. Hubert, H.B., M. Feinleib, P.M. McNamara, and W.P. Castelli: Obesity as an independent risk factor for cardiovascular disease: a 26-year follow-up of participants in the Framingham heart study. Circulation. 67:968–977, 1983.
27. Insel, P.M., and W.T. Roth: Health in a Changing Society. Palo Alto, Calif.: Mayfield, 1976.
28. Jahoda, M.: Current Concepts of Positive Mental Health. Joint Commission of Mental Illness and

Health, Monograph Series, No. 1. New York: Basic Books, 1958.

29. Keim, H.A.: Low back pain. Clin. Symp. *25*:2–32, 1973.

30. Keys, A., H.L. Taylor, and F. Grande: Basal metabolism and age of adult men. Metabolism. *22*:579–587, 1973.

31. Koop, C.F.: A smoke-free society by the year 2000. N.Y. State J. Med. *85*:302–306, 1985.

32. Kraus, H.: The Causes, Prevention and Treatment of Sports Injuries. New York: Playboy Press, 1981, pp. 126–38.

33. Kristein, M.M., C.B. Arnold, and E.L. Wynder: Health economics and preventive care. Science. *195*:457–462, 1977.

34. Lapidus, L., et al.: Distribution of adipose tissue and risk of cardiovascular disease and death: a 12-year follow-up of participants in the population study of women in Gothenburg, Sweden. Br. Med. J. *289*:1257–1261, 1984.

35. LaPlace, J.: Health. 2nd ed. Englewood Cliffs, N.J.: Prentice-Hall, 1976.

36. Larsson, B. et al.: Abdominal adipose tissue distribution, obesity, and risk of cardiovascular disease and death: 13 year follow-up of participants in the study of men born in 1913. Br. Med. J. *288*:1401–1404, 1984.

37. Leon, A.S., and H. Blackburn: The relationship of physical activity to coronary heart disease and life expectancy. Ann. N.Y. Acad. Sci. *301*:561–578, 1977.

38. Lew, E.A., and L. Garfinkel: Variations in mortality by weight among 750,000 men and women. J. Chron. Dis. *32*:563–576, 1979.

39. Martin, R.P., W.L. Haskell, and P.D. Wood: Blood chemistry and lipid profiles of elite distance runners. Ann. N.Y. Acad. Sci. *301*:346–360, 1977.

40. Mayer, J.: Exercise and weight control. In Exercise and Fitness. Edited by S.C. Staley, T.K. Cureton, L.J. Huelster, and A.J. Barry. Chicago: Athletic Institute, 1960, pp. 110–122.

41. Mayer, J.: Genetic factors in human obesity. Ann. N.Y. Acad. Sci. *131*:412–421, 1965.

42. McArdle, W.D., F.I. Katch, and V.L. Katch: Exercise Physiology: Energy, Nutrition, and Human Performance. 3rd ed., Philadelphia: Lea & Febiger, 1991.

43. McCloy, C.H.: Fitness in later life. JOHPER. *16(1)*:18–20, and 48–51, 1945.

44. McCloy, C.H., and N.D. Young: Tests and Measurements in Health and Physical Education. 3rd ed. New York: Appleton-Century-Crofts, 1954.

45. National Center for Health Statistics. Weight by height and age of adults, United States, 1960–1962. Vital and Health Statistics. Public Health Service Publ. No. 1000-Series 11, No. 14, U.S. Government Printing Office, 1966.

46. National Center for Health Statistics. Plan and Operation of the National Health and Nutrition Survey, 1976–1980. Washington, D.C.: U.S. Public Health Service, 1981. DHHS publ. no. (PHS) 81-1317. (Vital and Health Statistics, series 1, no. 15).

47. National Institutes of Health Consensus Development Conference Statement. Health implications of obesity. Ann. Intern. Med. *103*:1073–1077, 1985.

48. National Safety Council. Accident Facts. 1979, p. 23.

49. Notkins, A.L.: The causes of diabetes. Sci. Amer. *241(5)*:62–73, 1979.

50. Pate, R.R.: A new definition of youth fitness. Physician Sportsmed. *11(4)*:77–83, 1983.

51. Report of Inter-Society Commission for Heart Disease Resources. Circulation. *70*:153A–205A, 1984.

52. Report of the Joint National Committee on Detection, Evaluation, and Treatment of High Blood Pressure. NIH Pub. no. 84-1088. Washington, D.C., 1984.

53. Rogot, E., and J.L. Murray: Smoking and causes of death among U.S. veterans: 16 years of observation. Public Health Rep. *95*:213–222, 1980.

54. Rosenberg, L., D.W. Kaufman, S.P. Helmrich, and S. Shapiro: The risk of myocardial infarction after quitting smoking in men under 55 years of age. N. Engl. J. Med. *313*:1511–1514, 1985.

55. Schneidman, E.S.: An overview: personality, motivation and behavior theories. In Suicide, Theory and Clinical Aspects. Edited by L.D. Lankoff and B. Einsidler. Littleton, Mass.: PSG Publ., 1979, pp. 143–163.

56. Selye, H.: The Stress of Life. New York: McGraw-Hill, 1976 (Revised edition).

57. Seltzer, C.C.: Some reevaluations of the Build and Blood Pressure Study, 1959 as related to ponderal index, somatotype and mortality. N. Engl. J. Med. *274*:254–259, 1966.

58. Sheldon, W.H., C.W. Dupertuis, and E. McDermott: Atlas of Men. New York: Harper & Bros., 1954.

59. Sinacore, J.C., and A.C. Sinacore: Health: A Quality of Life. 3rd ed. New York: Macmillan, 1982.

60. Stunkard, A.J., et al.: An adoption study of human obesity. N. Engl. J. Med. *314*:193–198, 1986.

61. Tall, A.R., and D.M. Small: Plasma high density lipoproteins. N. Engl. J. Med. *299*:1232–1236, 1978.

62. Terris, M.: Approaches to an epidemiology of health. Am. J. Pub. Health. *65*:1037–1045, 1975.

63. Trieff, N.M. (editor): Environment and Health. Ann Arbor, Mich.: Ann Arbor Science, 1980.

64. Trunkey, D.D.: Trauma. Sci. Amer. *249(2)*:28–35, 1983.

65. Van Itallie, T.B.: Obesity: adverse effects on health and longevity. Am. J. Clin. Nutr. *32*:2723–2733, 1979.

66. Van Itallie, T.B.: Health implications of over-

weight and obesity in the United States. Ann. Intern. Med. *103*:983–986, 1985.
67. Wamsley, J.R., and J.E. Roberts: Body composition of USAF flying personnel. Aerospace Med. *34*:403–405, 1963.
68. Warner, K.E.: The economics of smoking: dollars and sense. N.Y. State J. Med. *83*:1273–1274, 1983.
69. White, K.L.: Life and death and medicine. Sci. Amer. *229(3)*:23–33, 1973.
70. World Health Organization. Constitution. Geneva: World Health Organization, 1960.
71. World Health Organization Technical Report Series 686. Primary prevention of essential hypertension. Geneva: World Health Organization, 1983.
72. Zanchetti, A., and C. Bartorelli: Central nervous mechanisms in arterial hypertension: experimental and clinical evidence. *In* Hypertension. Edited by J. Genest, et al. New York: McGraw-Hill, 1977, pp. 59–76.

BIBLIOGRAPHY

1. Edlin, G., and E. Golanty: Health and Wellness: A Holistic Approach. 2nd ed. Boston: Jones & Bartlett, 1985.
2. Hoyman, H.S.: Our modern concept of health. J. School Health. *32(7)*:253–264, 1962.
3. Insel, P.M., and W.T. Roth: Health in a Changing Society. Palo Alto, Calif.: Mayfield, 1976.
4. LaPlace, J.: Health. 2nd ed. Englewood Cliffs, N.J.: Prentice-Hall, 1976.
5. Sinacore, J.C., and A.C. Sinacore: Health: A Quality of Life. 3rd ed. New York: Macmillan, 1982.

9

EXERCISE AND CHRONIC DISEASE

INTRODUCTION

The development of major chronic diseases with advancing age was examined in the previous chapter. It was stated that, in essence, such development represents lifestyle diseases, since the way a person lives his/her life with regard to dietary habits, physical activity level, smoking and stress management, greatly influences occurrence and development. The role of each of these factors—except exercise—in contributing to a healthy lifestyle and thus, retarding the effects of chronic disease, was also examined. In this chapter, the effect of exercise training on certain chronic diseases is examined. The importance of medical screening and selection of appropriate activities to minimize the risks from overexertion are also discussed.

OSTEOPOROSIS

Since osteoporosis and the resultant increased incidence of fracture is most common in post-menopausal Caucasian women, interest in the role of physical activity levels has recently centered on this population.[117] Suggestive evidence that prolonged recreational athletic activity (primarily tennis) resulted in significantly higher radial content and density in postmenopausal women, ages 55 to 75 years, compared to an age-matched nonathletic control group, was observed by Jacobson and co-workers.[62] In an early non-randomized longitudinal study, Aloia et al.[1] observed that postmenopausal women who exercised at a moderate intensity for 1 hour, 3 times per week, for 1 year, had an increase in total body calcium, while the control group experienced a decreased total body calcium.

Smith et al.[118] studied the effects of various weightbearing activities performed 3 days per week, 45 minutes per day, for 3 years in women aged 35 to 65 years. The exercise group, when performing upper body strength training, increased bone mineral content of the radius by 3%, while the sedentary control group lost 4% of radius bone mineral content. Simkin and co-workers[112] examined the effect of diverse dynamic loading exercises of the distal forearm in postmenopausal women and observed a 3.8% increase in radius bone density over 1 year, while the sedentary control group showed a 1.9% decrease. Smith and Raab[117] concluded that prophylactic effects of exercise on bone mass in the total skeleton may require a total fitness program that places stress on various bones, with emphasis on those most susceptible to fracture.

Dalsky et al.[28] examined the effect of progressive weightbearing exercise training for 1 hour per day, 3 days a week on postmenopausal women, ages 55 to 70 years. The lumbar mineral content increased significantly within 9 months and was maintained over the 22-month exercise training program. Upon cessation of exercise, the women's bone mineral content reverted toward baseline. Chow and colleagues[23] conducted a randomized group trial to determine if weightbearing strength and aerobic training in postmenopausal women, ages

50 to 62 years, performed for 45 minutes, 3 times per week for 1 year, yielded a greater effect on bone mass of the trunk and upper thigh than weightbearing aerobic training alone. No significant difference in bone mass increases in the trunk and upper thighs was observed between the two training groups, while the sedentary control group showed a decreased bone mass in these areas.

Nelson et al.[89] suggest that greater bone mineral density may result from increased mechanical strain and endocrine changes due to exercise, as well as differences in nutrient intake, which lead to differences in calcium absorption and excretion, and bone formation. Lindsay[75] concluded from his review that effective prevention of osteoporosis consists of dietary and lifestyle alterations—primarily increases in calcium intake and exercise—and the judicious use of estrogens.

OBESITY

The effect of obesity on increased incidence of hypertension and an enhanced mortality rate from diabetes and coronary heart disease were examined in Chapter 8. Also discussed was the etiology of obesity, including genetic predisposition and, in brief, the influence of nutrition and other environmental/behavioral factors.

OVERVIEW OF DIETARY CALORIC RESTRICTION ON WEIGHT REDUCTION IN THE OBESE

Properly prescribed and medically supervised diets of obese patients can effect sufficient caloric restriction to result in body weight losses of 3 to 5 lbs per week over several months. Further, the amount of weight loss tends to be greater in those with greater excess weight at the beginning of a very low calorie diet.[77] However, with very low calorie diets, up to 40% of the weight loss during the first several weeks is water and lean tissue.[17,145] Even after several months, as much as 20% of the total weight loss is lean tissue and water.[145,147]

The most persistent problem, however,

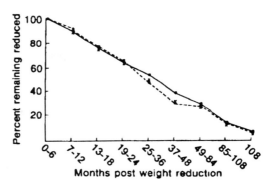

FIG. 9–1. Obese patients who lose a significant amount of body weight via caloric restriction usually fail to maintain that weight loss for more than 3 years. In this study, less than 10 percent were able to maintain their initial weight loss for 9 years. (From Johnson, D., and E.J. Drenick: Therapeutic fasting in morbid obesity. Arch. Intern. Med. 137:1381–1382, 1977, as modified by McArdle, W.D., F.I. Katch, and V.L. Katch: Exercise Physiology: Energy, Nutrition, and Human Performance. 2nd ed. Philadelphia: Lea & Febiger, 1986, p. 547.)

in the clinical treatment of obesity via dietary caloric restriction is the recidivism that occurs. In an early report,[124] 95% of obese subjects returned to their initial weight following significant dietary caloric restriction weight loss within 2 years. Figure 9–1 shows the results of an interesting 9-year follow-up of morbidly obese patients' ability to maintain their initial dietary caloric restriction weight loss. In this study,[63] about 50% of the 121 patients were able to maintain their initial weight reduction for 2 to 3 years, but only 7 patients were able to maintain it over the full 9 years. More recently, Brownell[18] concluded that if "cure" from obesity is defined as reduction to ideal weight and maintenance for 5 years, a person is more likely to recover from many forms of cancer than from obesity.

There appear to be two primary explanations for why dietary caloric restriction weight reduction does not result in effective long-term weight control in the initially overweight. It was mentioned in previous chapters that obesity has a strong genetic component, but that either diet or exercise can alter the total number of fat cells significantly until adulthood (perhaps 25%), whereupon there is essentially no change,[55] unless obesity is particularly severe.[46] The importance of enhanced fat cell number relative to the maintenance of weight loss accomplished by the obese patient, is that their fat cell number is about 3 times greater than the normal adults' 30 billion, while their fat cell size is only about 35% greater.[55] When obese adults lose large amounts of weight, there is essentially no change in fat cell number, but fat cell size can be reduced to a level less than one-fourth their original size, and less than one-half the size of normal weight adults.[54] There is also evidence, both from animal models and from clinical observations, that the body responds to enhance hunger and appetite in order to induce increased caloric intake to return fat cells toward their original size following weight loss induced by caloric restriction.[68]

A related phenomenon to the body's apparent drive to maintain a particular level of body fat is the set point theory. That is, when one undergoes prolonged dietary caloric restriction, there is a substantial reduction in basal metabolic rate.[16,67] Conversely, when normal weight individuals attempt to induce weight gain above their normal weight by force-feeding, the basal metabolic rate increases.[113] In one study of 3000 kilocalories (kcal) caloric restriction per day for 24 days, 6 obese patients averaged a 17% decrease in basal metabolic rate which resulted in only 7% loss in body weight, as compared to a 12½% loss if no change in basal metabolic rate had occurred.[16]

EFFECT OF EXERCISE ON WEIGHT REDUCTION IN THE OBESE

Simply stated, in order to lose a pound of body fat, one must decrease energy intake by 3,500 kcal and/or increase energy expenditure by an amount that results in a net deficit of 3,500 kcal. For many years, exercise was not ascribed a significant role in weight reduction programs because it takes considerable time when engaged in moderate activity to expend 3,500 kcal,

e.g., about 6 hours for a 220-lb person playing tennis.[83] However, the caloric expenditure effects of exercise are cumulative, and our overweight tennis player would use about 3,500 kcal in 6 daily 1 hour sessions of tennis. This would result in a loss of about 1 pound of body fat within a week, provided that caloric intake remained constant.

Regular aerobic exercise has been found to result in significant weight reduction and loss of body fat in obese adults, even without caloric restriction.[9,48,74] In one study,[74] 6 sedentary obese men exercised 5 days per week for 16 weeks by walking vigorously on a treadmill for 90 minutes per day. Their mean body weight loss was 5.7 kg., with percent body fat decreasing from 23.5 to 18.6, but with no significant change in lean body weight. In another study, obese women who walked at least 30 minutes per day, 5 days per week, lost an average of 20 lb at the end of 1 year.[48] Other studies have confirmed the maintenance of lean body weight in exercise-induced weight loss programs and, in some instances a slight increase.[39,133,147]

Exercise effects on obesity appear even more important in terms of coping with disadvantages associated with weight loss achieved via dietary caloric restriction alone. For example, increased daily activity can utilize a portion of fat stored in cells of obese patients who have achieved fat cell size levels below those of normal weight individuals. Also, exercise induces a higher fat metabolism that persists for periods of 18 hours, or more.[7] Presumably, this could reduce the previously described drive to return fat cell size to original levels, at least if exercise is undertaken on a regular daily basis.

While dietary caloric restriction appears to have little, if any, effect on the body fat set point, exercise training seems to lower it so that body weight loss is maintained at a new somewhat lower level than pretraining. Experimental evidence supporting this contention is still sparse but, one study[86] is particularly notable. When 5 obese subjects were placed for 2 weeks on a 500-kcal/day diet, they experienced a gradual reduction in resting metabolic rate to 91% of their predieting level. They then exercised for 20 to 30 minutes per day at about 60% of their $\dot{V}O_{2max}$, whereupon resting metabolic rate increased to control values within 3 to 4 days, and continued to increase over 2-weeks to 105% of control. Conversely, two continuously sedentary individuals who maintained the same 500 kcal/day diet for 4 weeks experienced a reduction in resting metabolic rate that reached 81% of the predieting control level.[121] More research is needed to determine if this distinct difference in basal metabolic rate effected by dietary caloric restriction and exercise is directly associated with an altered set point which influences the efficacy of each for long-term weight control.

SPOT REDUCTION. A persistent objective of some who attempt weight loss regimens is the selective loss of excessive fat stores in particular regions of the body. From regional fat biopsy studies, it is clear that localized exercise, for example sit ups, does not result in a greater loss of fat in the abdominal region than in other areas. Katch and colleagues[64] examined the effects of a 4-week sit up training program to determine the effects on fat cell size in the abdomen, gluteal and subscapular regions, as well as total body fat, skinfold and girth measurements at several locations on the body. They concluded that the conventional sit up exercise does not preferentially reduce adipose cell size or subcutaneous fat thickness in the abdominal region to a greater extent compared to other adipose sites. Despres et al.[30] observed that 20 weeks of intense aerobic training in previously sedentary young adult males produced a body weight loss of 5 lbs, a reduction in body fat from 17.3 to 14.6%, and significant reductions in suprailiac fat cell size and skinfolds at 7 sites. These authors concluded that the training program reduced subcutaneous body fat in the same proportion as total body fat. There was a tendency for a greater percent loss in the trunk skinfold than for skinfold sites in the arms and legs, but this observation has not been confirmed by others.[39,83]

EXERCISE AND FOOD INTAKE

There is no doubt that workers and athletes expending large amounts of energy each day consume diets with significantly higher caloric content than do sedentary individuals, yet routinely maintain below average percent body fat.[83] This observation leads to the conclusion that physical activity level is not uniformly related to caloric expenditure across the full continuum existent in humans. Indeed, there is abundant evidence that the relationship of activity level and caloric intake is not linear, especially in the sedentary range in which man's hypothalamic appetite control mechanism is not as sensitive as that which evolved during a previously enforced vigorous activity regimen before recent industrialization and technologic advancement.[81,135]

In a classic study, Mayer and colleagues[82] exercised free-eating groups of animals, accustomed to a sedentary existence, on a treadmill for periods extending from 20 minutes to 8 hours. As shown in Figure 9–2, the animals who exercised for 20 to 60 minutes each day actually experienced a reduction in caloric intake in this range, with a concurrent decrease in body weight. Between 1 and 6 hours of exercise per day (range of proportional response) resulted in a progressive increase of daily caloric intake, but with constant body weight (i.e., a zone of proportional response and thus, weight control). When daily exercise was extended beyond 6 hours, the animals lost body weight, accompanied by decreased caloric intake and a deteriorated appearance. Passmore[100] confirmed Mayer et al.'s observations in animal experiments, when he demonstrated that food consumption during sedentary periods exceeded food consumption during a period of light exercise. Stevenson et al.[122] observed that single or repeated bouts of exercise in male rats caused an appetite suppression compared to the sedentary control condition. Dohm and colleagues[32] trained three groups of rats at different intensities for 1 hour per day, 6 days per week for 6 weeks, and observed that all ate less and had significantly less body fat than a sedentary control group.

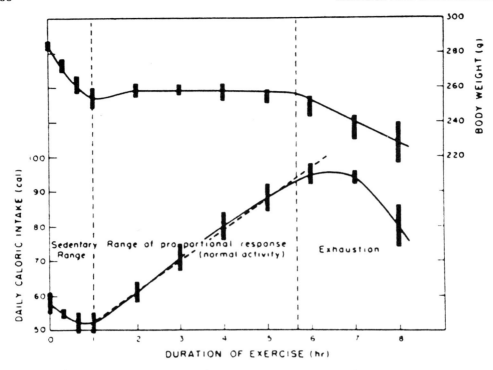

FIG. 9–2. Voluntary caloric intake and body weight as functions of exercise in normal rats. Note that decreased activity in the sedentary range resulted in an increase in caloric intake and body weight. (From Mayer, J. et al.: Exercise, food intake and body weight in normal rats and genetically obese adult mice. Am. J. Physiol. *177*:544–548, 1954.)

Mayer and colleagues[81] essentially confirmed their observations on animals in an epidemiologic study of an industrial population in India engaged in a wide range of physical activity, as depicted along the horizontal axis of Figure 9–3. The diet was nearly uniform in composition within groups and from group to group. It is apparent that those groups who were engaged in moderate to heavy work demonstrated a greater daily caloric intake associated with increased physical activity and a substantially decreased body weight. Experimental evidence suggesting that physical activity may regulate energy balance in humans by affecting energy intake as well as expenditure, is inconclusive. For example, Woo and colleagues[142] found no significant difference in caloric intake over 19 days in 6 obese women randomly assigned to (1) normal sedentary activity, (2) mild treadmill exercise requiring 281 kcal/day (10% above sedentary level), and (3)

moderate treadmill exercise requiring 694 kcal/day (25% above sedentary level). The latter activity level did increase the rate of fat loss significantly. In a study previously cited,[74] it was observed that 6 obese men engaged in vigorous exercise (1,100 kcal/day for 90 minutes), 5 days per week for 16 weeks, experienced a reduced caloric intake during the latter stage of training, though no attempt was made by the investigators to influence food intake.

DIET AND EXERCISE AS THE MOST EFFECTIVE MEANS OF WEIGHT LOSS AND MAINTENANCE

Following review of experimental and clinical research, the American College of Sports Medicine developed a position statement regarding proper and improper weight loss programs.[2] They defined desirable weight loss programs as those that

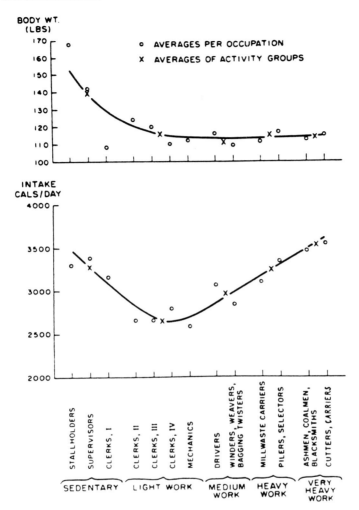

FIG. 9–3. Body weight and caloric intake as functions of physical activity level in an industrial male population, illustrating that sedentary activity is associated with increased caloric intake and body weight in humans. (From Mayer, J., P. Roy, and K.P. Mitra: Relation between caloric intake, body weight, and physical work: studies in an industrial male population in West Bengal. Am. J. Clin. Nutr. 4:169–175, 1956.)

are nutritionally sound and result in maximum losses in fat weight and minimal losses of fat-free tissue. Further, they identified the primary components of a desirable weight loss program as:

1. Provides a caloric intake not lower than 1200 kcal/day for normal adults in order to get a proper blend of foods to meet nutritional requirements. (Note: this requirement may change for children, older individuals, athletes, etc.)

2. Includes foods acceptable to the dieter from viewpoints of sociocultural background, usual habits, taste, cost, and ease in acquisition and preparation.

3. Provides a negative caloric balance (not to exceed 500 to 1000 kcal/day lower than recommended), resulting in gradual weight loss without metabolic derangements. Maximal weight loss should be 1 kg/week.

4. Includes the use of behavior modification techniques to identify and eliminate dieting habits that contribute to improper nutrition.

5. Includes an endurance exercise program of at least 3 days/week, 20 to 30 minutes in duration, at a minimum intensity of 60% of maximum heart rate.
6. Provides that the new eating and physical activity habits can be continued for life in order to maintain the achieved lower body weight.[2;x]

These ACSM guidelines would seem to be most appropriate for the vast majority of obese women (90.5%), as classified by Stunkard.[123] As shown in Table 9–1, Stunkard has identified three classifications of obesity: (1) mild, (2) moderate, and (3) severe, according to the percentage of overweight. In addition to the prevalence of each among obese women, he has identified the type of obesity with regard to increased fat cell size (hypertrophic) and/or increased fat cell number (hyperplastic), treatment methods, and potential for complications. Surgical treatment is advocated only for the most severely obese who have evidence of unusually high fat cell number and a history of repeated failures to lose substantial amounts of weight upon medically supervised very low calorie diets.[123]

Treatment of moderate obesity (41 to 100% above average body weight) consists first of a medically supervised very low calorie diet therapy to effect substantial initial weight loss.[123] Experience, however, has shown that losses of 100 lbs, or more, via very low calorie diets, alone, are poorly maintained. For example, Wadden et al.[138] found that 56% of their patients had regained more than half their initial weight loss within 2 years. Significantly improved persistence in maintaining weight loss in moderately obese patients has been reported when behavior modification, nutrition education, and exercise were added to a very low calorie diet to reach target weight loss.[5] Garrow[44] maintains that exercise is likely to have only minimal impact during the initial stages of treatment in the moderately obese (especially those 65 to 100% above average body weight), because their tolerance for even light to moderate exercise is limited.

For the mildly obese (20 to 40% above average body weight), a combination of caloric restriction plus exercise has been found to facilitate a satisfactory rate of body weight loss, with optimal body composition changes. Zuti and Golding[147] compared the relative effects of diet and exercise on weight loss in moderately obese women. They randomly assigned subjects to 1 of 3 groups for a period of 16 weeks, with each being subjected to a 500 kcal/day deficit. The diet only group continued normal activity with 500 kcal/day caloric restriction. The exercise group engaged in 500 kcal/day of increased activity, over control levels with no change in caloric intake. The third group incorporated 250 kcal/day caloric restriction, together with 250 kcal/day enhanced activity over sedentary control levels. The results are summarized in Figure 9–4; it is readily apparent that all groups experienced no significant difference in the amount of weight loss. However, both the exercise only and the com-

Table 9–1.   A Classification of Obesity, Together With Prevalence, Pathology, Complications, Anatomy, and Treatment of the Three Types*

	Classification of Obesity		
	Mild	Moderate	Severe
Percentage overweight	20–40%	41–100%	>100%
Prevalence (among obese women)	90.5%	9.0%	0.5%
Pathology	Hypertrophic	Hypertrophic, hyperplastic	Hypertrophic, hyperplastic
Complications	Uncertain	Conditional	Severe
Treatment	Behavior therapy (lay)	Diet and behavior therapy (medical)	Surgical

*From Stunkard, A.J.: The current status of treatment for obesity in adults. In Eating and Its Disorders. Edited by A.J. Stunkard and E. Stellar. New York: Raven, 1984, p. 158.

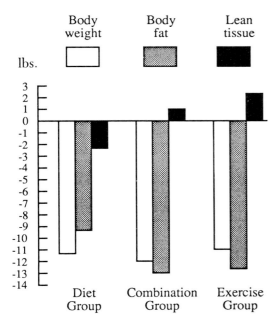

FIG. 9–4. Comparison of the relative effects of diet and/or exercise at the same 500 kcal per day deficit for 16 weeks in moderately obese women. (From Zuti, W.B., and L.A. Golding: Comparing diet and exercise as weight reduction tools. Physician Sportsmed. *4(1):*49–53, 1976.)

bined diet and exercise group demonstrated significantly greater body fat loss, and experienced a slight increase in lean body weight, while the diet only group lost about 2 lbs of lean tissue. The latter could not be attributed to reduced protein intake, per se, as these women had an average protein intake of 71 g/day. Other studies in which diet only caloric restriction and the same dietary caloric restriction with added exercise were compared, have shown a greater weight loss effect, with reduced, or no loss in lean body mass for the added exercise regimen.[140,142]

An even more important value of exercise as an adjunct to dietary caloric restriction is the observed improvement in weight loss maintenance compared to caloric restriction alone. In a review of 105 reports of the effects of weight loss programs (with subsequently high recidivism), Le Bow[73] found that 80% of these studies taught clients to change eating habits, but failed to teach them about the importance of increasing energy expenditure. Subsequently, the vital importance of increased physical activity on the persistence of weight loss has been demonstrated in numerous studies.[19,24,27,120,125] Colvin and Olson[24] concluded from their study and review of results from other studies that exercise is systematically identified as a fundamental component for the majority of individuals who have successfully maintained significant weight loss for 1 to 5 years.

Brownell[18] has astutely noted that ordinarily advocated exercise intensity and duration are not well tolerated by many obese patients. However, starting with low levels of exercise, together with persistent admonition to increase their physical activity throughout the day, can significantly aid in weight loss and result in enhanced weight loss maintenance for most obese individuals. The value of commitment to an eventually substantial increase in exercise over time has been reported by Tremblay et al.[132] Five formerly obese male runners (average initial body weight of 236 lbs) had a mean body weight of 149 lbs after an average of 5.2 years of endurance running and competition. Their mean percent body fat at the time of study (mean age = 32.6 yrs.) was 14.3; if it is assumed that there was no change in lean body mass, their initial body fat 5.2 years previous would have been 46.4%. While 3 of the 5 formerly obese runners had also made adjustments in their diet, their average weight loss on a mean weekly training dose of 60 miles at the time of study was not different than the 2 runners who had made no conscious change in their diet. The formerly obese runners' mean fat cell size was 33% lower than a group of sedentary controls.

Also of concern is the use of vigorous aerobic exercise to alleviate the gradual weight gain through middle age (i.e., creeping obesity) that is characteristic of most of the adult population in Western countries. Utilizing a similar retrospective technique as Tremblay et al.,[132] we (Adams, unpublished observations) found that a group of 7 middle-aged males (mean age = 40 years at the time of study), weighed 165 lbs following an average of 6.8 years of

5 to 6 days of aerobic running (mean distance = 38 miles per week). Their measured percent body fat was 15.2%, compared to 23.5% for a sedentary control group of similar age. Assuming no change in lean body mass with training, the runners' mean body fat percent at age 33 years (when their body weight was 185 lbs) would have been 24.3%, which is slightly above the 23.0% average value reported by Durnin and Womersley.[34]

COMPLEXITY OF TREATMENT FOR OBESITY AND WEIGHT CONTROL

While previous discussion has underlined the high recidivism of obese patients following substantial weight loss via dietary caloric restriction, even programs incorporating behavior modification, including attention to energy expenditure via increased physical activity, are far from totally successful.[123] Van Itallie has reviewed this fundamental problem and states:

One explanation for the recidivism of reduced obese patients could turn out to be the same as the explanation for the existence of much obesity in the first place; namely, our culture predisposes to obesity by providing us with unlimited quantities of readily available food that is calorically concentrated (high in fat and sugar), palatable, and varied. On the other hand, our culture does not provide us with an environment that requires us to expend many calories; indeed, we are encouraged to be sedentary. The recent preoccupation with jogging, running, tennis, etc., is certainly an antisedentary trend, but nationwide those involved in such activities remain a small minority. In any case, it is widely recognized that, although obese individuals drastically reduce calorie intake during weight reduction, few really learn how to make appropriate changes in their eating and exercise behavior. And of those who do learn, few manage to apply what they have learned so as to avoid weight regain at some later time.[135:111]

Van Itallie[135] concludes that while it is not impossible for many formerly obese patients with adipose tissue hyperplasia to maintain weight loss, it is exceedingly difficult. Thus, more attention should be given to preventing obesity, rather than investing too high a proportion of available resources in seeking new treatment strategies. de Vries concurs with this notion, advising the early development of appropriate life-long habits as the most effective means of long-term weight control, and states:

It should be emphasized that weight is best controlled as a matter of childhood habit formation, which then automatically takes care of the long haul. This habit formation should include the development of physical skills that will permit, indeed encourage and motivate, regular participation in vigorous activity. Individuals who develop these skills and participate in them regularly—at least twice and preferably three or four times a week—will seldom have to be unduly concerned about their diet.[31:352]

HYPERTENSION

It was mentioned in Chapter 8 that hypertension is of particular health importance because of its association as a primary risk factor for enhanced heart attack and stroke mortality rates. Further, it was stated that, though genetics was a principal predisposing factor, lifestyle factors, viz., obesity, salt intake, and stress-induced psychologic tension, were also of substantial importance.

Results from large clinical trials in several countries have clearly demonstrated the efficacy of reducing elevated blood pressure in terms of cardiovascular morbidity and mortality.[60] Most hypertension can be treated with drugs (primarily beta-blockers or diuretics) that either reduce cardiac output and/or total peripheral resistance. While this therapy is quite effective for severe, persistent hypertension, there are side effects, cost, and compliance considerations.[49,127] For these reasons, numerous studies have examined the efficacy of non-pharmacologic therapy to manage hypertension. Most of these studies suggest effective management via reduced body weight, lower salt intake, stress reduction, and/or enhanced physical activity.[84,131] Exercise appears to present an attractive intervention, particularly for one with mild hypertension.[11,49] Further, though weight reduction in the obese clearly results in decreased blood pressure in hypertensive individuals, there is evidence of a separate effect of exercise beyond that induced by weight loss alone.[58]

All types of exercise intervention, extending from stretching to aerobics and strength training, could potentially provide the same chronic effect on blood pressure.[128] However, of particular concern is the disparate acute blood pressure response of isometric and heavy resistance, low repetition strength training regimens that induce extremely high blood pressures[78] in contrast to the more moderate elevations seen with moderate resistance, high repetition aerobic training loads.[127] Because of the extreme acute blood pressure response induced by heavy resistance exercise, it is not recommended as exercise therapy for hypertensive patients.[83,127]

Aerobic exercise training results in lower blood pressure at any given submaximal workload due to reduced heart rate and usually, reduced cardiac output.[83,131] This reduced work of the heart during exercise occurs through a reduction of sympathetic tone and/or an increased vagal tone. Since hypertension is determined on the basis of resting blood pressures, there have been numerous studies of the effects of exercise training on both normotensive and hypertensive subjects. There is no clear evidence of any effect of exercise training on resting blood pressures in young adults with pretraining values of 125/85 mmHg, or lower.[131]

In 1986, Hagberg and Seals[49] reviewed 16 published studies in which the effects of exercise training on patients with mild to moderate hypertension had been examined. The average reduction in blood pressures over the course of exercise training was 11 mmHg for resting systolic pressure and 8 mmHg for diastolic pressure. Unfortunately, many of these studies had design and methodologic problems, including lack of a non-exercising control group, use of only a small group of subjects, and most usually, middle-aged males of varied hypertension levels.[111]

Duncan and colleagues[33] studied the effects of 16 weeks of aerobic fast walking and jogging for 60 minutes, 3 days per week in 44 adult males (mean age, 30.4 years) with mild hypertension. Their systolic pressure decreased significantly from

146 to 134 mm Hg, while diastolic pressure decreased from 94 to 87 mm Hg, with the sedentary control group experiencing no significant change in either. Roman et al.,[108] utilizing subjects as their own controls, examined the effects of varied activity levels in 27 female adult hypertensive subjects (mean age, 37 years). Three months of aerobic training, 3 days per week for 30 minutes per day, at 70% of maximum heart rate, resulted in a decrease of systolic pressure from 182 to 161 mmHg, while diastolic pressure fell from 113 to 96 mmHg. After 3 months of detraining, blood pressures had returned to pretraining levels (i.e., 179/113 mmHg). Following a second training period of 1 year, the group's blood pressures fell to 159/95 mmHg.

Hagberg and Seals[49] contend that the threshold intensity for eliciting reduced blood pressures in hypertensives may be below that necessary to produce increased cardiorespiratory endurance. Kiyonaga et al.[69] observed that hypertensive subjects (mean age, 46 years) experienced a significant reduction in resting blood pressures after 10 weeks training at a moderate intensity (less than 40% of $\dot{V}O_{2max}$), 3 times per week for 60 minutes per session.

There is now increasingly impressive evidence from large epidemiologic studies that routine vigorous exercise is related to a lower risk of developing hypertension.[11] Paffenberger and colleagues[99] followed a cohort of 15,000 Harvard alumni for up to 10 years, 16 to 50 years after entering college. They found that those who participated regularly in vigorous sports, such as running, swimming, handball, and cross-country skiing, had a 35% lower risk of developing hypertension than those who were sedentary. This relationship was independent of other predictors of increased risk of hypertension, such as high weight to height ratio, weight gain since college, and history of parental hypertension. In another study, 6,000 healthy normotensive males and females (mean age, 41 years) were followed for 1 to 12 years (median of 4 years) to determine if their initial level of physical fitness—assessed by maximal treadmill testing—was related to the development of hypertension.[13] Those individuals with low levels of initial fitness were found to evidence a 52% greater incidence of developing hypertension (i.e., 140/90 mmHg) than the high fitness group. This relationship appeared to be independent of sex, age, follow-up interval, and initial blood pressure and weight to height ratio. Following review of exercise and hypertension studies, McKinney and Mellion[84] concluded that the results suggest a preventive role for exercise, and that it may be useful as a prophylactic measure for persons at risk for developing hypertension.

Physiologic mechanisms associated with the depressor effect of aerobic exercise training on hypertensives are currently under investigation.[49,66] Since blood pressure is equal to the product of cardiac output (blood flow) and total peripheral resistance, research interest has been directed toward both central and peripheral changes. Reduced heart rate is a near universal resultant of exercise training, with only a modest increase in stroke volume, thus resulting in decreased cardiac output.[49,83,131] There is also evidence of reduced peripheral resistance which, together with reduced cardiac output, suggests reduced central and peripheral sympathetic nervous system activity. The latter is associated with reduced resting catecholamine levels and/or reduced receptor sensitivity.[33,49,131] There is also evidence of enhanced parasympathetic nervous system activity accounting for decreased resting heart rate. Exercise training of hypertensives appears to influence renal function, such that the adverse effects of sodium retention are reduced.[10,90,131]

DIABETES

While physical activity has been considered beneficial for individuals with diabetes mellitus for centuries, some patients experience clinical deterioration following heavy exercise. Hence, it has become apparent that the effects of exercise differ among the spectrum of patients with diabetes, and that the benefits (and risks) of exercise are dependent on the specific type

of diabetes and the individual patient's state of metabolic control.[136]

Two main forms of diabetes have been identified: (1) Type I, which is characterized by a deficiency of insulin production and usually manifested before adulthood; and (2) Type II, formerly called "maturity-onset diabetes," which arises in the middle-aged and elderly, particularly in those who are obese, and is characterized by insulin receptor site loss or insensitivity. Type I (insulin-dependent) diabetes, fortunately, represents less than 10% of all cases. Type II (noninsulin-dependent) diabetes is found in more than 80% of diabetics and is strongly associated with obesity.[35] The latter is amenable to diet, exercise, and oral drug therapy.

Effective treatment of diabetes depends on the control of blood glucose levels in the absence of insulin production, receptor site loss and/or insensitivity. The insulin dependent patient seeks to maintain blood glucose levels at near normal levels via periodic insulin injections. This can be effectively managed by Type I diabetics if diet and activity are maintained near constant on a daily basis. De Fronzo and colleagues[29] have demonstrated that exercise training induces an enhanced insulin sensitivity in Type I diabetics which is similar to that observed in normal individuals following training. This usually results in the need to decrease insulin by up to 50%.[105] However, this does not automatically result in improved blood glucose control. In fact, some diabetics experience a significant (and potentially dangerous) hypoglycemic response upon undertaking vigorous exercise due to the elevated skeletal muscle glucose utilization and simultaneous increase in insulin supply from the increased circulation rate induced by exercise.[139] Kemmer and Berger[65] have observed that small amounts of carbohydrate taken before, during and/or after exercise, such as jogging for 1 to 2 miles or cycling for 30 minutes, can usually prevent hypoglycemia.

Exercise training is not recommended in insulin dependent patients unless blood glucose levels can be effectively maintained by a combination of insulin reduction and dietary manipulation. Once this is achieved, Virtug et al.[136] recommend aerobic exercise of 20 to 40 minutes duration at 50 to 60% of $\dot{V}O_{2max}$, 4 to 7 days per week, performed in the morning. Though this generally does not improve blood glucose control in diabetics, under appropriate medical supervision, exercise training can enhance exercise capacity in these patients, thus permitting participation in sports and other active leisure-time activities available to the normal individual. Other benefits of exercise training for the Type I diabetic include possible reduction in the development of atherosclerosis[136] and as an aid in reducing obesity.[35]

The importance of physical activity in Type II (noninsulin-dependent) diabetes is more readily apparent. Whereas about 7% of individuals, age 20 to 74 years, have diabetes in the United States, the Pima Indians in Arizona and some Micronesian and Melanesian populations in the Pacific region now have a 20% incidence in the adult population, though the disease was relatively rare several decades ago. Ekoe[35] contends that, though diabetes is strongly genetically determined, heredity cannot totally explain this high rate. Rather, lack of physical activity, superimposed on overnutrition, plays a fundamental role. Taylor and co-workers[129] have found double the incidence of Type II diabetes in sedentary Melanesian and Indian men in the Fiji Islands, compared to their physically active counterparts, which could not be ascribed simply to differences in body weight. It was observed in another study[61] that Sumo wrestlers, who are well known for their extremely large body weight, experience a high rate of diabetes upon cessation of training at an age of about 35 to 40 years.

In addition to exercise's role in preventing or diminishing the likelihood of Type II diabetes developing, there is also increasing evidence that exercise training can improve the noninsulin dependent diabetic's condition. One important role is to reduce other cardiovascular disease risk factors (such as hypertension and obesity) which occur with greater frequency in diabetics.[105] Another role is as an important adjunct in achieving effective metabolic control without medication in non-insulin dependent patients, many of whom had previously maintained serum glucose levels only via oral hypoglycemic agents or insulin.[6] A combination of 26 days of intensive dietary modification (increased complex-carbohydrate and fiber, and reduced fat) and exercise resulted in significantly reduced fasting blood glucose (from 195 to 145 mg/100 dl) in 60 noninsulin dependent patients, with 34 of 40 patients taking oral hypoglycemic agents or insulin able to achieve similar fasting glucose levels without continuing medication.[6]

Other studies of the effects of exercise without intensive dietary modification in patients with Type II diabetes have shown only modest changes in plasma insulin levels and glucose tolerance.[105] Further, in one study in which metabolic control in Type II patients was improved by diet and weight loss, addition of exercise resulted in only a slight additional effect.[14] Rogers[106] has observed that most previous studies of the effects of exercise training on glucose tolerance in Type II diabetics, utilized relatively low intensity exercise and measured glucose tolerance 3 to 7 days following the last training session. Schneider et al.[110] observed that 6 weeks of training, 3 times per week for 30 minutes at 60% of $\dot{V}O_{2max}$, resulted in lower fasting glucose levels and improved glucose tolerance at 12 hours, but not 72 hours following the last exercise session.

Holloszy and colleagues[56] have shown that cardiac rehabilitation patients with Type II diabetes and impaired glucose tolerance were able to normalize their glucose tolerance (despite a marked blunting of their insulin response to the glucose load) following 12 months of aerobic exercise training, including the last 6 months at 5 days per week for 50 to 60 minutes each, at an intensity of 70 to 85% of $\dot{V}O_{2max}$. They performed their final glucose tolerance test within 18 hours following the last training session. These results, together with the observations of Rogers et al.[107] that 7 consecutive days of 50 to 60 minutes exercise at 68% of $\dot{V}O_{2max}$ significantly improved glucose tolerance and insulin resistance in 10 patients with mild Type II diabetes, suggest that exercise training must be performed regularly and vigorously to produce improved metabolic control in these patients.

CORONARY HEART DISEASE

EPIDEMIOLOGIC EVIDENCE OF THE ROLE OF PHYSICAL ACTIVITY IN THE INCIDENCE OF CORONARY HEART DISEASE

The American Heart Association[3] has identified cigarette smoking, high blood cholesterol, and hypertension as major risk factors associated with increased incidence of coronary heart disease that can be changed. Upon review of relevant evidence, Oberman[92] concluded that by 1983, the role of physical activity as an important risk factor for coronary heart disease had not been firmly established, though there was strong evidence from multiple sources supporting this contention.

In 1987, Powell and colleagues[104] conducted a critical review of 121 studies published in English obtained from a computerized search of the literature on physical activity and the incidence of coronary heart disease. They examined these studies with respect to consistency of findings, strength of the association, appropriate temporal sequence, dose-response relationship, biologic coherence, and experimental evidence (i.e., the criteria used to establish the causal relationship of smoking and cancer). These authors concluded that observations in the literature supported the inference that physical activity is inversely and causally related to the incidence of coronary heart disease. Of particular interest was the strength of this association in terms of a median relative risk of 1.9 between physical inactivity and coronary heart disease. This value was closely comparable to risk ratios for elevated systolic blood pressure (2.1 for >150 mm Hg versus those with <130 mm Hg), 2.4 for serum cholesterol (>268 mg/dl versus <218 mg/dl), and 2.5 for smoking (>1 pack of cigarettes/day versus no smoking) determined from a pooling of data from 5 large clinical trials.[130] Of further interest is that the estimate of adult prevalence for each of the three primary risk factors at the upper levels given above was much less than that for physical in-

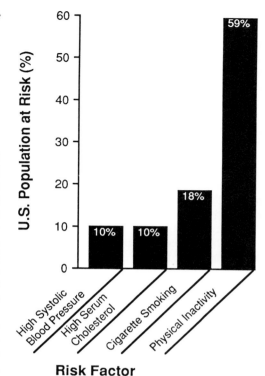

Risk Factor

FIG. 9–5. Percentage of U.S. adult population at risk for recognized major risk factors of coronary heart disease vs. that for physical inactivity. (From Casperson, C.J.: Physical inactivity and coronary heart disease. Physician Sportsmed. *15(11)*:43–44, 1987.)

activity, compared to one who exercises for 20 minutes 3 times per week (Fig. 9–5).

The observed inverse association between physical inactivity and the incidence of coronary heart disease could indicate either a direct protective effect of exercise, or that exercise indirectly reduces the risk of coronary heart disease by its effect on other risk factors, or both. Evidence for the effect of exercise training on obesity, hypertension, and diabetes (all associated with enhanced incidence of coronary heart disease) was reviewed earlier in this chapter. Powell et al.[104] found that studies which accounted for age, sex, blood pressure, smoking status, serum cholesterol, and obesity were just as likely to find an association between physical inactivity and coronary heart disease as those that did not make these adjustments, though the risk ratio for physical inactivity was reduced somewhat. In their review, Siscovick et al.[114] observed that the difference in incidence related to habitual activity was greatest for persons who were older, hypertensive, or obese, suggesting that habitually active people with other risk factors may benefit the most.

In addition to accounting for the effect of other risk factors on the inverse relationship of physical activity and coronary heart disease incidence, more recent studies have sought to isolate inactive versus active group pre-selection in arriving at whether habitual activity level has a protective effect. These have included (1) starting with a screened healthy population, thus minimizing the potential confounding that results from sick persons who tend to be less active; (2) examining whether those in the inactive group develop coronary heart disease earlier during follow-up because of subclinical manifestations not identified in initial screening; and (3) examining whether changes in job classification altered the relationship between activity level and coronary heart disease. Morris et al.[88] concluded that excluding cases of coronary heart disease that occurred early in the follow-up period did not alter the inverse relationship with physical activity among those who survived for longer periods. Further, they found that the misclassification produced by minimally ill persons shifting to the inactive group was not large enough to affect the inverse relationship for the cohort studied. Brand et al.[15] also observed that changes in job classification did not significantly affect the inverse relationship between job activity level and coronary heart disease incidence.

Studies utilizing the above methods to attenuate the potential preselection bias in the comparison of activity level and coronary heart disease indicate that the relationship exists for both occupational and leisure-time activity. Paffenbarger and Hale[97] followed about 4,000 San Francisco longshoremen over 21 years, keeping accurate, detailed records of job assignments, some of which required 3 to 4 times more energy (heavy) than others (light). The longshoremen were surveyed annually for job transfers and changes in work energy output. The heavy energy expenditure work group experienced an age-adjusted mortality rate of less than 60% that of the light energy expenditure group. When deceased workers were classified on the basis of the job they held 6 months before death, excluding men with job transfers did not significantly alter the otherwise observed risk ratio.

Few occupations today necessitate a significant energy expenditure demand. Thus, Morris and colleagues[87] hypothesized that contributions to health from exercise would occur primarily during leisure time. These authors studied nearly 18,000 middle-aged male office workers in the English Civil Service, beginning in 1968. After 8½ years, they found that the men who had engaged in regular vigorous exercise—defined as 7.5 kcal/min, or about 1.5 liters/min of $\dot{V}O_2$—had a relative risk of coronary heart disease of less than ½ that of their sedentary counterparts. As depicted in Figure 9–6, the most marked difference was observed in the older age groups. The effect of physical activity on the incidence of coronary heart disease was found to be independent of obesity and cigarette smoking.

Slattery et al.[116] followed 2,600 white male railroad workers, initially screened for absence of cardiovascular disease, for 17 to 20 years. These authors surveyed the leisure-time activity of the men, and categorized them from sedentary (equivalent to less than 10 minutes of light activity per day) to very active (equivalent to about 45 minutes per day of activity at moderate intensity). The workers' jobs were categorized as either sedentary or active. The authors found that after adjustment for age, those men who were sedentary had a 1.39 times greater risk for coronary heart disease than did the most active leisure time group. Even when adjusted for the effects of smoking, high blood pressure, and cholesterol levels, the effect of leisure time activity remained independent and significant. The authors also noted that high leisure time activity reduced the risk for men with sedentary jobs more than for those with active jobs.

In an ongoing study of 17,000 Harvard

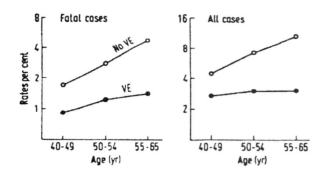

FIG. 9–6. Civil servants who exercised vigorously (VE) during leisure-time demonstrated significantly lower rates of fatal and nonfatal coronary heart disease events than did those who did no vigorous exercise (No VE). (From Morris, J.N., R. Pollard, M.G. Everitt, and S.P.W. Chave: Vigorous exercise in leisure-time: protection against coronary heart disease. Lancet. 2:1207–1210, 1980.)

University alumni, Paffenbarger et al.[98] have addressed the consideration of whether "constitutional" factors associated with college athletic participation (versus post-college exercise levels) were associated with coronary heart disease incidence. The group of alumni studied during 12 to 16 years of follow-up were aged 35 to 74 years at the initiation of the study. In addition to determining whether they had participated in athletics during college, the alumni were surveyed to determine postgraduate hours per week of sports activity, stairs climbed, and walking, which were categorized as <500, 500 to 2,000, and >2,000 kcal per week of exercise (the latter represents about 20 miles per week of walking or jogging for a man of average size). The authors found that the more sedentary alumni had 49% excess risk for coronary heart disease than did the group with high habitual post-college exercise. The varsity athletes who became sedentary had a similar elevated risk as sedentary nonathletes, compared to sedentary students who became physically active following graduation.

Though the study by Paffenbarger et al.[98] showed significantly lower risk of coronary heart disease in alumni who expended greater than 2,000 kcal per week in walking, climbing stairs, and sports play, they maintain that the types and amount of exercise likely to achieve optimum cardiovascular health are uncertain. Haskell[52] has observed that most exercise training regimens have been primarily evaluated according to their effect on the subject population's aerobic power or endurance. He concludes that health benefits of exercise may occur in conjunction with improvement in physical performance capacity, but that there is accumulating evidence suggesting that some health benefits appear to be achieved by exercise that does not necessarily result in improved physical fitness. However, constancy of habit, i.e., regular sustained exercise during 9 or more months of the year, appears necessary to maintain cardiovascular health.[79]

PHYSIOLOGIC MECHANISMS BY WHICH EXERCISE CAN PROTECT AGAINST CORONARY HEART DISEASE

In addition to reducing the impact of risk factors previously discussed, viz., hypertension, obesity, diabetes, and stress, there is also evidence that exercise may retard the atherosclerotic process, improve myocardial function, and improve the ratio of myocardial oxygen supply versus demand.

EFFECT ON ATHEROGENIC DEVELOPMENT. Coronary heart disease arises from the gradual buildup of fatty deposits (largely cholesterol and triglycerides) on the inner arterial walls. Kramsch and co-workers[70] studied the effects of 3 to 4 years of exercise equivalent to 1 hour of jogging, 3 times per week, on Malaysian monkeys fed an atherogenic diet. At the end of the experiment, these authors observed significantly less atherosclerotic development in the coronary arteries of the exercise group than in the sedentary control group. Similarly, Link et al.[76] observed that pigs who performed daily treadmill running for 10 minutes at 10 mph, 5 days per week, for 22 months, had substantially less fatty deposits in their coronary arteries than did the sedentary controls. Few comparisons of the development of coronary atherosclerosis in active and sedentary humans have been made, with no substantive difference observed in one postmortem study.[119]

EFFECT ON BLOOD LIPIDS. One means of retarding the rate of atherosclerotic buildup is the reduction of blood lipids, primarily cholesterol and triglycerides. Following review of studies examining the effects of exercise therapy on cholesterol. Superko and Haskell[126] concluded that cholesterol level does not change appreciably unless accompanied by diet alterations and/or body weight (fat) loss.

However, Haskell[51] contends that the lack of any substantial change in total cholesterol directly attributable to exercise training may obscure changes in the concentrations of cholesterol transported as part of the specific lipoprotein carriers, viz., low density lipoprotein, associated with transport and deposition of fat on the arterial wall, and high density lipoprotein, which has been shown to transport cholesterol out of the arterial wall to the liver for excretion and is the lipid subfraction inversely associated with coronary heart disease incidence.[21]

High density lipoprotein levels are higher in middle-aged male runners[143] and are generally increased in sedentary men who undertake aerobic endurance training.[126,144] Evidence suggests that a threshold of greater than the equivalent of 10 miles per week of jogging for several months is required before significant increases in high density lipoprotein levels occur, with somewhat larger changes induced with increasing levels of exercise.[51]

While fasting triglyceride concentration is not considered an independent risk factor for coronary heart disease, the triglyceride-rich very low density lipoprotein may be atherogenic.[146] Endurance exercise usually decreases triglyceride levels when the pretraining values are elevated, but not when pretraining values are relatively low.[51] The triglyceride lowering effect appears to have an acute component that is more apparent following vigorous exercise.[25]

INCREASED MYOCARDIAL OXYGEN SUPPLY. Atherosclerotic buildup in the coronary arteries can eventually result in inadequate oxygen supply to the myocardium. Limited evidence suggests that exercise training can improve myocardial oxygen supply by one, or more, of several means. Kramsch et al.,[70] in a study previously cited, observed larger coronary artery size in monkeys following prolonged exercise training. Similar observations have been obtained in other animal models, but there is only limited evidence that exercise training in humans induces a similar effect. Currens and White[26] reported interesting observations on Clarence DeMar, who was a champion marathon runner and continued training and competition into later life. Upon death from cancer at age 69, an autopsy performed on DeMar revealed only a mild degree of atherosclerosis, and that his coronary arteries were 3 times larger than normal for a man his age and size. Though one cannot presume cause and effect on the results from study of one individual, the authors speculated that their autopsy findings were, at least in part, a result of DeMar's prolonged vigorous endurance training.

Coronary collaterals, which are small vessels that connect coronary arteries and/or their branches, can provide alternate routes of myocardial blood supply when usual routes are restricted by atherosclerotic buildup. Exercise training in animal models, in which partial coronary occlusion is surgically induced, has been shown to enhance coronary collateral development.[41] However, angiographic studies of coronary heart disease patients following 3 to 13 months of exercise training have not revealed collateral vessel development. The latter may be due, in part, to the angiographic technique not being sensitive enough to detect meaningful changes in coronary collateral development.[92]

Exercise may also enhance fibrinolytic capacity of the blood, which improves dissolution of blood clots. Exercise training has been shown to augment the fibrinolytic response to venous occlusion in healthy adults[141] and might reduce the incidence of coronary thrombosis.[104]

DECREASED MYOCARDIAL WORK AND OXYGEN DEMAND. Aerobic exercise training induces decreased heart rate and systolic blood pressure at rest and during submaximal work. Since the product of heart rate and systolic blood pressure is well related to the oxygen demand of the myocardium, this means that there is less cardiac work for a given amount of total body work. This is of particular importance to an older person with reduced oxygen supply due to atherosclerotic buildup, in that it results in an increased exercise tolerance and higher values for heart rate and systolic blood pressure before lack of adequate myocardial oxygen supply develops.[91] There is also suggestive evidence that aerobic exercise training enhances the myocardial contractile process in rats,[85,109] although human echocardiographic data from longitudinal and cross-sectional studies do not reveal significant training effects on myocardial contractile performance.[101]

ENHANCED MYOCARDIAL ELECTRICAL STABILITY. Aerobic exercise training increases cardiac parasympathetic tone, which has been shown to modify cardiac electrostability, such that reduced incidence of ventricular fibrillation during cardiac ischemia was observed in dogs that were identified as susceptible to sudden cardiac death.[8] Epstein et al.[36] found that middle-aged males engaged in a sedentary occupation, but who engaged in vigorous leisure-time activity, had significantly less evidence of cardiac dysrhythmias than those who were not vigorously active during leisure time.

USE OF EXERCISE STRESS TESTING IN THE DETECTION OF CORONARY HEART DISEASE

Typically, an exercise stress test entails progressive work intensity increments to maximal voluntary effort, or to a symptom limited endpoint (Fig. 9–7). An enhanced myocardial oxygen demand is effected which, in persons with significant coronary atherosclerosis, often reveals inadequacies in oxygen supply that results in ischemia. This procedure has been used successfully in combination with electrocardiographic response as a prominent noninvasive diagnostic means to identify subtle signs of coronary heart disease not evident at rest. Also assessed is the occurrence of effort-induced angina pectoris, a temporary but painful condition that indicates myocardial oxygen deficiency. This condition represents a 30% incidence of initially identifiable manifestation of coronary heart disease.[4]

Electrocardiographic response to exercise stress indicative of coronary heart disease is evaluated in terms of myocardial oxygen deficiency (ischemia) and certain cardiac rhythm abnormalities. Exercise-induced ischemia[42] and ventricular arrhythmias[45] have both been found to correlate well with more sophisticated invasive methods of determining the existence of significant atherosclerosis in one or more coronary arteries (usually assessed by coronary angiography, a technique requiring injection of an opaque fluid via catheterization into the coronary circulation so that a series of x rays reveal specific sites of arterial narrowing). The occurrence of exercise-induced premature ventricular contractions have been associated not only with the degree of coronary atherosclerosis, but with enhanced mortality and sudden death.[12] The latter is of particular importance, since the incidence of sudden death in one study was about 8 times higher in a group with frequent ventricular arrhythmias, compared to other individuals with evidence of coronary disease but without these arrhythmias.[22]

Exercise stress testing in the detection of coronary heart disease in asymptomatic individuals is subject to error, in that it identifies about 40% of individuals as having coronary heart disease when subsequent, more precise tests do not indicate this (i.e., false-positive), and vice versa (false-negative).[40] Nonetheless, exercise stress testing remains an extremely valuable cost-effective, non-invasive method of detecting coronary heart disease in asymptomatic persons. For example, with the electrocardiographic response, it provides a much better prediction of individuals at greater risk of evidencing angina, sudden death,

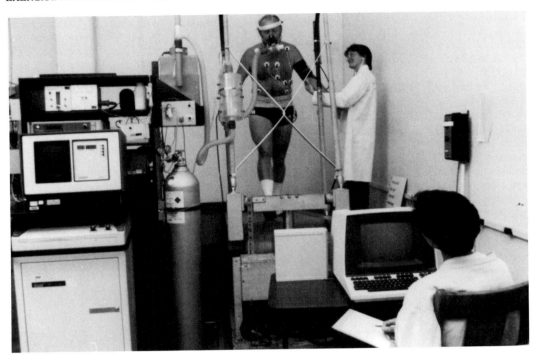

FIG. 9–7. Illustration of an exercise stress test on a motor-driven treadmill, in which work intensity is progressively increased while blood pressure response is monitored, together with electrocardiographic (upper left monitor) and respiratory metabolism response.

or myocardial infarction than does any of the primary risk factors (hypertension, hyperlipidemia, and smoking) discussed previously. Froelicher et al.[42] observed an enhanced risk ratio of 14.3 during a 6-year follow-up in otherwise asymptomatic men evidencing a positive exercise stress test response. Further, Bruce and colleagues[20] have shown that exercise stress test response, together with primary risk factors, resulted in a better prediction of primary coronary heart disease events in healthy men over a 5.6-year follow-up, than did risk factors alone.

EXERCISE THERAPY AND CARDIAC REHABILITATION

While the focus of this section is on the role of exercise training in the rehabilitation of appropriately screened cardiac patients, such programs are increasingly multifaceted in their approach, including applica-

tion of continuing education and behavior modification to effect smoking cessation, better nutritional management with regard to reducing hyperlipidemia and achieving effective weight control, and stress management.[37] Major objectives of cardiac rehabilitation programs include not only improving the patients' functional capacity and quality of life, but also reduction of morbidity and mortality.[96]

Not all patients with cardiovascular disease are appropriate candidates for inclusion in a cardiac rehabilitation program entailing exercise training.[38] This necessitates medical screening which, if not contraindicated, includes an exercise stress test with a physician monitoring the patient's electrocardiographic response. The stress test serves first as an additional means of screening patients for referral to an exercise training program, and also as an objective means of quantitating the intensity of exercise for each patient.[47]

The exercise prescription entails slow but rhythmical, aerobic activities, such as walking, jogging, cycling, skating, swimming, rowing, rope skipping, and rhythmic calisthenics. In initiating exercise training in a medically monitored outpatient program, the patient with low exercise tolerance might start with as little as 10 minutes of exercise at an intensity set as low as 40 to 60% of functional capacity (Fig. 9–8). Duration of exercise should be gradually increased to as much as 30 to 60 minutes as the patient's functional capacity and clinical status improve. Many patients will eventually be able to exercise safely at an intensity of 65 to 90% of maximal heart rate (which may be symptom limited), with 5- to 10-minute periods for lighter warmup and cool-down activity. Frequency of exercise training usually ranges between 3 to 5 days per week.[47]

Aerobic exercise training at the typically prescribed intensity, duration, and frequency, generally increases the coronary heart disease patient's maximal work capacity.[57,72] Further, the patient's myocardial oxygen demand at any given submaximal workload is reduced with the decrease in both heart rate and systolic blood pressure following training. This reduces cardiac work in proportion to total body work and lessens circulatory demands.[94] Peripheral adaptations to training result in increased oxygen pick-up in the trained musculature, and there is suggestive evidence that patients with ischemic exercise response experience improvement in their myocardial oxygen supply-demand ratio following training.[43,71] Also, available data suggest that psychologic benefits occur consequent to cardiac rehabilitation although, in part, they may accrue from the program participation, rather than the physical training alone.[72]

As discussed earlier, exercise training can modify coronary heart disease risk factors, but patients in exercise only cardiac rehabilitation programs have exhibited little improvement in reducing major risk factors.[93] Nonetheless, there is now evidence from the combined analysis of available randomized trials of cardiac rehabilitation

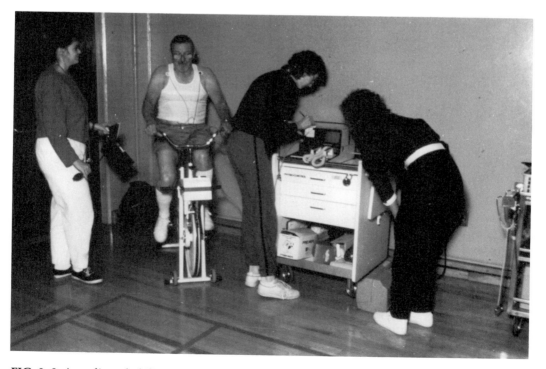

FIG. 9–8. A cardiac rehabilitation patient exercises at a carefully prescribed and monitored workrate in an outpatient medically supervised program.

after myocardial infarction that participation in exercise based programs reduced the 3-year follow-up mortality from all causes by 20% and mortality from reinfarction by 25%. No significant differences were seen between the morbidity (i.e., nonfatal infarction) incidence for the cardiac rehabilitation group and the control group.[95]

CARDIOVASCULAR RISKS OF EXERCISE

It is essential to understand that though an enhanced habitual activity level appears to protect against coronary heart disease, it does not preclude the possibility that there is a transient increase in the risk of sudden cardiac death during exercise.[114] In children and young adults, sudden cardiac death is most often caused by congenital or structural anomaly of the heart or the coronary vessels.[137] In middle-aged and older adults, however, sudden cardiac death is almost always due to advanced coronary heart disease, as revealed in postmortem studies.[102]

In a retrospective survey of 40 exercise facilities over 5 years, Vander et al.[134] found 1 cardiac death per 887,000 man-hours of exercise. Vuori[137] has emphasized that though the absolute risk of cardiovascular complications is low, the risk of cardiac sudden death in jogging has been found to be 7 times greater than in sedentary activity and 5 times higher in prolonged cross-country skiing than during the rest of the day. Siscovick et al.[115] also observed that habitually active men had a 5 times greater incidence of cardiac arrest while engaged in vigorous exercise than during other times of the day. However, the risk of cardiac arrest in men with the lowest levels of habitual activity during unusual exercise was several times higher. These authors also examined the effect of the enhanced transient cardiac arrest effect during vigorous exercise on the habitually active group's overall risk, compared to the rate experienced by sedentary men during the whole day. As shown in Figure 9–9, the 5 times greater occurrence in habitually active men during exercise only raises their overall rate marginally above that at other

times. Thus, overall, the habitually active men still had a 24-hour cardiac arrest rate that was only 40% of that experienced by the sedentary men. This suggests that the short-term increased risk of cardiac arrest during vigorous exercise is outweighed by the long-term beneficial effects of habitual vigorous activity levels.[114]

The risk of cardiac arrest during exercise is obviously higher in persons who have documented coronary heart disease, but the risk of sudden cardiac death can be kept relatively low if the exercise program is individualized and medical supervision is provided.[50] Further, May and colleagues[80] have reviewed the balance of benefits and risks of exercise training in 6 cardiac rehabilitation programs, with an average follow-up from 1 to 4 years. When the results were pooled, the total mortality was 19% lower in the exercise trained patients than in those who did not exercise.

REDUCTION OF EXERCISE TRAINING RISKS

Fundamental to reducing exercise training risks in adults varying widely in age, fitness, and chronic disease state is appropriate medical screening. The American College of Sports Medicine guidelines for exercise testing[47] state that apparently healthy persons (i.e., no symptoms) under age 45, can usually initiate exercise training without exercise testing as long as the program begins at a moderate level and progresses gradually in intensity. However, it is recommended that other individuals undergo medical screening, including a medical history, physical examination, and appropriate laboratory tests, to determine whether one is: (1) apparently healthy, with no major coronary risk factors; (2) at higher risk, with symptoms suggestive of possible coronary disease and/or at least one major coronary risk factor (Table 9–2); or (3) a person with known cardiac, pulmonary, or metabolic disease. A physician-monitored maximal exercise stress test is recommended for apparently healthy persons over 45 years, those at higher risk with symptoms (over age 35 years) and,

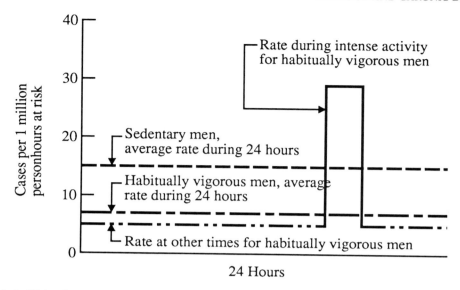

FIG. 9–9. Risk of primary cardiac arrest during vigorous physical activity and at other times, by level of habitual physical activity. Note that though the 1 hour per day rate is "momentarily" high for those who exercise vigorously, their average rate for 24 hours is only 40% of that of sedentary men. (From Siscovick, D.S., N.S. Weiss, R.H. Pletcher, and T. Lasky: The incidence of primary cardiac arrest during vigorous exercise. N. Engl. J. Med. *311*:874–877, 1984.)

Table 9–2.   Major Coronary Risk Factors*

1. History of high blood pressure (above 145/95).
2. Elevated total cholesterol/high density lipoprotein cholesterol ratio (above 5).
3. Cigarette smoking.
4. Abnormal resting ECG—including evidence of old myocardial infarction, left ventricular hypertrophy, ischemia, conduction defects, dysrhythmias.
5. Family history of coronary or other atherosclerotic disease prior to age 50.
6. Diabetes mellitus.

*From Guidelines for Exercise Testing and Prescription. 3rd ed. (American College of Sports Medicine.) Philadelphia: Lea & Febiger, 1986, p. 2.

unless contraindicated, in individuals with disease.

In addition to its role in the medical screening process, the exercise stress test response serves as the basis for developing an appropriate individual exercise prescription. Guidelines for use with apparently healthy persons, and modifications appropriate for cardiac rehabilitation patients, have been described previously. Exercise training is currently being used also as an adjunct treatment for numerous other chronic diseases, including obstructive pulmonary disease, hypertension, diabetes, peripheral vascular disease, and arthritis, as well as for obesity. Because vigorous exercise can be potentially dangerous for people with these diseases, the exercise prescription is modified to enable these persons to make the best physiologic and psychologic adjustment to the training program while minimizing risks.[47]

Haskell[52] has examined the long-held contention that physical fitness (performance capacity) and health are synonymous, particularly with reference to exercise training effects in older adults. He contends that, though a high level of fitness is usually associated with good health, an improvement in one's physical performance capacity with exercise training does not insure an increase in resistance to disease or its clinical consequences. Exercise training can improve both physical fitness and clinical health status, but the improvement in health may be due to biologic changes different from those responsible for improved fitness. Haskell[52] emphasizes that an exercise training program which fails to induce an increase in maximal aerobic power can still effect many biologic and psychologic benefits. For example, low intensity dynamic activity (i.e., performed at <50% of $\dot{V}O_{2max}$) may reduce stress, contribute to weight loss, or selected peripheral biochemical reactions. Indeed, there is strong evidence that regular activity of moderate intensity (e.g., walking, climbing steps, and yardwork) is associated with reduced coronary heart disease morbidity and mortality.[98] Further, Hurley et al.[59] have observed that resistive training performed by apparently healthy middle-aged males at an average intensity of 45% of $\dot{V}O_{2max}$, 3 to 4 times per week for 16 weeks, resulted in significant reduction of some coronary heart disease risk factors without altering maximal aerobic power or percent body fat.

These observations highlight the importance of health related benefits (especially for the older adult and in other individuals with significant chronic disease) of exercise training programs at moderate intensity. Indeed, Haskell et al.[53] contend that health benefits attributable to exercise appear relatively greater at lower to moderate levels of increased physical activity. The improvement seems greatest when the least-active middle-aged and older adults are compared with moderately active persons (i.e., expenditure of 200 to 300 kcal/day, or roughly equivalent to walking/jogging 2 to 3 miles). The difference in health related benefits between moderately active and the few very active persons seem much less apparent. While the dose-response relationship of exercise intensity and health benefits is not precisely apparent,[53] it does seem likely that, in older persons, physical activity of rather low intensity (such as walking and flexibility exercise), is well advised. Haskell[52] contends that exercise programs of low to moderate intensity reduce the risk of sudden cardiac death and musculoskeletal injury, and are likely to increase compliance. Powell and Paffenbarger[103] have summarized these notions in Figure 9–10, in which the theoretical relationship of benefits and risks with increasing levels of physical activity is depicted. That is, the increase in health related benefits appears greatest at low to moderate levels, with the rate diminishing

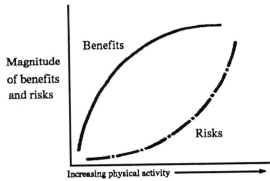

FIG. 9–10. Qualitative illustration of the magnitude of health benefits to risk ratio with increasing physical activity. Note that health related benefits appear to plateau at a moderate activity level, while risks increase disproportionally thereafter. (From Powell, K.E., and R.S. Paffenbarger: Workshop on epidemiological and public health aspects of physical activity and exercise: a summary. Public Health Rep. *100*:118–126, 1985.)

at higher levels. Risks, however, are low for up to moderate levels of physical activity, and only become increasingly more frequent and severe at higher levels of activity.

SUMMARY

1. Prevention of osteoporosis and the resultant increased incidence of fracture, most common in postmenopausal Caucasian women, consists of dietary and life-style alterations—primarily increased calcium intake and exercise—and the judicious use of estrogen.

2. Regular aerobic exercise, in combination with caloric restriction in a diet which maintains essential amounts of nutrients, produces a satisfactory rate of body weight loss (with a greater portion being fat tissue) in the moderately obese person.

3. An even more important value of exercise as an adjunct to caloric restriction in the treatment of moderate obesity, is the observed improvement in weight loss maintenance compared to that achieved by caloric restriction alone.

4. Aerobic exercise training in middle-

aged adult patients with mild to moderate hypertension usually results in significant reductions of both systolic and diastolic blood pressures during rest and at any specific submaximal workload.

5. There is now impressive evidence from large epidemiologic studies that participation in regular vigorous exercise is associated with a lower risk of developing hypertension.

6. Following appropriate medical screening, exercise training can improve the diabetic patient's condition by increasing exercise tolerance, thus enabling participation in an array of activities similar to that of persons without diabetes. Additional improvement may also occur due to reduction of other cardiovascular disease risk factors, particularly obesity and hypertension.

7. There is strong evidence that elevated habitual physical activity is inversely related to the incidence of coronary heart disease; this association is evident even when age, sex, blood pressure, smoking status, serum cholesterol, obesity, and family history of heart disease have been accounted for.

8. Studies designed to attenuate the potential preselection bias in the comparison of physical activity level and coronary heart disease indicate that the relationship exists for both occupational and leisure-time activity.

9. In addition to its role in reducing the impact of principal risk factors on the incidence of coronary heart disease, there is evidence that exercise training can retard the atherosclerotic process, improve the ratio of myocardial oxygen supply versus demand, and probably improve myocardial function.

10. The exercise stress test, with appropriate medical screening, has become a useful non-invasive means for detecting evidence of coronary heart disease. It also provides quantitative information used to design individual presciptions for exercise training.

11. Exercise training has become a vital component of effective cardiac rehabilitation programs, which aim to improve the patient's functional capacity and quality of life, as well as reducing subsequent morbidity and mortality.

12. The short-term increased risk of cardiac arrest during moderately vigorous exercise is significantly outweighed by the long-term beneficial effects achieved by those who regularly participate in similar activity.

13. Fundamental to reducing exercise training risks in adults varying widely in age, fitness, and chronic disease state is appropriate medical screening. This process is further facilitated in most older adults by a physician-monitored exercise stress test.

14. Health-related benefits, in previously sedentary middle-aged and older adults appear to be initiated with regular activity of low to moderate intensity, which also reduces the incidence of musculoskeletal injury and the risk of cardiac arrest. At higher activity intensity, health-related benefits appear to level off, while exercise-induced risks increase rapidly.

15. The best exercise training programs for middle-aged and older adults employ individualized activity prescription, are varied and fun, and of low to moderate intensity, thus increasing health-related benefit to risk ratio and habitual activity adherence.

REFERENCES

1. Aloia, J.F., et al.: Prevention of involutional bone loss by exercise. Ann. Intern. Med. 89:356–358, 1978.

2. American College of Sports Medicine. Position statement on proper and improper weight loss programs. Med. Sci. Sports Exer. 15(1):ix–xiii, 1983.

3. Amer Heart Association. Heart Facts. Dallas: 1990.

4. Amsterdam, E.A., and D.T. Mason: Coronary artery disease: pathophysiology and clinical correlations. In Exercise in Cardiovascular Health and Disease. Edited by E.A. Amsterdam, J.H. Wilmore, and A.N. DeMaria. New York: Yorke Medical, 1977, pp. 13–34.

5. Atkinson, R.L., et al.: A comprehensive approach to outpatient obesity management. J. Am. Dietet. Assoc. 84:439–446, 1984.

6. Barnard, R.J., et al.: Response of non-insulin-dependent diabetic patients to an intensive pro-

gram of diet and exercise. Diabetes Care. 5:370–374, 1982.

7. Bielinski, R., Y. Shutz, and E. Jequier: Energy metabolism during the postexercise recovery in man. Am. J. Clin. Nutr. 42:69–82, 1985.

8. Billman, G.E., R.J. Schwartz, and H.L. Stone: The effects of daily exercise on susceptibility to sudden cardiac death. Circulation. 69:1182–1189, 1984.

9. Bjorntorp, P.: Exercise in the treatment of obesity. Clin. Endocrinol. Metab. 5:431–453, 1976.

10. Bjorntorp, P.: Hypertension and exercise. Hypertension. 4 (Suppl. III):56–59, 1982.

11. Blackburn, H.: Physical activity and hypertension. J. Clin. Hyperten. 2:154–162, 1986.

12. Blackburn, H., et al.: Premature ventricular complexes induced by stress testing. Their frequency and response to physical conditioning. Am. J. Cardiol. 31:441–449, 1973.

13. Blair, S.N., N.N. Goodyear, L.W. Gibbons, and K.H. Cooper: Physical fitness and incidence of hypertension in healthy normotensive men and women. JAMA. 252:487–490, 1984.

14. Bogardus, C., et al.: Effect of physical training on carbohydrate metabolism in patients with glucose intolerance and non-insulin-dependent diabetes mellitus. Diabetes. 33:311–318, 1984.

15. Brand, R.J., R.S. Paffenbarger, R.I. Sholtz, and J.P. Kampert: Work activity and fatal heart attack studied by multiple logistic risk analysis. Am. J. Epidemiol. 110:52–62, 1979.

16. Bray, G.A.: Effect of caloric expenditure in obese patients. Lancet. 2:397–398, 1969.

17. Brown, M.R., et al.: Low calorie liquid diet in the treatment of very obese adolescents: long-term effect on lean body mass. Am. J. Clin. Nutr. 38:20–31, 1983.

18. Brownell, K.D.: The psychology and physiology of obesity: implications for screening and treatment. J. Am. Dietet. Assoc. 84:406–413, 1984.

19. Brownell, K.D., and A.J. Stunkard: Physical activity in the development and control of obesity. In Obesity. Edited by A.J. Stunkard. Philadelphia: Saunders, 1980, pp. 300–324.

20. Bruce, R.A., T.A. DeRouen, and K.F. Hossack: Value of maximal exercise tests in risk assessment of primary coronary heart disease events in healthy men. Am. J. Cardiol. 46:371–378, 1980.

21. Castelli, W.P., et al.: HDL cholesterol and other lipids in coronary heart disease. The cooperative lipoprotein phenotyping study. Circulation. 55:767–772, 1977.

22. Chiang, B.N., et al.: Relationship of premature systoles to coronary heart disease and sudden death in the Tecumseh epidemiological study. Ann. Intern. Med. 70:1159–1166, 1969.

23. Chow, R., J.E. Harrison, and C. Notorius: Effect of two randomised exercise programmes on

bone mass of healthy postmenopausal women. Br. Med. J. 295:1441–1444, 1987.

24. Colvin, R.H., and S.B. Olson: A descriptive analysis of men and women who have lost significant weight and are highly successful at maintaining the loss. Addict. Behav. 8:287–295, 1983.

25. Cullinane, E., S. Siconolfi, A. Saritelli, and P.D. Thompson: Acute decrease in serum triglycerides with exercise: is there a threshold for an exercise effect? Metabolism. 31:844–847, 1982.

26. Currens, J.H., and P.D. White: Half a century of running—clinical, physiologic, and autopsy findings in the case of Clarence DeMar (Mr. Marathon). N. Engl. J. Med. 265:988–993, 1961.

27. Dahlkoetter, J., E.J. Callahan, and J. Linton: Obesity and the unbalanced energy equation: exercise versus eating habit change. J. Consult. Clin. Psych. 47:898–905, 1979.

28. Dalsky, G.P., et al.: Weight bearing exercise training and lumbar bone mineral content in postmenopausal women. Ann. Intern. Med. 108:824–828, 1988.

29. De Fronzo, R.A., et al.: Synergistic interaction between exercise and insulin on peripheral glucose uptake. J. Clin. Invest. 68:1468–1474, 1981.

30. Despres, J.P., et al.: Effects of aerobic training on fat distribution in male subjects. Med. Sci. Sports Exer. 17:113–118, 1985.

31. deVries, H.A.: Physiology of Exercise for Physical Education and Athletics. 4th ed. Dubuque, Iowa: Wm. C. Brown, 1986.

32. Dohm, G.L., G.B. Beecher, T.P. Stephenson, and M. Womack: Adaptations to endurance training at three intensities of exercise. J. Appl. Physiol. 42:753–757, 1977.

33. Duncan, J.J., et al.: The effects of aerobic exercise on plasma catecholamines and blood pressure in patients with mild essential hypertension. JAMA. 254:2609–2613, 1985.

34. Durnin, J.V.G.A., and J. Womersley: Body fat assessed from total body density and its estimation from skinfold thickness: measurements on 481 men and women aged from 16 to 72 years. Br. J. Nutr. 32:77–97, 1974.

35. Ekoe, J-M.: Overview of diabetes mellitus and exercise. Med. Sci. Sports Exer. 21:353–355, 1989.

36. Epstein, L., J. Miller, F.W. Stitt, and J.N. Morris: Vigorous exercise in leisure time, coronary risk factors, and resting electrocardiogram in middle-aged male civil servants. Br. Heart J. 38:403–409, 1976.

37. Fardy, P.S., F.G. Yanowitz, and P.K. Wilson: Cardiac Rehabilitation, Adult Fitness, and Exercise Testing. 2nd ed. Philadelphia: Lea & Febiger, 1988, pp. 365–378.

38. Faulkner, J.A.: Cardiac rehabilitation: major concerns in basic physiology. In Heart Disease and Rehabilitation. Edited by M.L. Pollock and D.H.

Schmidt. Boston: Houghton Mifflin, 1979, pp. 663–677.

39. Franklin, B.A., and M. Rubenfire: Losing weight through exercise. JAMA. 244:377–379, 1980.

40. Froelicher, V.F.: Use of the exercise electrocardiogram to identify latent coronary atherosclerotic disease. In Exercise in Cardiovascular Health and Disease. Edited by E.A. Amsterdam, J.H. Wilmore, and A.N. DeMaria. New York: Yorke Medical, 1977, pp. 188–208.

41. Froelicher, V.F., and P. Brown: Exercise and coronary heart disease. J. Cardiac. Rehabil. 1:277–288, 1981.

42. Froelicher, V.F., M.M. Thomas, C. Pillow, and M.C. Lancaster: Epidemiologic study of asymptomatic men screened by maximal treadmill testing for latent coronary artery disease. Am. J. Cardiol. 34:770–776, 1974.

43. Froelicher, V.F., et al.: Cardiac rehabilitation: evidence for improvement in myocardial perfusion and function. Arch. Phys. Med. Rehabil. 61:517–522, 1980.

44. Garrow, J.S.: Effect of exercise on obesity. Acta Med. Scand. Suppl. 711:67–73, 1986.

45. Goldschlager, N., D. Cake, and K. Cohn: Exercise-induced ventricular arrhythmias in patients with coronary artery disease. Their relation to angiographic findings. Am. J. Cardiol. 31:434–440, 1973.

46. Greenwood, M.R.C.: Adipose tissue: cellular morphology and development. Ann. Intern. Med. 103:996–999, 1985.

47. Guidelines for Exercise Testing and Exercise Prescription. American College of Sports Medicine. 4th ed. Philadelphia: Lea & Febiger, 1991.

48. Gwinup, G.: Effect of exercise alone on the weight of obese women. Arch. Intern. Med. 135:676–680, 1975.

49. Hagberg, J.M., and D.R. Seals: Exercise training and hypertension. Acta Med. Scand. Suppl. 711:131–136, 1986.

50. Haskell, W.L.: Cardiovascular complications during medically supervised exercise training of cardiac patients. Circulation. 57:920–924, 1978.

51. Haskell, W.L.: Exercise-induced changes in plasma lipids and lipoproteins. Prev. Med. 13:23–36, 1984.

52. Haskell, W.L.: Physical activity and health: need to define the required stimulus. Am. J. Cardiol. 55:4D–9D, 1985.

53. Haskell, W.L., H.J. Montoye, and D. Orenstein: Physical activity and exercise to achieve health-related physical fitness components. Public Health Rep. 100:202–212, 1985.

54. Hirsch, J.: Adipose cellularity in relation to human obesity. In Advances in Internal Medicine. Vol. 17. Edited by G.H. Stollerman. Chicago: Year Book Medical, 1971, pp. 289–300.

55. Hirsch, J., and J. Knittle: Cellularity of obese and non-obese adipose tissue. Fed. Proceed. 29:1516–1521, 1970.

56. Holloszy, J.O., et al.: Effects of exercise on glucose tolerance and insulin resistance. Acta Med. Scand. Suppl. 711:55–65, 1986.

57. Holly, R.G., E.A. Amsterdam, R.H. Dressendorfer, and H.R. Superko: Effects of cardiac rehabilitation on maximal and symptom limited work capacity. Clin. Research. 31(2):297A, 1983.

58. Horton, E.S.: The role of exercise in the treatment of hypertension in obesity. Int. J. Obesity. 5(Suppl. I):165–171, 1981.

59. Hurley, B.F., et al.: Resistive training can reduce coronary risk factors without altering $\dot{V}O_{2max}$ or percent body fat. Med. Sci. Sport Exer. 20:150–154, 1988.

60. Hypertension Detection and Follow-up Program Cooperative Group. Five year findings. 1. Reduction in mortality of persons with high blood pressure including mild hypertension. JAMA. 242:2562–2571, 1979.

61. Irie, M., T. Hyodo, and T. Togane: Summary of previous studies in Sumo wrestlers. In Proceedings of the International Symposium on Epidemiology of Diabetic Microangiopathy. Edited by H. Abe and M. Hoshi. Basel: S. Karger, 1983, pp. 397–403.

62. Jacobson, P.C., et al.: Bone density in women: college athletes and older athletic women. J. Orthopaed. Research. 2:328–332, 1984.

63. Johnson, D., and E.J. Drenick: Therapeutic fasting in morbid obesity. Arch. Intern. Med. 137:1381–1382, 1977.

64. Katch, F.I., et al.: Effects of sit up exercise training on adipose cell size and adiposity. Res. Quart. Exer. Sport. 55:242–247, 1984.

65. Kemmer, F.W., and M. Berger: Exercise and diabetes mellitus. Int. J. Sports Med. 4:77–88, 1983.

66. Kenney, W.L., and E.J. Zambraski: Physical activity in human hypertension: a mechanisms approach. Sports Med. 1:459–473, 1984.

67. Keys, A., et al.: The Biology of Human Starvation. Minneapolis: University of Minnesota Press, 1950.

68. Kissileff, H.R., and T.B. Van Itallie: Physiology of the control of food intake. Ann. Rev. Nutr. 2:371–418, 1982.

69. Kiyonaga, A., K. Arabawa, H. Tanaka, and M. Shindo: Blood pressure and hormonal responses to aerobic exercise. Hypertension. 7:125–131, 1985.

70. Kramsch, D.M., et al.: Reduction of coronary atherosclerosis by moderate conditioning exercise in monkeys on an atherogenic diet. N. Engl. J. Med. 305:1483–1489, 1981.

71. Laslett, L., L. Paumer, and E.A. Amsterdam: Increase in myocardial oxygen consumption indexes by exercise training at onset of ischemia

in patients with coronary artery disease. Circulation. 71:958–962, 1985.

72. Laslett, L., L. Paumer, and E.A. Amsterdam: Exercise training in coronary artery disease. Cardiol. Clinics. 5:211–225, 1987.

73. Le Bow, M.D.: Can lighter become thinner? Addict. Behav. 3:116–120, 1977.

74. Leon, A.S., J. Conrad, D.B. Hunninghake, and R. Serfass: Effects of a vigorous walking program on body composition, and carbohydrate and lipid metabolism of obese young men. Am. J. Clin. Nutr. 33:1776–1787, 1979.

75. Lindsay, R.: Prevention of osteoporosis. Clin. Orthopaed. Related Research. 222:44–59, 1987.

76. Link, R.P., W.M. Pedersoli, and H.H. Safanie: Effect of exercise on development of atherosclerosis in swine. Atheroscl. 15:107–122, 1972.

77. Lockwood, D.H., and J.M. Amatruda: Very low calorie diets in the management of obesity. Ann. Rev. Med. 34:373–381, 1984.

78. MacDougall, J.D., et al.: Arterial blood pressure response to heavy resistance exercise. J. Appl. Physiol. 58:785–790, 1985.

79. Magnus, K., A. Matroos, and J. Strackee: Walking, cycling, or gardening with or without seasonal interruption in relation to acute coronary events. Am. J. Epidemiol. 110:724–733, 1979.

80. May, G.S., et al.: Secondary prevention after myocardial infarction: a review of long-term trials. Proc. Cardiovas. Dis. 24:331–352, 1982.

81. Mayer, J., P. Roy, and K.P. Mitra: Relation between caloric intake, body weight, and physical work: studies in an industrial male population in West Bengal. Am. J. Clin. Nutr. 4:169–175, 1956.

82. Mayer, J., et al.: Exercise, food intake, and body weight in normal rats and genetically obese adult mice. Am. J. Physiol. 177:544–548, 1954.

83. McArdle, W.D., F.I. Katch, and V.L. Katch: Exercise Physiology: Energy, Nutrition, and Human Performance. 3rd ed. Philadelphia: Lea & Febiger, 1991.

84. McKinney, M.E., and M.B. Mellion: Exercise and hypertension. In Office Management of Sports Injuries and Athletic Problems. Edited by M.B. Mellion. St. Louis: Mosby, 1988, pp. 98–109.

85. Molé, P.A.: Increased contractile potential of papillary muscles from exercise-trained rat hearts. Am. J. Physiol. 234:H421–H425, 1981.

86. Molé, P.A., et al.: Exercise reverses depressed metabolic rate produced by severe caloric restriction. Med. Sci. Sports Exer. 21:29–33, 1989.

87. Morris, J.N., R. Pollard, M.G. Everitt, and S.P.W. Chave: Vigorous exercise in leisure-time: protection against coronary heart disease. Lancet. 2:1207–1210, 1980.

88. Morris, J.N., et al.: Exercise and the heart (letter). Lancet. 1:267, 1981.

89. Nelson, M.E., C.N. Meredith, B. Dawson-Hughes, and W.J. Evans: Hormone and bone mineral status in endurance trained and sedentary postmenopausal women. J. Clin. Endocrinol. Metab. 66:927–933, 1988.

90. Nomura, G., et al.: Physical training in essential hypertension: alone and in combination with dietary salt restriction. J. Cardiac. Rehab. 4:469–475, 1984.

91. Oberman, A.: Rehabilitation of patients with coronary artery disease. In Heart Disease: A Textbook of Cardiovascular Medicine. 2nd ed. Edited by E. Braunwald. Philadelphia: Saunders, 1983, pp. 1384–1398.

92. Oberman, A.: Exercise and the primary prevention of cardiovascular disease. Am. J. Cardiol. 55:10D–20D, 1985.

93. Oberman, A.: Rehabilitation of patients with coronary artery disease. In Heart Disease: A Textbook of Cardiovascular Medicine. 3rd ed. Edited by E. Braunwald. Philadelphia: Saunders, 1988, pp. 1395–1409.

94. Oberman, A.: Does cardiac rehabilitation increase long-term survival after myocardial infarction? Circulation. 80:416–418, 1989.

95. O'Connor, G.T., et al.: Rehabilitation with exercise after myocardial infarction. Circulation. 82:234–244, 1989.

96. Oldridge, N.B., G.H. Guyatt, M.E. Fischer, and A.A. Rimm: Cardiac rehabilitation after myocardial infarction. JAMA. 260:945–950, 1988.

97. Paffenbarger, R.S., and W.F. Hale: Work activity and coronary heart mortality. N. Engl. J. Med. 292:545–550, 1975.

98. Paffenbarger, R.S., R.T. Hyde, A.L. Wing, and C.H. Steinmetz: A natural history of athleticism and cardiovascular health. JAMA. 252:491–495, 1984.

99. Paffenbarger, R.S., A.L. Wing, P.T. Hyde, and D.L. Jung: Physical activity and incidence of hypertension in college alumni. Am. J. Epidemiol. 117:245–256, 1983.

100. Passmore, R.: A note on the relation of appetite to exercise. Lancet. 1:29, 1958.

101. Peronnet, F., et al.: Echocardiography and the athlete's heart. Physician Sportsmed. 9(5):102–112, 1981.

102. Perper, J.A., L.H. Kuller, and M. Cooper: Atherosclerosis of coronary arteries in sudden unexpected deaths. Circulation. 52(Suppl. 3):27–33, 1975.

103. Powell, K.E., and R.S. Paffenbarger: Workshop on epidemiological and public health aspects of physical activity and exercise: a summary. Public Health Rep. 100:118–126, 1985.

104. Powell, K.E., P.D. Thompson, C.J. Caspersen, and J.S. Kendrick: Physical activity and the incidence of coronary heart disease. Ann. Rev. Public Health. 8:253–287, 1987.

105. Richter, E.A., and H. Galbo: Diabetes, insulin and exercise. Sports Med. 3:275–288, 1986.

106. Rogers, M.A.: Acute effects of exercise on glucose tolerance in non-insulin-dependent diabetes. Med. Sci. Sports Exer. 21:362–368, 1989.

107. Rogers, M.A., et al.: Improvement in glucose tolerance after one week of exercise in patients with mild NIDDM. Diabetes Care. 11:613–618, 1988.

108. Roman, O., A.L. Canuzzi, E. Villalon, and C. Klenner: Physical training program in arterial hypertension: a long-term prospective follow-up. Cardiol. 67:230–243, 1981.

109. Schaible, T., F. Penpargkul, and J. Scheuer: Cardiac responses to exercise training in male and female rats. J. Appl. Physiol. 50:112–117, 1981.

110. Schneider, S.H., L.F. Amarosa, A.K. Khachadurian, and N.B. Ruderman: Studies on the mechanism of improved glucose control during regular exercise in type 2 (non-insulin-dependent) diabetes. Diabetologia. 26:355–360, 1984.

111. Seals, D.R., and J.M. Hagberg: The effect of exercise training on human hypertension: a review. Med. Sci. Sports Exer. 16:207–215, 1984.

112. Simkin, A., J. Ayalon, and I. Leichter: Increased trabecular bone density due to bone-loading exercises in postmenopausal osteoporotic women. Calcif. Tissue Intern. 40:59–63, 1987.

113. Sims, E.A., and E.S. Horton: Endocrine and metabolic adaptation of obesity and starvation. Am. J. Clin. Nutr. 1:455–470, 1968.

114. Siscovick, D.S., R.E. LaPorte, and J.M. Newman: The disease-specific benefits and risks of physical activity and exercise. Public Health Rep. 100:180–188, 1985.

115. Siscovick, D.S., N.S. Weiss, R.H. Pletcher, and T. Lasky: The incidence of primary cardiac arrest during vigorous exercise. N. Engl. J. Med. 311:874–877, 1984.

116. Slattery, M.L., D.R. Jacobs, and M.Z. Nickaman: Leisure time physical activity and coronary heart disease. The U.S. railroad study. Circulation. 79:304–311, 1989.

117. Smith, E.L., and D.M. Raab: Osteoporosis and physical activity. Acta Med. Scand. Suppl. 711:149–156, 1986.

118. Smith, E.L., P.E. Smith, C.J. Ensign, and M.M. Shea: Bone involution decrease in exercising middle-aged women. Calcif. Tissue Intern. 36(Suppl):129–138, 1984.

119. Spain, D.M., and A.V. Bradess: Occupational physical activity and the degree of coronary atherosclerosis in "normal" men. A postmortem study. Circulation. 22:239–242, 1960.

120. Stalonas, P.M., W.G. Johnson, and M. Christ: Behavior modification for obesity: the evaluation of exercise, contingency management, and program adherence. J. Consult. Clin. Psych. 46:463–469, 1978.

121. Stern, J.S.: Is obesity a disease of inactivity? In Eating and Its Disorders. Edited by A.J. Stunkard and E. Stellar. New York: Raven, 1984, pp. 131–139.

122. Stevenson, J.A.F., B.M. Box, V. Feleki, and J.R. Beaton: Bouts of exercise and food intake in the rat. J. Appl. Physiol. 21:118–122, 1966.

123. Stunkard, A.J.: The current status of treatment of obesity in adults. In Eating and Its Disorders. Edited by A.J. Stunkard and E. Stellar. New York: Raven, 1984, pp. 157–173.

124. Stunkard, A.J., and M. McLaren-Hume: The results of treatment for obesity. Arch. Intern. Med. 103:79–85, 1959.

125. Stunkard, A.J., and S.B. Renick: Behavior modification in the treatment of obesity. The problem of maintaining weight loss. Arch. Gen. Psychiat. 36:801–806, 1979.

126. Superko, H.R., and W.L. Haskell: The role of exercise training in the therapy of hyperlipoproteinemia. Cardiol. Clinics. 5:285–310, 1987.

127. Tanji, J.L.: Exercise for hypertensives. Consultant. 28(9):123–130, 1988.

128. Tanji, J.L.: Exercise prescription. West. J. Med. 145:676–677, 1986.

129. Taylor, R., et al: Physical activity and prevalence of diabetes in Melanesian and Indian men in Fiji. Diabetologia. 27:578–582, 1984.

130. The Pooling Project Research Group. Relationship of blood pressure, serum cholesterol, smoking habit, relative weight and ECG abnormalities to incidence of major coronary events: final report of the Pooling Project. J. Chron. Dis. 31:202–306, 1978.

131. Tipton, C.M.: Exercise, training, and hypertension. In Exercise and Sport Sciences Reviews. Vol. 12. Edited by R.L. Terjung. Lexington, Mass: Collamore, 1984, pp. 245–306.

132. Tremblay, A., J-P. Despres, and C. Brouchard: Adipose tissue characteristics of ex-obese long-distance runners. Int. J. Obes. 8:641–648, 1984.

133. Tremblay, A., J.P. Despres, and C. Brouchard: The effects of exercise training on energy balance and adipose tissue morphology and metabolism. Sports Med. 2:223–233, 1985.

134. Vander, L., B. Franklin, and M. Rubenfire: Cardiovascular complications of recreational physical activity. Physician Sportsmed. 10(6):89–97, 1982.

135. Van Itallie, T.B.: The enduring storage capacity for fat: implications for treatment of obesity. In Eating and Its Disorders. Edited by A.J. Stunkard and E. Stellar. New York: Raven, 1984, pp. 109–119.

136. Virtug, A., S.H. Schneider, and N.B. Ruderman: Exercise and type 1 diabetes mellitus. In Exercise and Sport Sciences Reviews. Vol. No. 16. Edited by K.B. Pandolf. New York: Macmillan, 1988, pp. 285–304.

137. Vuori, I.: The cardiovascular risks of physical activity. Acta Med. Scand. Suppl. *711*:205–214, 1986.

138. Wadden, T.A., A.J. Stunkard, and K.D. Brownell: Very low calorie diets: their efficacy, safety, and future. Ann. Intern. Med. *99*:675–683, 1983.

139. Wallberg-Henriksson, H.: Acute exercise: fuel homeostasis and glucose transport in insulin-dependent diabetes mellitus. Med. Sci. Sports Exer. *21*:356–361, 1989.

140. Weltman, A., S. Matter, and B.A. Stamford: Caloric restriction and/or mild exercise: effects on serum lipids and body composition. Am. J. Clin. Nutr. *33*:1002–1009, 1980.

141. Williams, R.S., et al.: Physical conditioning augments the fibrinolytic response to venous occlusion in healthy adults. N. Engl. J. Med. *302*:987–991, 1980.

142. Woo, R., Y.S. Garrow, and F.X. PiSunyer: Effect of exercise on spontaneous calorie intake in obesity. Am. J. Clin. Nutr. *36*:470–477, 1982.

143. Wood, P.D., et al.: The distribution of plasma lipoproteins in middle-aged male runners. Metabolism. *25*:1249–1257, 1976.

144. Wood, P.D., et al.: Increased exercise level and plasma lipoprotein concentrations: a one-year randomized controlled study in sedentary middle-aged men. Metabolism. *32*:31–39, 1983.

145. Yang, M., and T.B. Van Itallie: Composition of weight loss during short-term weight reduction: metabolic responses of obese subjects to starvation and low-calorie ketogenic and nonketogenic diets. J. Clin. Invest. *58*:722–730, 1976.

146. Zilversmit, D.B.: Atherogenesis: a postprandial phenomenon. Circulation. *60*:473–485, 1979.

147. Zuti, W.B., and L.A. Golding: Comparing diet and exercise as weight reduction tools. Physician Sportsmed. *4(1)*:49–53, 1976.

BIBLIOGRAPHY

1. Astrand, P-O., and G. Grimby (editors): Physical activity in health and disease. Acta Med. Scand. Suppl. *711*:1–244, 1986.

2. Public health aspects of physical activity and exercise. Public Health Rep. *100*:118–224, 1985.

3. Skinner, J.S. (editor): Exercise Testing and Exercise Prescription for Special Cases: Theoretical Basis and Clinical Application. Philadelphia: Lea & Febiger, 1987.

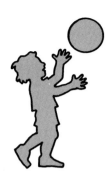

INDEX

Page numbers followed by f indicate figures; those followed by t indicate tables.